T0332188

Clinics in Developmental Medicine No. 160
HIP DISORDERS IN CHILDHOOD

© 2003 Mac Keith Press
High Holborn House, 52–54 High Holborn, London WC1V 6RL

Senior Editor: Martin C.O. Bax
Editor: Hilary M. Hart
Managing Editor: Michael Pountney
Sub Editor: Pat Chappelle

First published in this edition 2003

British Library Cataloguing-in-Publication data:
A catalogue record for this book is available from the British Library

ISSN: 0069 4835
ISBN: 1 898683 33 6

Printed by The Lavenham Press Ltd, Water Street, Lavenham, Suffolk
Mac Keith Press is supported by Scope

Clinics in Developmental Medicine No. 160

Hip Disorders
in
Childhood

Edited by

JOHN V. BANTA
University of Connecticut School of Medicine
Farmington, CT
USA

and

DAVID SCRUTTON
Institute of Child Health
University College London
England

2003
Mac Keith Press

Distributed by 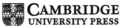 **CAMBRIDGE**
UNIVERSITY PRESS

ACKNOWLEDGEMENTS

The editors would like to recognize those individuals without whose time and effort this book would not have been possible. In the USA: Laurie MacNeil, MD, for research in the radiology files of the Children's Hospital; Linda Kaczmsrczyk for her invaluable assistance in the medical library at Hartford Hospital; and Michael McCarter and Patrick Reilly for their excellent medical photography. In the UK: Prof. Richard Robinson, Dr Lewis Rosenbloom and Dr Jean-Pierre Lin for reviewing some of the chapters.

CONTENTS

AUTHORS' APPOINTMENTS

John V. Banta — Professor of Orthopaedic Surgery, University of Connecticut School of Medicine, Farmington, CT; *and* Surgeon-in-Chief, Emeritus, Connecticut Children's Medical Center, Hartford, CT, USA

Bruce E. Bowman — Instructor, University of Connecticut School of Medicine, Farmington, CT; *and* Senior Physician Assistant, Newington Department of Orthopaedic Surgery, Connecticut Children's Medical Center, Hartford, CT, USA

Peter A. DeLuca — Connecticut Orthopaedic Specialists, New Haven, CT; *and* Associate Professor of Orthopaedic Surgery, University of Connecticut School of Medicine, Farmington, CT, USA

Christopher Foley — Director, Department of Pediatric Radiology, Connecticut Children's Medical Center, Hartford, CT, USA

Janet E. McDonagh — Senior Lecturer in Paediatric Rheumatology, Institute of Child Health, Diana, Princess of Wales Children's Hospital, Birmingham, England

Christopher Morris — Principal Orthotist, Department of Orthotics, Nuffield Orthopaedic Centre NHS Trust; *and* Honorary Research Associate, National Perinatal Epidemiology Unit, University of Oxford, Oxford, England

Durgesh Nagarkatti — Chief Resident, Department of Orthopedics, University of Connecticut, Farmington, CT, USA

Sylvia Õunpuu

Director and Kinesiologist, Center for Motion Analysis, Connecticut Children's Medical Center, Hartford, CT; *and* Assistant Professor, University of Connecticut School of Medicine, Farmington, CT, USA

J. Mark H. Paterson

Consultant Paediatric Orthopaedic Surgeon, The Royal London Hospital, London, England

Kristan A. Pierz

Assistant Professor of Orthopaedics, University of Connecticut School of Medicine, Farmington, CT, *and* Newington Department of Orthopaedic Surgery, Connecticut Children's Medical Center, Hartford, CT, USA

David Scrutton

Honorary Senior Lecturer, Institute of Child Health, University College London; and Guy's, King's College and St Thomas' Hospitals, King's College, London, England

Brian G. Smith

Associate Professor, Department of Orthopaedic Surgery, University of Connecticut School of Medicine, Farmington, CT, *and* Newington Department of Orthopaedic Surgery, Connecticut Children's Medical Center, Hartford, CT, USA

Jeffrey D. Thomson

Associate Professor, Department of Orthopaedic Surgery, University of Connecticut School of Medicine, Farmington, CT, *and* Director, Newington Department of Orthopaedic Surgery, Connecticut Children's Medical Center, Hartford, CT, USA

Jayesh Trivedi

Consultant Orthopaedic Surgeon, Robert Jones and Agnes Hunt Orthopaedic Hospital, Oswestry, England

FOREWORD

All health professionals who work in the field of paediatrics frequently find themselves concerned about the hips not only of children with disabilities such as cerebral palsy but also in the 'child without a disability' who may get a hip pathology at any time. It is worrying when, as a general physician or paediatrician, you see such cases: how serious a problem is the limp and the pain; how do you decide without reference to an orthopaedic surgeon—and not all orthopaedic surgeons are expert in children's hips—whether the child needs to be seen by someone else, or if you can reassure the family that there is no disease at the hip? What do we need? We need to know the normal development of the hip, and we need to know how to examine it—this was always something that worried me because it was buried away and difficult to palpate. Then we need to know, at the different ages, the common conditions in children that involve the hip, and be aware of the less common ones that may have a very serious significance.

It is these problems that Banta and Scrutton have addressed in this book on the hip, and it is splendidly practical, starting with the normal developmental anatomy of the hip, clinical and radiological examination, and then the common problems: congenital dislocation of the hip, limps, dysplasias, Perthes' disease, and the neuromuscular disorders of cerebral palsy and muscular dystrophy. In addition, we learn about the application of the gait laboratory and, very practically, we get advice on orthoses for the hip. Clear practical descriptions of how to examine and what one will see are backed up with extensive illustration.

The volume is one that all practitioners, therapists, paediatricians and, I suspect, many orthopaedic surgeons will want to have on their shelves in their clinical practice. Indeed, I wish I had had it by me during my years of clinical practice and I am sure that it is just the first edition of a book that will become a standby for all clinicians.

Martin C.O. Bax

1
ANATOMY OF THE HIP JOINT

John V. Banta

This chapter outlines the essential components of the embryology and developmental anatomy of the child's hip in order to give the reader a fundamental understanding of the various growth factors which contribute to the unique pathologic conditions that are described in more detail in subsequent chapters.

Embryology

The limb bud first appears as an elevation on the lateral wall of the embryo at approximately four weeks after ovulation. The lower limb bud develops approximately one to two days after the appearance of the upper limb bud and the hip joint becomes fully formed within the first two months, which comprises the embryonic period of development. Its origin is at the junction of the lumbar and first sacral levels. This structure is composed of mesoderm covered with ectoderm. The ectodermal cells elongate to form the apical ectodermal ridge, which is thought to be induced by the underlying mesoderm (Stevenson and Meyer 1993) (Fig. 1.1). The limb bud forms a flattened plate and undergoes progressive development into the limb segments in a proximal to distal fashion. As described by Stevenson and Meyer, "the cephalocaudal polarity of the limb depends on the zone of polarizing activity identified at the caudal junction of the early limb bud and the body wall" (Fig. 1.2). Numerous induction agents including such morphogens as transforming growth factor-β stimulate the mesenchymal cells. The primitive mesenchyme condenses and produces type II collagen that gives rise to the cartilage, which forms the primitive bone model (Thorogood 1983).

Remarkable advances in the understanding of the genetic control of limb development have shown that 10 gene families are critical in directing limb bud growth. These range from fibroblast growth factors that influence growth in the apical ectodermal ridge, to homeobox genes that act as transcription factors controlling positional limb development (Lovett *et al.* 1997). Much of the understanding of the genetic control of limb bud development in the higher vertebrates has evolved from study of the fruit fly, mouse and chick. These fundamental gene families have evolved in multiple numbers and some divergence in the higher vertebrates, for example the T-box genes first described in mice, in which a mutant resulted in mice with shortened tails and vertebral defects. Recently mutations in the human TBX-5 were found to cause the heart–hand genetic disorder Holt–Oram syndrome where phocomelia is noted as one phenotype (Lovett *et al.* 1997). Further research in the genome project will undoubtedly lead to greater understanding of the various congenital and developmental anomalies in the human hip.

As the limb bud elongates, the four extremities evolve in a ventral fashion from their lateral origin and rotate toward one another. Distally the limb bud tapers and flattens to

1

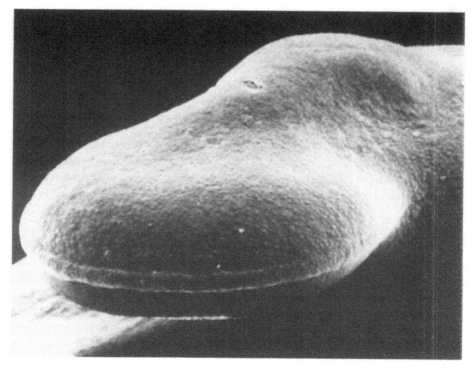

Fig. 1.1. Elongating limb bud of a mouse embryo showing the apical ectodermal ridge along its distal border. (Reproduced by permission from Kelley 1985.)

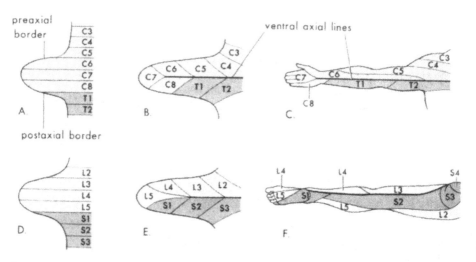

Fig. 1.2. Schematic diagram of the development of the proximal and distal limb buds from embryonic to mature fetal development illustrating the mature dermatomal innervation. (Reproduced by permission from Moore 1977.)

2

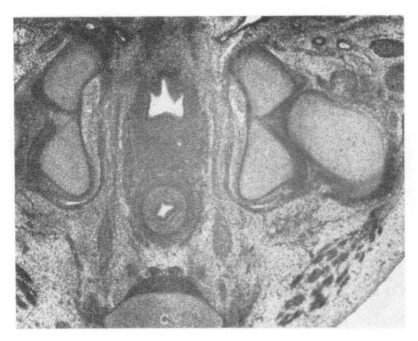

Fig. 1.3. Human embryo, 22.8 mm. Transverse section depicting the ischio-pubic recess forming the acetabulum. The femoral neck is anteverted 30° from the midline of the embryo. (Reproduced by permission from Strayer 1971.)

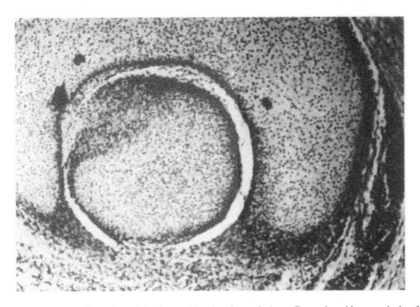

Fig. 1.4. Spherical configuration of the femoral head and acetabulum. (Reproduced by permission from Watanabe 1974.)

3

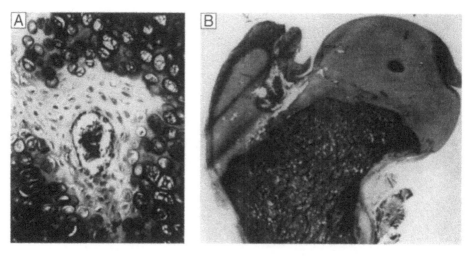

Fig. 1.5. (A) Calcified zone round the vessels in the midst of mature cartilage (×130). (B) Central nucleus of ossification in the human femoral head at the age of 4–6 months. (Reproduced by permission from Trueta 1968.)

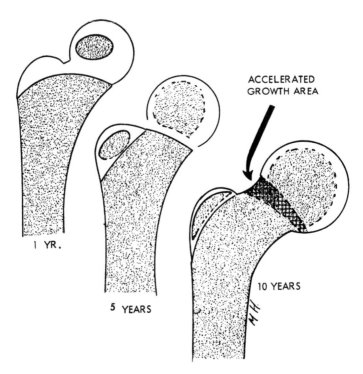

Fig. 1.6. The common growth plate separates with the lateral half providing growth to the greater trochanter while the medial half through accelerated growth causes elongation as well as varus orientation of the femoral neck. (Reproduced by permission from Tronzo 1973.)

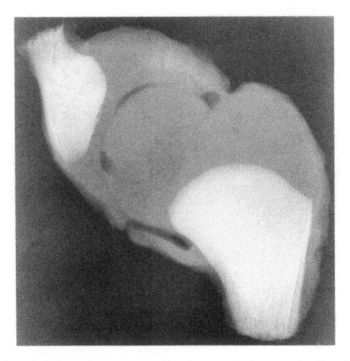

Fig. 1.7. Radiograph of a neonatal necroscopy specimen demonstrating the extent of cartilage tissue forming the acetabulum, femoral head, neck and greater trochanter. (By courtesy of M.B. Ozonoff, Newington Children's Hospital.)

develop into the future foot and toes. At six weeks the primitive cartilage model of the femur develops from the cellular blastema, resulting in a club-shaped femur (Chung 1981). In the blastema of the innominate the early depression indicates the development of the future acetabulum (Fig. 1.3). At the 17 mm stage of embryonic development a zone of demarcation between the future femoral head and acetabulum begins to develop, and by the late embryonic period the hip joint space begins to develop through a process of cellular degeneration in the zone between the two future opposing articular cartilage surfaces. According to studies by Chung the femoral head undergoes major change in size with respect to the developing acetabulum, representing 80% of a sphere in the embryo but reducing to 50% at birth (Fig. 1.4). Thus the coverage of the femoral head decreases from nearly 100% in early fetal development to only 65% at birth. By five months of fetal growth the hip joint as well as the surrounding capsule and adjacent muscles are fully developed (Ozonoff 1992).

The femoral head is entirely cartilagenous at birth, and the growth plate of the femoral head and greater trochanter are one continuous line of physeal growth (Fig. 1.5). It is of interest that John Hunter in the mid-18th century was the first to describe this basic anatomic fact in his experiments with the pig by studying the effect of red madder upon the developing proximal femoral growth plate (Dobson 1948). As noted by Chung, proximal femoral growth occurs in four regions: the capital growth plate, the trochanteric growth plate, the

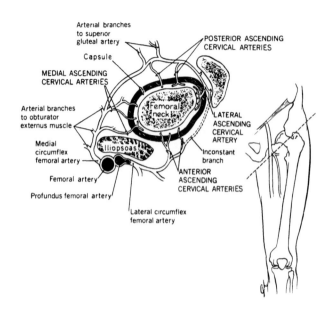

Fig. 1.8. Oblique transverse drawing at the base of the femoral neck demonstrating the anastamotic ring forming the blood supply for the proximal femur. (Reproduced by permission from Chung 1981.)

pre-osseous femoral head cartilage, and the greater trochanter pre-osseous cartilage. There is a differential rate of growth in the growth plate with the greatest rate of growth occurring in the central region, which results in the progressive elongation and varus angulation of the femoral neck (Fig. 1.6). The ossific nucleus of the femoral head does not appear until between 2 and 6 months of age in girls and between 3 and 7 months in boys (Stewart *et al.* 1986, Ozonoff 1992) (Fig. 1.5). Thus evaluation for developmental hip dysplasia in the period from birth to 5 months of age is best analyzed by ultrasonography, which provides the most detailed image of the non-ossified femoral head (Fig. 1.7).

The acetabulum develops as a cup-shaped depression surrounding the developing femoral head and is composed of three bones: the ilium in the superior aspect, the ischium in the inferior lateral position, and the pubis forming the medial wall. A notch is formed in the depths of the inferior aspect of the acetabulum, which is spanned by the transverse acetabular ligament. It is through this region that the arteries of the ligamentum teres pass from the obturator artery to the developing femoral head. The outer edge of the articular surface of the acetabulum is blended into a tough fibrocartilagenous ring, the labrum, which further increases the capacity of the acetabulum. By five months of fetal growth the hip joint has developed with its enveloping capsular and muscular attachments, and the orientation of the femoral neck which was in relative retroversion in early fetal development is progressing to an average of 35° anteversion noted at birth.

The development of the arterial supply of the femoral head and neck is of great importance to understanding the critical issue of avascular necrosis in the child's hip. The arterial supply is derived from the medial and lateral femoral circumflex vessels that arise from

6

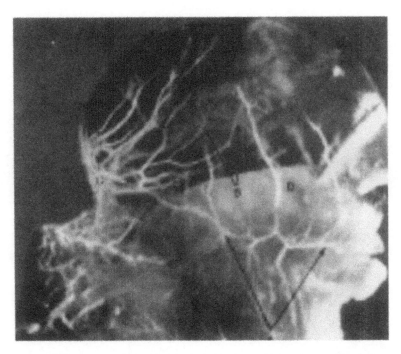

Fig. 1.9. Neonatal hip specimen following injection of barium sulfate to demonstrate the intracapsular vascular ring. (Reproduced by permission from Chung 1981.)

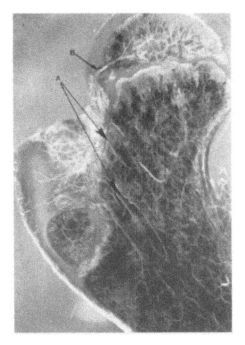

Fig. 1.10. Middle coronal section of the femur of a 6½-year-old female. (Reproduced by permission from Chung 1981.)

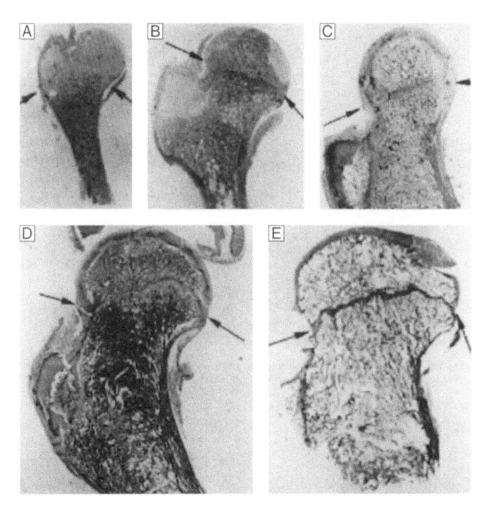

Fig. 1.11. Coronal sections of various femora demonstrating the groove of Ranvier and the perichondrial ring of Lacroix. (Reproduced by permission from Chung 1981.)

the femoral and profundus femoral artery (Fig. 1.8). These vessels form an anastamotic ring at the base of the femoral neck at the attachment of the capsule of the hip joint. Vessels pass through the capsule and ascend along the neck as metaphyseal vessels passing into the neck as well as epiphyseal branches to the ossification center of the femoral head (Fig. 1.9). In early life, prior to the development of the ossific nucleus of the femoral head, there are vessels from the femoral neck, which pass through the physeal plate to further supply the femoral head. After 15–18 months of life these penetrating vessels are blocked by the developing physeal plate, and the entire blood supply to the femoral head is dependent upon the medial and lateral circumflex vessels and their ascending posterior superior and posterior inferior epiphyseal vessels. A variable blood supply to the developing femoral head is

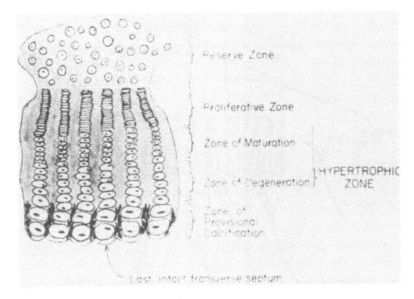

Fig. 1.12. The cartilaginous zones of the growth plate. (Reproduced by permission from Brighton 1978.)

provided by the artery in the ligamentum teres, but this is inconsistent (Chung 1981). Thus in the infant multiple posterior superior and posterior inferior epiphyseal vessels supply the femoral head from the medial and lateral femoral circumflex vessels. After the epiphyseal plate blocks the direct metaphyseal supply at the time of formation of the ossific nucleus, the femoral head is dependent totally upon the smaller lateral and posterior ascending cervical arteries that ascend upon the surface of the developing femoral neck (Ozonoff 1992) (Fig. 1.10). A circumferential groove called the perichondrial ring, located at the junction of the growth plate and the femoral metaphysis, provides mechanical support to the growth plate (Fig. 1.11).

The growth plate is composed of cartilage with five distinct zones (Fig. 1.12), the bony metaphysis situated immediately below the plate, and a peripheral fibrous band that surrounds these two structures, termed the groove of Ranvier and the perichondral ring of Lacroix (Brighton 1978). The most proximal of the five zones of cartilage, called the reserve zone, lies directly beneath the ossific nucleus in the developing femoral head. Beneath the reserve zone in descending order are the proliferative zone, the zone of maturation, the zone of degeneration and finally the zone of provisional calcification which is adjacent the developing metaphyseal bone. As seen in Figure 1.12, the cells of the reserve zone are spherical and surrounded by abundant extracellular matrix. The chondrocytes in the underlying proliferative zone divide and produce matrix which results in the longitudinal growth. In the hypertrophic zone the cells enlarge by a factor of five and then undergo degeneration in which hydroxyapatite crystal formation leads to calcification of the septae which becomes the zone of provisional calcification. The newly formed bone forms the metaphysis, which through remodeling with further growth elongates the femoral neck.

9

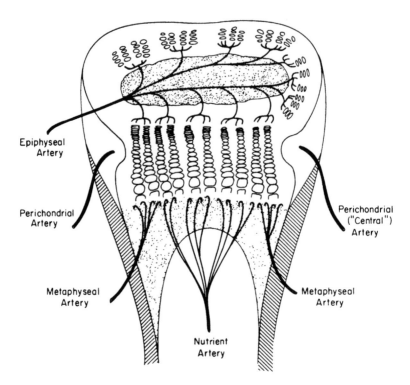

Fig. 1.13. Drawing of the blood supply of a typical growth plate. (Reproduced by permission from Brighton 1978.)

The blood supply to the growth plate initially includes the epiphyseal arteries, a perichondrial artery and the metaphyseal arteries (Fig. 1.13). As noted earlier, the blood supply of the proximal femur is unique since the entire femoral neck and head is intra-articular after the age of 2–3 years (Ozonoff 1992). The primary blood supply to the femoral head and neck arises from the medial and lateral femoral circumflex vessels in an anastamotic ring at the base of the femoral neck. There are arteriosinusoidal vessels, which penetrate the growth plate until the ossification of the epiphysis blocks them. Subsequent to the appearance of the ossification of the ossific nucleus of the epiphysis, the blood supply is entirely dependent upon the ascending lateral and posterior cervical vessels as the femoral head continues to grow. An ossification groove, first described by Ranvier in 1873 (see Brighton 1978), encircles the growth plate. Cells in this groove contribute to the peripheral growth of the growth plate leading to an increase in the circumference of the plate with further growth of the proximal femur. This groove is overlaid by a dense fibrous band with multidirectional collagen fibrous bands that provide the support to the growth plate (Lacroix 1951). This complex of collagen fibers is of particular relevance to the condition of slipped capital femoral epiphysis since the pathologic process occurs at this point with progressive instability between the epiphysis and the underlying metaphysis. It should also be remem-

10

bered that this is the same region where the metaphyseal and ascending cervical arteries can be compromised by vascular occlusion with a severe displacement of the epiphysis (Fig. 1.11).

Anatomic findings at birth

At birth the orientation of the acetabulum is facing anterior (anteverted) approximately 40°, the femoral neck is also anteverted approximately 35°, and the hip joint is most stable in the position of flexion and mild abduction. The orientation of the acetabulum does not change; however, there is a progressive decrease in femoral anteversion during the first 10 years of life until it reaches the adult range of 15°. Femoral anteversion refers to the plane of the femoral neck in relation to the bicondylar axis of the distal femur at the knee joint (Ruwe *et al.* 1992). Figure 1.14 demonstrates the ideal method of measurement of femoral anteversion by means of computerized axial tomography. Serial transverse sections are measured at the femoral head/greater trochanteric region and compared to the bicondylar axis of the distal femur. Perpendicular lines constructed from these two axes allow for direct measurement of the degree of anterior deviation (anteversion) or posterior deviation (retroversion) of the proximal femur. Many young children may demonstrate a relative increase in femoral anteversion resulting in an increase in internal rotation of the entire lower extremity in gait, because the femoral head seeks normal articulation with the acetabulum. The progressive increase in length as well as circumference of the femur is due to a combination of growth and remodeling of bone mediated by the capital and greater trochanteric physeal plates as well as the non-ossified cartilage of the femoral head. The subsequent growth and development of the femoral head and neck is dependent upon the forces applied across the joint (Nordin and Frankel 1989). In children with neuromuscular conditions the normal reduction in femoral anteversion with growth is retarded. This is explained by a combination of reduced strength in the abductor musculature resulting in relative valgus angulation of the femoral neck, reduced weight-bearing forces altering the remodeling of the femur with growth, and increased motor tone as well as contractures across the hip joint. This is evident from the comparison of the normal reduction of femoral anteversion in the normal child versus children with motor imbalance such as cerebral palsy as noted in Figure 1.15. In addition, when there is associated weakness of the gluteal muscles resulting in abductor weakness, less tension force is applied to the greater trochanter, which leads to an increased neck shaft angle. All subsequent growth and development of the hip joint is dependent upon the intimate concentric relationship between the femoral head and the acetabulum (see Chapter 4).

A thick fibrous capsule comprising an inner synovial layer reinforced by overlying ligaments encloses the hip joint. The ischiofemoral ligament envelops the posterior aspect of the joint, and the iliofemoral ligament, otherwise known as the Y ligament of Bigelow, extends over the anterior surface of the hip joint from the acetabular rim to insert on the inferomedial aspect of the femoral neck. Immediately overlying this structure is the tendon of the iliopsoas muscle, which crosses the anterior aspect of the joint to insert onto the lesser trochanter. The capsular and ligamentous structures are compressed with the normal hip in full extension and internal rotation, with the femoral head and acetabular cartilaginous

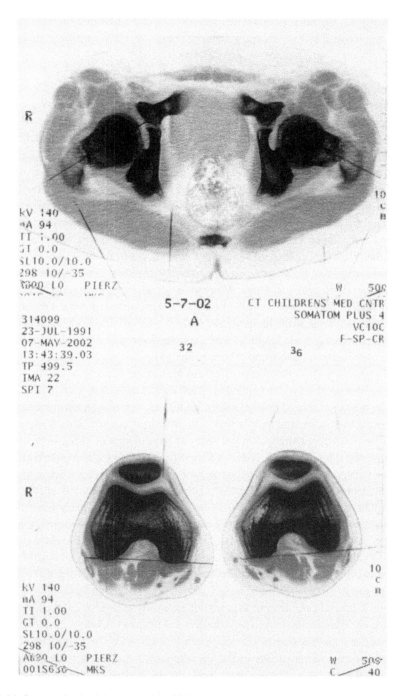

Fig. 1.14. Computerized axial tomography of the pelvis, hip and distal femur demonstrating the method of measuring femoral anteversion. Perpendiculars are erected from the mid-coronal axis of the femoral head/neck/greater trochanter and the bicondylar axis of the distal femur. In this example the femoral anteversion is measured as 32° in the right hip and 36° in the left hip.

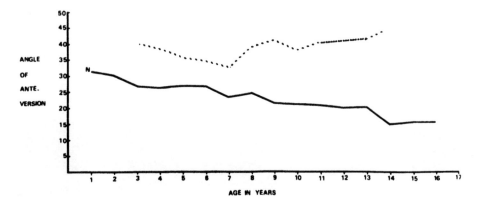

Fig. 1.15. Graph of the average measurements of femoral anteversion in relation to age *(solid line)* with comparison to the increased anteversion noted in patients with cerebral palsy *(dotted line)*. (Reproduced by permission from Hensinger 1986.)

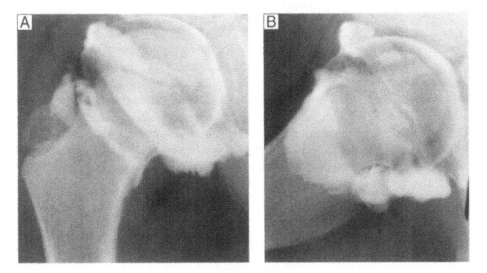

Fig. 1.16. Arthrogram in the (A) anteroposterior and (B) frog projections demonstrating the intracapsular space of a normal hip. Note the thin line of contrast outlining the articular surface of the femoral head, the clear demarcation of the lateral edge of the acetabulum, and the relative pooling of contrast in the inferior region of the neck in the frog projection when the hip is abducted and externally rotated.

surfaces in maximum contact. With abduction, flexion and external rotation the capsular and ligamentous structures are most relaxed thereby reducing the intracapsular pressure on the hip joint. The normal confines of the intra-articular space of the hip joint are illustrated in Figure 1.16). The overlying muscles further contribute to the stability of the hip joint and may be summarized as consisting of four quadrants in the sagittal and coronal plane providing flexion, extension, abduction and adduction of the lower limb. In the transverse

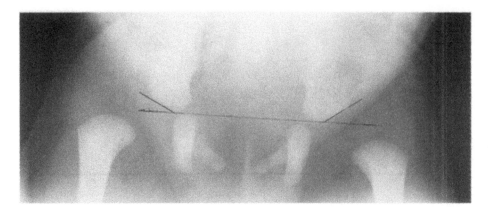

Fig. 1.17. Anteroposterior radiograph of a neonatal pelvis demonstrating bilateral dislocation of the femoral heads. The horizontal line drawn through the triradiate cartilage (Hilgenriger's line) is easily identified. The underdeveloped acetabular margins do not allow for accurate measurement of the acetabular index. The cartilaginous femoral head is not visible at this point of development but is laterally displaced from the underdeveloped acetabulum.

plane these muscles in coordination provide for internal and external rotation, with the femoral head and acetabulum serving as the fulcrum for all motion. The radiographic appearance at birth of the hip of a child with bilateral hip dislocation is shown in Figure 1.17. It is readily apparent from viewing the radiograph of the neonatal pelvis that the acetabular margins are not well demarcated, making accurate measurement of the acetabular index prone to error. The acetabular index, a, normally decreases from 25° in boys and 22° in girls to 18° and 19° respectively by 24 months of age (Scoles *et al.* 1987). Since the femoral capital epiphysis is not ossified and the lateral acetabular edge is also cartilaginous at this age, it is important to utilize ultrasonography to examine the newborn hip within the first five months.

Pathologic abnormalities
From the standpoint of the histology of the articular cartilage, the growth plate and the underlying bone, one can derive an understanding of many of the pathologic conditions that can affect the hip joint. Table 1.1 outlines the major histologic zones and the common abnormalities that can arise as a result of various pathologic conditions.

As noted by Warkany (1971), true congenital dislocation of the hip joint is rare, and the term "congenital dislocation of the hip" has now been superceded by "developmental dysplasia of the hip". There are, however, some instances in which a true teratologic dislocation of the hip is found. This is almost always associated with congenital syndromes or malformations such as arthrogryposis multiplex congenita, sacral agenesis (Duhamel 1961) and spinal dysraphism. In the teratologic dislocation the femoral head is totally dislocated during the later stages of fetal development. In a teratologic dislocation, not only is the femoral head totally dislocated, but the acetabulum in turn is underdeveloped with a shallow socket the superior aspect of which is flattened (Fig. 1.18).

14

TABLE 1.1
Major histologic zones of the hip and common abnormalities that can arise as a result of various pathologic conditions

Cellular region	Disease	Mechanism
Reserve zone of physis	Diastrophic dwarfism Pseudoachrondroplasia	Type II collagen defect Defective processing of proteoglycans
Proliferative zone of physis	Achondroplasia Gigantism	Deficient cell proliferation Excessive cell proliferation
Hypertrophic zone of physis	Mucopolysaccharidosis	Lysozomal enzyme defects
Zone of provisional calcification	Rickets	Calcium/VitaminD deficiency
Metaphyseal bone	Osteomyelitis Metaphyseal dysplasia	Bacterial invasion Hypertrophic cells extend into metaphysis

Adapted by permission from Staheli (1998).

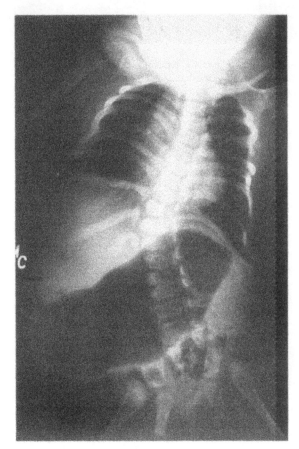

Fig. 1.18. Anterior view of the spine and pelvis of a newborn child with diabetic embryopathy. Note the bilateral teratogenic dislocation of both hips, the congenital scoliosis and the right-sided abdominal wall herniation.

15

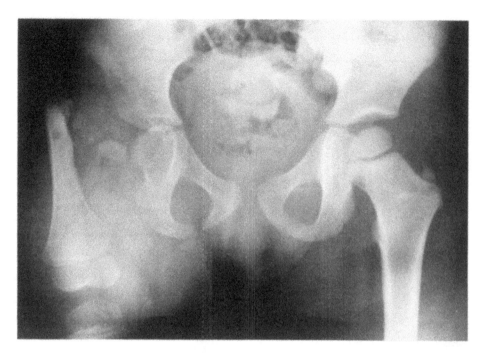

Fig. 1.19. Radiograph of the right hip demonstrating proximal femoral focal deficiency with severe femoral shortening, varus angulation at the fibrocartilaginous neck, and the underdeveloped fragment of the femoral head within the acetabulum.

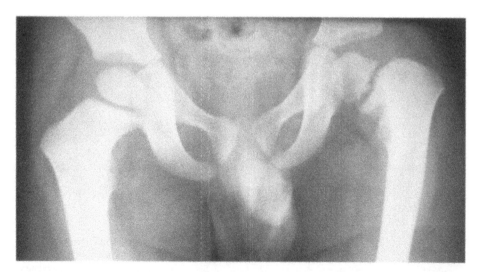

Fig. 1.20. Radiograph of congenital coxa vara of the femur. Note the inferomedial wedge-shaped fragment of bone at the base of the femoral neck. This results from a defect in or about the epiphyseal plate, and the triangular fragment may be thought of as a fragment broken away from the medial metaphysis.

16

The condition of proximal femoral focal deficiency refers to a spectrum of underdevelopment of the femur with femoral shortening and varying degrees of femoral head and neck deformity ranging from a pseudoarthrosis in the subtrochanteric area to total absence of the femoral head and neck (Gillespie 1997). Such cases are evident at birth as the child presents with shortening of the affected extremity, with varying degrees of instability of the hip depending upon the degree of involvement (Fig. 1.19). It has been hypothesized that various noxious stimuli may occur during early embryonic development, including irradiation, maternal diabetes and viral infection, leading to defective limb development. The rare condition of congenital short femur is related to thalidomide exposure (Hamanishi 1980).

A primary defect in the formation of the femoral neck may result in the condition of congenital coxa vara (Weinstein *et al.* 1984). The primary defect is one of a disturbance in the proximal femoral physeal plate leading to progressive decrease in the neck shaft angle, with disruption of the metaphyseal side of the plate with increasing varus deformation of the proximal femur (Fig. 1.20).

REFERENCES

Brighton, C.T. (1978) 'Structure and function of the growth plate.' *Clinical Orthopaedics and Related Research*, **136**, 22–32.

Chung, S.M.K. (1981) *Hip Disorders in Infants and Children.* Philadelphia: Lea & Febiger.

Dobson, J. (1948) Pioneers of osteology, John Hunter: 1728–1793.' *Journal of Bone and Joint Surgery, British Volume*, **30**, 361–364.

Duhamel, B. (1961) 'From the mermaid to anal imperforation: the syndrome of caudal regression.' *Archives of Diseases in Childhood*, **36**, 152–155.

Gillespie, R. (1997) 'Classification of congenital abnormalities of the femur.' *In:* Herring, J.A., Birch J.G. (Eds.) *The Child with a Limb Deficiency.* Rosemont, IL: American Academy of Orthopaedic Surgeons, pp. 63–72.

Hamanishi, C. (1980) 'Congenital short femur.' *Journal of Bone and Joint Surgery, British Volume*, **62**, 307–320.

Hensinger, R.N. (1986) *Standards in Pediatric Orthopedics: Tables, Charts and Graphs Illustrating Growth.* New York: Raven Press.

Kelley, R.O. (1985) 'Early development of the vertebrate limb: an introduction to morphogenetic tissue interactions using scanning electron microscopy.' *Scanning Electron Microscopy*, **2**, 827–836.

Lacroix, P. (1951) *The Organization of Bone.* New York: McGraw-Hill.

Lovett, M., Clines, G., Wise, C.A. (1997) 'Genetic control of limb development.' *In:* Herring J.A., Birch, J.G. (Eds.) *The Child with a Limb Deficiency.* Rosemont, IL: American Academy of Orthoapedic Surgeons, pp. 13–24.

Moore, K.L. (1977) *The Developing Human, 2nd Edn.* Philadelphia: W.B. Saunders.

Nordin, M., Frankel, V.H. (1989) *Basic Biomechanics of the Musculoskeletal System.* Philadelphia: Lea & Febiger.

Ozonoff, M.B. (1992) *Pediatric Orthopaedic Radiology, 2nd Edn.* Philadelphia: W.B. Saunders.

Ruwe, P.A., Gage, J.R., Ozonoff, M.B., DeLuca, P.A. (1992) 'Clinical determination of femoral anteversion.' *Journal of Bone and Joint Surgery, American Volume*, **74**, 820–830.

Scoles, P.V., Boyd, A., Jones, P.K. (1987) 'Roentgenographic parameters of the normal infant hip.' *Journal of Pediatric Orthopaedics*, **7**, 656–663.

Staheli, L.T (1998) *Fundamentals of Pediatric Orthopedics, 2nd Edn.* Philadelphia: Lipppincott-Raven.

Stevenson, R.E., Meyer, L.C. (1993) 'The limbs.' *In:* Stevenson, R.E., Hall, J.G., Goodman, R.M. (Eds.) *Human Malformations and Related Anomalies , Vol. 2. Oxford Monographs of Medical Genetics No. 27.* Oxford: Oxford University Press, pp. 699–702.

Stewart, R.J., Patterson, C.C., Mollan, R.A. (1986) 'Ossification of the normal femoral capital epiphysis.' *Journal of Bone and Joint Surgery, British Volume*, **68**, 653–654.

Strayer, L.M. (1971) 'Embryology of the human hip joint'. *Clinical Orthoapaedics and Related Research*, **74**, 221–240.

Thorogood, P. (1983) 'Morphogenesis of cartilage.' *In:* Hall, B.K. (Ed.) *Cartilage, Vol. 2. Development, Differentiation and Growth.* New York: Academic Press, pp. 223–239.

Tronzo (1973) *Surgery of the Hip Joint.* Philadelphia: Lea & Febiger.

Trueta, J. (1968) *Studies of the Development and Decay of the Human Frame.* Philadelphia: W.B. Saunders; Bath: Pitman.

Warkany, J. (1971) *Congenital Malformations: Notes and Comments.* Chicago: Year Book Medical.

Watanabe, R.S. (1974) 'Embryology of the human hip.' *Clinical Orthopaedics and Related Research*, **98**, 8–26.

Weinstein, J.N., Kuo, K.N., Millar, E.A. (1984) 'Congenital coxa vara: a retrospective review.' *Journal of Pediatric Orthopedics*, **4**, 70–77.

2
PHYSICAL EXAMINATION OF THE CHILD'S HIP

Bruce E. Bowman

Musculoskeletal examination of some joints is facilitated by the fact that there is little or minimal soft tissue overlying a given joint. The hip, however, is difficult to examine as it is more deeply located within overlying musculature and soft tissues. Disorders of infection, anatomic abnormality and vascularity that can affect a child's hip carry significant morbidity. Thus the clinician must maintain a *high index of suspicion for occult hip pathology* when examining a child with lower extremity complaints. There can be a wide variation in the presentation of symptoms. Referred pain patterns may make the clinician suspect that pathology originates in a location other than the hip, thus possibly delaying adequate evaluation and early treatment of morbid conditions.

By closely observing a child's gait and performing a careful systematic examination of the child's hip and related areas, any occult pathology should be revealed. As in all aspects in the physical examination, the child must be adequately disrobed to allow for a thorough observation, inspection and examination.

Anatomic considerations
Patients with a synovitis of the hip hold their limb in a slightly abducted, flexed and externally rotated position. Anatomically the iliofemoral, pubofemoral and ischiofemoral joint ligaments are wound tightly about the hip. The iliofemoral or "Y" ligament is at its greatest tension with the hip in extension. These ligaments are strong and act to support the stability of the hip joint especially in stance. The fibers are wrapped in a fashion that when the limb is in extension the femoral head is driven deeper into the acetabulum (Moore and Dalley 1999). Any effusion present in the hip will inhibit and block internal rotation and extension of the hip. With distention of the hip capsular space, the leg is held flexed, abducted and externally rotated in an attempt to reduce the intra-articular pressure and resultant pain. The use of ultrasound should be considered to help identify and document effusions.

The hip joint is innervated by multiple peripheral nerves. This includes the femoral nerve, the anterior division of the obturator nerve, the sciatic nerve and the superior gluteal nerve (Moore and Dalley 1999). Pain may be referred along the course of any of these nerves, which accounts for the consistent complaints of distal thigh and knee pain in the presence of hip pathology. Pain may be radiating from the patient's low back, abdomen, sacroiliac joint, knees or ankles. Each of these areas needs to be examined.

History

Obtain a detailed history that includes current presentation detailing the onset of symptoms, intensity, frequency and duration. Ask about traumatic versus insidious onset of pain, and any associated symptoms such as fever, rashes or loss of appetite. Are there endemic diseases that should be considered, such as Lyme disease in the northeastern USA, sickle cell disease in the Caribbean, etc.? Are there any aggravating or ameliorating factors? Is the pain reproducible? What is the location of the pain? Is there any lateral pain over the greater trochanter suggestive of a bursitis from the iliotibial band snapping over the greater trochanter? A sharp anterior groin pain may be suggestive of a labral tear. Is there night-time pain well relieved by nonsteroidal anti-inflammatory agents suggestive of an osteoid osteoma?

What is the sports participation history? Is the child involved in more than one team in the same sport at the same time, or on multiple teams for different sports at the same time? If the pain is of traumatic origin, what was the mechanism, and what forces were placed on the extremity? Constitutional symptoms and an index of suspicion are important in recognizing the potential of disorders such as leukemia. Approximately 20% of pediatric leukemia patients present with bone pain (Greene 2001).

Of equal importance is the past medical history including birth history. Was the child born preterm, or was there any difficulty with the delivery that may have provided an hypoxic insult? Is the developmental history normal? This information paired with subtle posturing of an upper extremity and gait asymmetries may suggest cerebral palsy.

Family history is relevant in the evaluation of limping children. Is there a family history of osteogenesis imperfecta, sickle cell disease, arthritis or hemophilia? Is there a family history of hip dislocations?

Child at risk

It is an unfortunate reality to have to consider the risk of child abuse. What is the social history? Who is the primary care giver? Do both parents work and who watches the child while they are away? Who else lives in the home? Are there any suspicions of child abuse given the presentation? Is the history of the event consistent over time? Are family members consistent in relating facts about the incident? Are there multiple bruises at various stages of resolving? Is there any inappropriate behavior on the part of caregivers that makes you suspicious? Is there any suggestion of substance abuse by the parents?

Physical Examination

THE ACUTELY ILL CHILD

The acutely ill child with a fever and gait disturbance or refusal to walk must always raise the concern of a potential pyarthrosis with its risk of chondrolysis (Morrisey 2001). This child may guard excessively and prevent adequate examination. When evaluating an acutely ill young child, gain their confidence by examining the uninvolved extremity first. Start with gentle maneuvers such as a *roll test* (Fig. 2.1.) Progress with a more thorough examination of the extremity once having obtained a sense of the degree of irritability.

When examining a patient's hips or lower extremities in a supine position the examiner

20

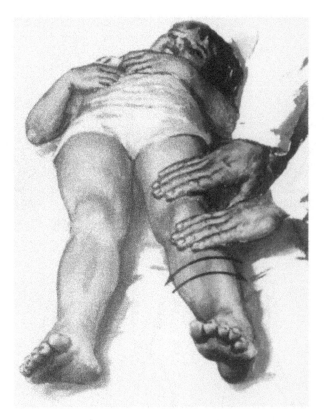

Fig. 2.1. Roll test. Gently roll the extremity back and forth to elicit guarding and/or pain. Begin with the uninvolved extremity. (Reproduced by permission from the *CIBA Collection of Medical Illustrations, Vol. 8, Part 2.*)

should check each extremity by standing on the same side as the extremity being examined. The examiner should stabilize the patient by placing a hand on the patients torso or pelvis. This allows the examiner to best appreciate end points in range of motion tests. The examiner will also be in a position to sense any subtle guarding by the patient and it allow for a more accurate measurement of range of motion. Careful examination and performing a thorough range of motion will help clarify the location of pathology.

OBSERVATION OF GAIT
The well child should be asked to walk utilizing the longest corridor available in your office. Have the child walk back and forth several times to get a representative appearance of their normal gait pattern. The child should have minimal clothing and be barefoot. Confirm with the child's parents that the gait pattern is reflective of what they see at home. Often children will perform for you and provide you with their "best" or "doctor's" gait. There are times when it is helpful to have the child run, as they may forgo their inhibitions

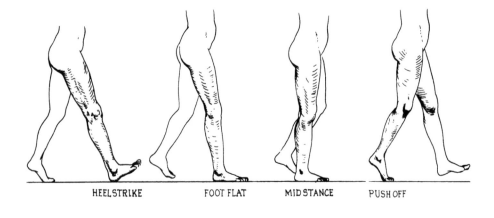

| HEELSTRIKE | FOOT FLAT | MID STANCE | PUSH OFF |

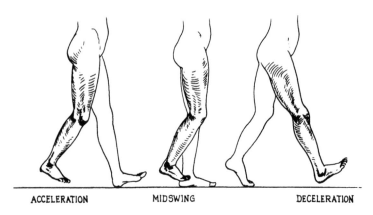

| ACCELERATION | MIDSWING | DECELERATION |

Fig. 2.2. Gait cycle: phases of stance and swing for the lower extremity. (Reproduced by permission from Hoppenfeld 1976.)

and more subtle nuances may be appreciated, such as posturing of an upper extremity in a mild hemiplegic. Have the child squat, stand on one leg, and then hop on one leg.

Observe the child's normal pattern of the gait cycle (stance phase: heel strike, foot flat, mid-stance, push-off; swing phase: acceleration, mid-swing, deceleration) (Fig. 2.2).

Look for deviations from the normal cadence, and lack of normal excursion at the hip, knee and ankle. Is the patient avoiding stressing a certain joint and exhibiting an antalgic gait? An antalgic gait is an asymmetric cadence characterized by reduced stance phase on one extremity secondary to pain inhibition with attempted weight-bearing on the affected limb.

Is there a reciprocal motion of the upper extremities? Observation of the sagittal plane motion of the lower extremity may reveal poor knee flexion as seen in children with diplegic cerebral palsy. Is there dorsiflexion at the ankle to allow adequate clearance of the toes during the swing phase? Or does the child walk with a drop foot, and drag the forefoot in swing

22

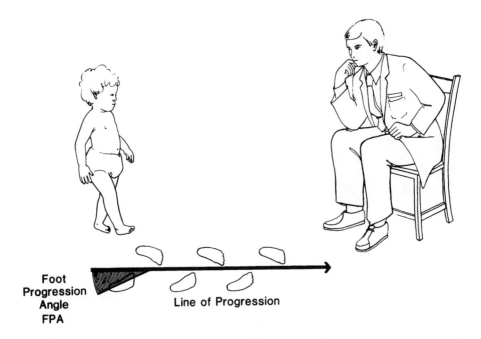

Fig. 2.3. The foot progression angle (FPA) is derived from the direction of travel and a bisector of the heel and second toe. (Reproduced by permission from Staheli 1986.)

phase? Does the patient circumduct the limb to avoid knee flexion? Is the child walking on his/her toes indicative of possible spasticity from cerebral palsy or is s/he an idiopathic toe walker? Is s/he up on the toes on one side because of a leg length discrepancy? A toddler presenting for a leg length discrepancy may have a unilateral hip dislocation. Have the child run.

The *foot progression angle* (FPA) is the angle derived from the direction of the gait and the long axis of the foot drawn from the second toe and bisecting the heel (Fig. 2.3). Thus one can describe the FPA as internal or external, and be able to qualify its extent. For example, an adolescent with slipped capital femoral epiphyses may exhibit an antalgic gait and an external foot progression pattern.

STANDING EXAMINATION
When examining the torso, pelvis and upper thighs observe any cutaneous abnormalities such as: café au lait spots, scars, nodules, erythema, swelling, increased skin temperature, asymmetry of skin folds, or masses. Note any postural abnormalities, such as a trunk shift, asymmetry of the waist line, asymmetry between the waist and the dependent arms, asymmetric positioning of either the posterior superior iliac spines or anterior iliac spines suggestive of leg length discrepancy (Fig. 2.4), or scoliosis. Apparent scoliosis may be compensatory postural changes seen because of a limb length discrepancy and not a structural scoliosis. What are the sagittal contours of the spine? Is there a normal thoracic kyphosis

23

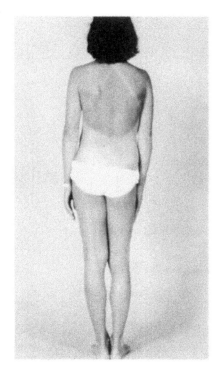

Fig. 2.4. Leg length discrepancy with apparent scoliosis. There is slight shoulder asymmetry, scapular prominence on left, and asymmetry of triangle formed by dependent arms and trunk. Note asymmetry in markers placed over the posterior superior iliac spines.

and lumbar lordosis? With forward flexion of the spine does the sagittal contour of the thoracic spine sharply angulate as found in Scheuermann's kyphosis? Loss of lumbar lordosis may reflect lumbar paravertebral muscle spasm in a patient with back pain, bilateral hip flexion contractures, or an advanced case of spondylolisthesis. Observe the lower extremities in stance. Is there any atrophy, or malalignment of the limb? The normally aligned limb has the weight of the body passing through the center of the hip, knee and ankle. Does the child easily stand erect with both feet in a plantar grade position with knees at full extension?

PELVIC STATION

Assess any pelvic obliquity by having the patient stand erect *with knees locked*. Place your hands on the top of the iliac crests and maintain your thumbs at the same level. If there is any difference in the height of your thumbs, then level the pelvis with blocks to determine the difference in leg lengths. Pelvic station can also be determined by observing any differential height between the posterior superior iliac spine (PSIS) or the anterior superior iliac spine (ASIS). The level of the PSIS is characterized by the presence of the overlying dimples in the non-obese child.

SOFT TISSUE AND BONE PALPATION

Palpation of soft tissue structures in the hip area can be principally divided into four regions: posterior, lateral, medial, and anterior. To examine the posterior aspect place the patient in

24

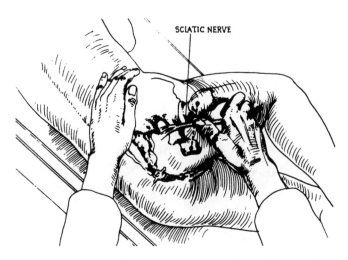

SCIATIC NERVE

Fig. 2.5. Sciatic notch palpation. Locate the greater trochanter and the ischial tuberosity. The sciatic nerve will run between these two landmarks. Firm pressure in this location will cause pain in the presence of sciatic nerve irritability. (Reproduced by permission from Hoppenfeld 1976.)

a lateral position. In this position you can appreciate the cutaneous dimpling over the PSIS. The iliac crest can be readily palpated from the PSIS, along the crest, to the ASIS. Orient yourself to anatomic landmarks. The PSIS is level with the spinous process of S2, as is the middle of the sacroiliac joint. The iliac crests are level with the L4–L5 disk space (Moore and Dalley 1999).

The sacroiliac joint is not accessible to palpation due to the posterior extension of the ilium beyond its articulation with the sacrum. The body of the sacrum can be palpated along the natal cleft. In the presence of concern regarding the coccyx, the coccyx can be palpated between the examiner's gloved index finger in the rectum and the thumb over the posterior part of the sacrum.

Laterally palpate the iliac crest. Bring your fingers more distal below the iliac crest and palpate the greater trochanter. Patients with a greater trochanteric bursitis will have localized tenderness at this level. The ischial tuberosity can be palpated inferior and medial to the greater trochanter. The ischial tuberosity is the site of origin of the biceps femoris, adductor magnus, semitendinosus and semimembranosus. Using the ischial tuberosity and the greater trochanter as landmarks, palpate deeply between them with your thumb to elicit any sciatic nerve tenderness (Fig. 2.5). The sciatic nerve will have exited the pelvis superiorly at the sciatic notch and may be compressed by the firm pressure of your thumb.

Anteriorly the ASIS is easily found on the anterior edge of the iliac crest. The inguinal ligament traverses from the ASIS inferiorly and medially to the pubic tubercle at the superior lateral edge of the pubic symphysis. This is the superior border to the *femoral triangle* (Fig. 2.6). The contents of the femoral triangle from lateral to medial are the femoral nerve, artery and vein. The lateral border of the femoral triangle is the sartorius. The medial border is the adductor longus muscle. In the medial aspect of the femoral triangle are the lymph

25

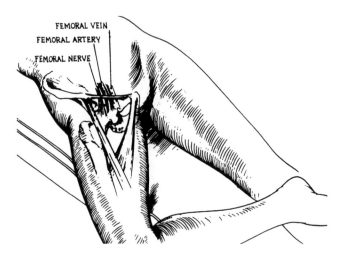

Fig. 2.6. Femoral triangle/figure 4. Place the extremity in a figure 4 position by flexing, externally rotating and abductng the leg. The "femoral triangle" has a superior border of the inguinal ligament, medial border of the adductor longus, and lateral border of the sartorius. The content of the femoral triangle from lateral to medial is: femoral nerve, femoral artery, femoral vein and lymphatics. (Reproduced by permission from Hoppenfeld 1976.)

nodes that drain the lower extremity, lower abdominal wall, perineum and portions of the rectum.

The lateral femoral cutaneous nerve exits the pelvis superficially just medial to the ASIS. This nerve is easily injured on surgical exposure of the hip and may be traumatized by wearing tight belts and clothing. Meralgia paresthetica is an irritation of this nerve.

RANGE OF MOTION

Alterations in range of motion are the indicators of hip pathology. Loss of internal rotation is the most sensitive for pathology such as transient or toxic synovitis, pyarthrosis, Legg–Calvé–Perthes disease or slipped capital femoral epiphysis. The longer standing the hip pathology is, the more fixed contractures will develop. Range of motion can be assessed actively and passively. Always compare the range of motion between the afflicted joint or extremity to the contralateral "normal" side. The passive range of motion should be greater than active range of motion. By asking the patient to perform active tests against manual resistance, one can test motor strength.

Flexion (0–120°)

With the patient supine, maximally flex the hip not being examined to stabilize the pelvis and reduce the lumbar lordosis. Then assess the tested hip in neutral rotation from maximum extension to maximal flexion. The normal range is 0–120°. By 3 months of age the typical mean neonatal hip flexion contracture of 20° has resolved to a mean of 7° (Coon *et al.* 1975). Observe any limitations (Fig. 2.7).

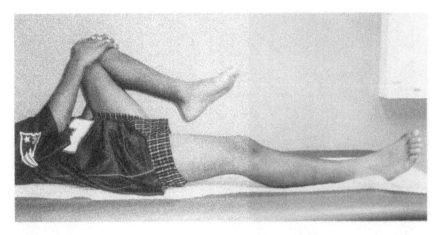

Fig. 2.7. Hip flexion. The patient may actively flex the hip (as here), or a passive examination may be done. With the patient in a supine position flex the hip until the pelvis start to tilt. Patients generally have approximately 120° of hip flexion.

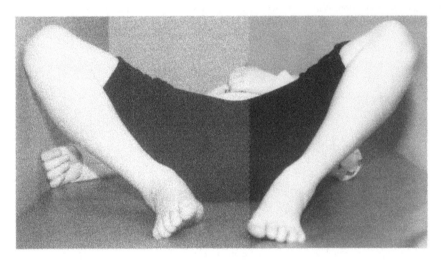

Fig. 2.8. Hip abduction. Hip abduction may be checked with the legs extended or with the hips flexed at 90°. When checking with the legs extended, place a hand on the pelvis to appreciate the end-point of the motion before the pelvis starts to tip.

Abduction (45–50°)

In testing hip abduction in extension it is helpful for the examiner to place their hand on the child's pelvis spanning the ASIS with thumb and little finger. This allows the examiner to better determine the end-point in the range of motion. For examiners with smaller hands the whole forearm may be placed across the pelvis (Fig. 2.8).

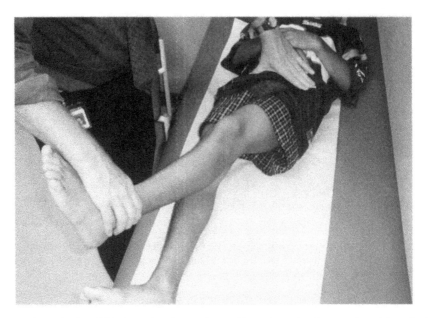

Fig. 2.9. Hip adduction. With the patient in a supine position, place a hand across the pelvis and bring the limb being tested across the midline to its maximal extent.

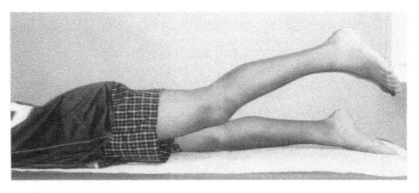

Fig. 2.10. Hip extension. Have the patient lie prone. The patient may actively extend the hip (as here), or a passive examination may be done. Stabilize the pelvis with one hand and flex the knee to 90°, while with the other hand grasp the ankle and lift the leg, extending the hip to its fullest extent.

Adduction (20–30°)
Stabilize the pelvis with hand or forearm as described above. Adduct the limb to its fullest extent (Fig. 2.9).

Extension (0–30°)
Have the patient lie prone. They may actively extend the hip (Fig. 2.10), or a passive

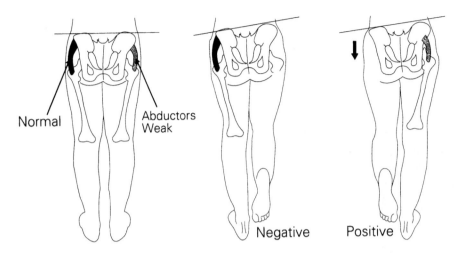

Normal

Abductors Weak

Negative   Positive

Fig. 2.12. Trendelenburg test. To determine if there is any weakness in the hip abductors have the patient stand on one leg. Lowering of the contralateral hemipelvis constitutes a positive test. (Reproduced by permission from Staheli 1992.)

Maneuvers

Trendelenburg Test

To determine if there is any weakness in the hip abductors have the patient stand on one leg. Lowering of the contralateral hemipelvis constitutes a positive test. In patients with normal strength and no hip pathology the non-stance hemipelvis is elevated or is maintained level. This test requires normal strength in the patient's stance-side hip abductors (gluteus medius and minimus) (Fig. 2.12). Patients with bilateral positive Trendelenburg tests will ambulate with an alternating lateral trunk shift with each step. A waddling gait with bilateral trunk shifts in a toddler may be indicative of bilateral hip dislocations, or bilateral coxa vara.

Palpable Version—Craig Test

The plane of the neck shaft is angled anteriorly relative to the transcondylar axis of the femur by 15° in a normal adult hip. Excessive internal rotation of the hip is termed anteversion. Conversely, excessive external rotation of the hip is termed retroversion. Infants are born with approximately 30–40° of anteversion. In children with normal muscle tone the femoral neck version recedes at the rate of 2–3° per year (Staheli 1980). The version can be determined by having the child lay prone. Place one hand over the greater trochanter. With the other hand grasp the tibia above the ankle. As you gently internally and externally rotate the limb, feel the greater trochanter for the position with the maximal lateral prominence. Palpable version is the degree of leg rotation at the time you feel the maximal degree of version or inclination of the femoral neck. One vector of this angle is the starting point of zero degrees of internal rotation with the flexed knee and the tibia perpendicular to the examining table (Fig. 2.13).

31

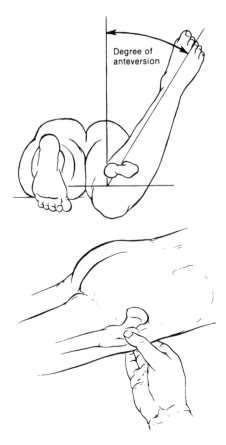

Fig. 2.13. Palpable version. Version can be determined by having the child lie prone. Place one hand over the greater trochanter. With the other hand grasp the tibia above the ankle. As you gently internally and externally rotate the limb, feel the greater trochanter for the position with the maximum lateral prominence. (Reproduced by permission from Chung 1981.)

Hip rotation ranges change as the child develops. Initially there are physiologic external rotation contractures about the hip. Thus, the infant's anteversion is masked until approximately 3 years of age when the physiologic contractures resolve.

THOMAS TEST

Hip flexion contracture is measured by the Thomas test. A patient's normal lumbar flexibility can mask a restricted range of motion in the hip. This flexibility is evidenced by the examiner being able to place his or her hand between the examining table and the patient's lumbar spine. In order to measure the hip flexion contracture, the pelvis must be stabilized. This is accomplished by having the patient maximally flex both hips. This places the pelvis in an anatomically neutral position with the ASIS and PSIS aligned perpendicular to the examining table. It is easy to over or under compensate the position of the pelvis. While maintaining one hip in flexion, and aligned ASIS and PSIS, allow the other hip to lower to a "hip neutral" position. If the hip being lowered cannot be lowered to the examining table then the angle subtended by the long axis of the femur and that of the table is the amount of hip flexion contracture (Fig. 2.14).

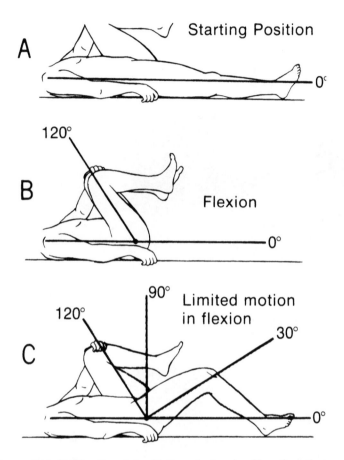

A Starting Position

0°

B 120°

Flexion

0°

C 90° Limited motion in flexion

120°

30°

0°

Fig. 2.14. Thomas Test. Stabilize the pelvis with the patient supine. Have the patient maximally flex both hips. This places the pelvis in an anatomically neutral position with the anterior and posterior superior iliac spines aligned perpendicular to the examining table. This eliminates the lumbar lordosis. While maintaining one hip in flexion, and leveling the pelvis, allow the other hip to lower to a "hip neutral" position. If the hip being lowered cannot be lowered all the way to the examining table then the angle subtended by the long axis of the femur and the table is the amount of hip flexion contracture.

FIGURE 4 TEST (PATRICK OR FABER TEST)

With the patient in a supine position, place the lower extremity in a figure 4 position. In doing so the limb will have been flexed, abducted and externally rotated. The examiner's hands are then placed on the child's contralateral iliac crest and flexed knee. A downward force is placed across the knee, compressing the sacroiliac joint posteriorly. This same maneuver places a stretch on the femoral nerve (see Fig. 2.7) This is as shown for the femoral triangle.

OBER TEST

The Ober test is performed to assess pathologic tightness of the fascia lata and iliotibial

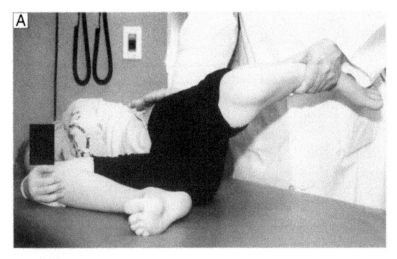

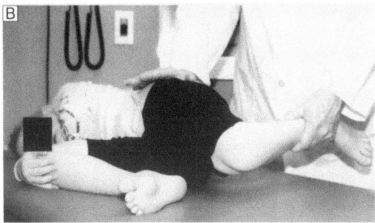

Fig. 2.15. Ober Test. The patient is placed in a lateral position. Flex the downside hip to 90° and hold it in place with the patient's hands. Flex the knee on the hip being tested, and bring the femur to a hip neutral position. Stabilize the hip with your opposite hand. Hold the patient's limb in an abducted position (A), and gently lower the knee toward the examining table (B). In a patient with a contracture of the iliotibial band, the knee on the side being tested cannot be lowered to the table secondary to the contracture.

band. The patient is placed in a lateral position. Have the patient flex the downside hip to 90° and hold it in place with their hands. Flex the knee on the hip being tested, and bring the femur to a hip neutral position. Stabilize the hip with your opposite hand. Hold the patient's limb in an abducted position, and gently lower the knee toward the examination table. In a patient with a contracture of the iliotibial band, the knee on the side being tested cannot be lowered to the table secondary to the contracture (Fig. 2.15). This test may be positive in patients with muscular dystrophy, myelomeningocele or polio.

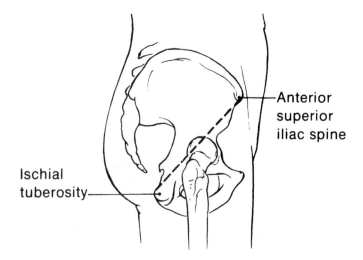

Anterior
superior
iliac spine

Ischial
tuberosity

Fig. 2.16. Nealton's line. Draw an imaginary line between the anterior superior iliac spine and the ischial tuberosity with the patient supine. The greater trochanter should be below this line. If the greater trochanter is superior to this line the femoral head is subluxated or dislocated. (Reproduced by permission from Chung 1981.)

NEALTON'S LINE

Nealton's line is an imaginary line drawn between the ASIS and the ischial tuberosity. The greater trochanter is felt to be below this line when palpating it in an infant. If the greater trochanter is superior to this line the femoral head is subluxated or dislocated (Fig. 2.16).

ELY TEST

Test the rectus femoris for spasticity by placing the patient prone on the examining table. Place one hand on the sacrum to stabilize the pelvis and flex the knee. In a positive test resistance is encountered as the knee is flexed, and then the resistance diminishes. In a very spastic and/or contracted patient the pelvis may be felt to rise on the side being tested (Fig. 2.17).

GALEAZZI TEST

This is used as a test for asymmetric leg length. Flex the patient's hips to 90°. Look for asymmetric heights to the patellae indicative of a leg length discrepancy in the femur (Fig. 2.18). Have the patient lie prone and flex the knees to 90°. Look for asymmetric heights of the calcaneal fat pads.

GAENSLEN'S SIGN (TEST FOR SACROILIAC PATHOLOGY)

Have the patient lie supine and flex both hips up to their chest. Shift the patient to the edge of the table so that one buttock extends over the edge. Allow the leg on the side off the table to come into extension and rest below the level of the table. Pain with this maneuver in the sacroiliac joint region is indicative of pathology at this location (Fig. 2.19).

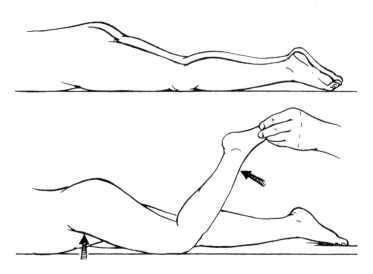

Fig. 2.17. Ely test. Place the patient prone on the examining table. Place one hand on the sacrum to stabilize the pelvis, and flex the knee. In a positive test resistance is encountered as the knee is flexed, and then the resistance diminishes. In a very spastic and/or contracted patient the pelvis may be felt to rise on the side being tested. (Reproduced by permission from Chung 1981.)

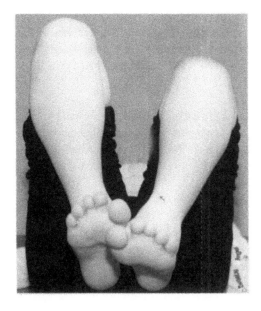

Fig. 2.18. Galeazzi test. Have the patient lie supine. Flex both knees to 90°. Look for a height asymmetry of the knees. Take care to not rock or tilt the pelvis to either side causing a false positive test.

NEONATAL HIP EXAMINATION

Developmental dysplasia of the hip is better appreciated and more readily treated the earlier that it is diagnosed. In the first six weeks of life the *Ortolani maneuver* (Fig. 2.20A) can be utilized to see if a dislocated hip will reduce. One hip is examined at a time with the

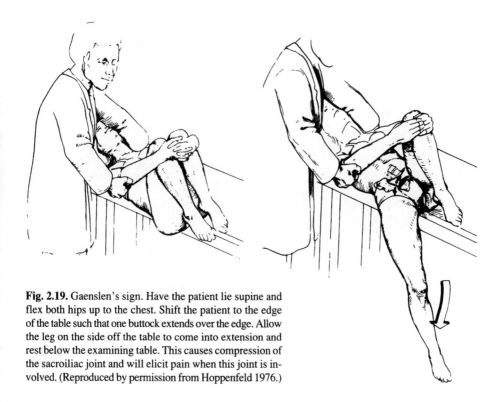

Fig. 2.19. Gaenslen's sign. Have the patient lie supine and flex both hips up to the chest. Shift the patient to the edge of the table such that one buttock extends over the edge. Allow the leg on the side off the table to come into extension and rest below the examining table. This causes compression of the sacroiliac joint and will elicit pain when this joint is involved. (Reproduced by permission from Hoppenfeld 1976.)

infant supine. Place the palm of your hand at the flexed knee, with the index and long fingers overlying the greater trochanter. Flex the hip being examined to 90°, then as you abduct the hip, push medially and superiorly on the greater trochanter. If the hip is dislocated, you will feel the femoral head ride over the posterior lip of the acetabulum and reduce.

The *Barlow maneuver* (Fig. 2.20B) is a provocative test to see is there is sufficient capsular laxity to allow the femoral head to dislocate. This maneuver is done in the reverse fashion from the Ortolani test. The hand position is the same as for the Ortolani test. The hip is flexed to 90°, and is adducted. As the hip is adducted place a downward force on the knee and feel for the femoral head gliding over the posterior rim of the acetabulum and dislocate. These examinations must be performed in infants who are not extremely irritable. If the examiner cannot adequately control the child's extremities it may be best to pause, let the infant nurse or eat, and then reexamine when the child is more relaxed. Both maneuvers are often combined in a fluid motion of the examiner's wrist attempting to reduce a dislocated hip and then attempting a redislocation.

After the first six weeks of life a dislocated hip will begin to develop contracture. An asymmetry to abduction may be the first physical examination finding encountered after losing the ability to perform the Ortolani and Barlow tests of a hip at risk. Look for loss of hip abduction with the development of an adduction contracture. Asymmetric thigh folds may be a suggestion of an underlying hip dislocation, but more often are a physiologic variant.

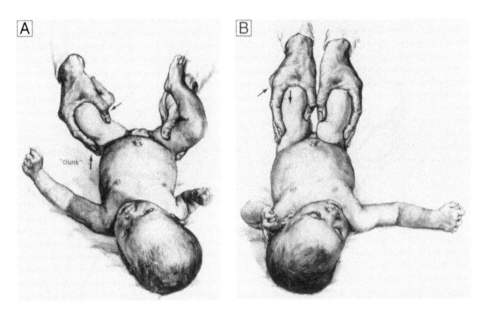

Fig. 2.20. Ortolani and Barlow tests. (Reproduced by permission from *CIBA Collection of Medical Illustrations, Vol. 8, Part 2.*)

(A) Ortolani: Place the infant in a supine position. Flex the knees to 90°. Examine one hip at a time. Grasp the knee in your palm and place index and long fingers over the greater trochanter. Gradually abduct the hip while placing an upward force over the greater trochanter with your index and long finger. Feel for the dislocated femoral head gliding over the posterior rim of the acetabulum and reduce.

(B) Barlow: A provactive test for instability. Place the infant in a supine position. Flex the knees to 90°. Examine one hip at a time. Gently adduct the hip being tested as a downward force is placed over the knee. Feel for the femoral head gliding out of the acetabulum and ride over the posterior rim and dislocate.

The examiner can attempt to feel for excessive motion within the hip capsule by pistoning or telescoping the flexed knee and hip up and down. The more contracted the infant's muscles become because of an altered resting length, the less motion may be encountered with this maneuver.

Conclusion

In summary, having a *high index of suspicion* is the key to not missing potentially significant pathology.

REFERENCES

Chung, S.M.K. (1981) *Hip Disorders in Infants and Children.* Philadelphia: Lea & Febiger.
Coon, V., Donato G., Houser, C., Bleck E.E. (1975) 'Normal ranges of motion in infants – six weeks, three months, and six months of age.' *Clinical Orthopedics and Related Research,* **110,** 256–260.
Greene, W.B. (2001) 'Diseases related to the hematopoetic system.' In: Morrissey, R.T., Weinstein, S.L.(Eds.) *Lovell and Winter's Pediatric Orthopaedics. 5th Edn.* Philadelphia: Lippincott, Williams & Wilkins, pp. 416–426.

Hoppenfeld, S. (1976) *Physical Examination of the Spine and Extremities.* Norwalk, CT: Appleton & Lange.

Moore, K.L., Dalley, A.F. (1999) 'Lower limb.' *In: Clinically Oriented Anatomy. 4th Edn.* Philadelphia: Lippincott, Williams & Wilkins, pp. 504–663.

Morrisey, R.T. (2001) 'Bone and joint sepsis.' *In:* Morrissey, R.T., Weinstein, S.L. (Eds.) *Lovell and Winter's Pediatric Orthopaedics. 5th Edn.* Philadelphia: Lippincott, Williams & Wilkins, pp. 465–466.

Staheli, L.T. (1986) 'Torsional deformity.' *Pediatric Clinics of North America*, **33**, 1373–1383.

3
RADIOLOGY

Christopher Foley

Imaging plays a central role in the assessment of the pediatric hip. There are multiple modalities available for these evaluations. Choosing the best test, or the test most likely to provide the correct diagnosis in a given clinical setting is always the challenge. The goal of this imaging should be the most accurate diagnosis for the least patient risk and expense.

Plain films are the mainstay of the radiographic evaluation of hip disease. They enjoy wide availability, ease of performance, relatively low radiation risk and low cost. These radiographs can be quite sensitive for the detection of hip disease, and should be obtained first in most instances. Unfortunately, plain films are not specific, and may not exclude disease in many instances. However, even when the results of the test are equivocal, they will usually provide some direction for the next best test.

Ultrasound displays soft tissue and cartilage not visible on plain radiographs. Additionally, it employs no ionizing radiation and is performed without the need for sedation. Consequently, it is the examination of choice in the evaluation of the infant hip for developmental dysplasia. Ultrasound can also display joint effusions in the older child. However, it does not show bone, and in fact the ultrasound beam is blocked by bone and air, so its usefulness in older children is limited.

Computed tomography (CT) displays bone in exquisite detail. The tomographic techniques allow separation of complex and overlying body parts. Resolution of soft tissues is good, and improves significantly with the injection of contrast material. Current scanners allow reformation of data in almost any plane, along with three-dimensional reconstruction and display. Modern scanners are quite fast, imaging large volumes in seconds. This has eliminated the need for sedation in all but the most active children. All of these improvements come at the cost of increasing radiation dose. CT is moderately expensive as well, so the modality should be applied judiciously.

Nuclear scintigraphy with bone radiotracer is very sensitive to increases in bone metabolic rate, almost invariably seen in bone pathologic states. Consequently, it is quite valuable in the assessment of patients with symptoms and signs of bone disease without overt plain film findings. The examination requires meticulous attention to detail. Sedation may be required in young patients, since any motion will degrade the image. Radiation doses are moderate, predominately to the bone itself. Because of the time involved, as well as isotope cost, the method is moderately expensive.

Magnetic resonance imaging (MRI) shows soft tissue anatomy and pathology in exquisite detail without the use of ionizing radiation. It also displays pathologic changes in bone marrow. It does not display bone structure as well as CT. Image acquisition times remain long, so that sedation or anesthesia is required in many children. Because of the high cost of equipment and the time required to perform these examinations, MRI remains expensive and consequently should be used judiciously.

The usefulness of all these imaging modalities is well documented in almost all of the diseases that affect the pediatric hip. Unfortunately, the conditions affecting patients at presentation are usually unknown. Consequently, an algorithm that accurately discriminates among the likely diseases in the differential at the time of presentation will provide the most accurate diagnosis for the least risk and cost, the goal of diagnostic imaging. The order of studies, including imaging, is determined by the initial history and physical examination (McBeath 1985, Eich *et al.* 1999, Fischer and Beattie 1999, Maroo 1999). In general, the age of the patient will help limit the list of possible diseases.

In the newborn period, the most common abnormality encountered is developmental dysplasia of the hip (DDH), with some degree of laxity identified in around 1% of live births. Sixty per cent of these hips normalize within the first week of life (Mandel 1990). Consequently, although confirmation of subluxation or dislocation is important, imaging investigation should be delayed until after the first week of life. In addition to those patients with persistent abnormal physical examinations, babies with a clinical history of breech presentation, or with a family history of DDH are at risk for dislocation (MacEwan and Bassett 1984). Dynamic ultrasound of the hip is now the standard initial imaging procedure in these cases (Harcke *et al.* 1984, Harcke and Grissom 1986). This method allows evaluation of the cartilagenous femoral head and its relationship to the cartilagenous acetabulum, as well as the stability of the femoral head in the acetabulum with stress. Once the diagnosis of developmental dysplasia is confirmed, serial ultrasonographic evaluations will allow documentation of normal hip development during therapy (Grissom *et al.* 1988, Polaneur *et al.* 1990). Occasionally, ultrasound will reveal an unexpected abnormality, usually some form of skeletal dysplasia, requiring additional imaging, usually plain radiographs of the hip. In 1–2 per thousand cases, delayed hip subluxation will be encountered. Because of the patient's size and the progressive ossification of the femoral head, ultrasound evaluation becomes impossible. In fact, after 4–6 months of age, ultrasound evaluation of the hip for subluxation becomes unreliable. In these delayed cases, plain films of the pelvis are most effective for evaluation of the hip.

Skeletal dysplasias, including proximal focal femoral dysplasia, are usually clinically evident and best evaluated initially with plain radiographs. In addition to radiographs of the pelvis, skeletal survey may help in diagnosis.

In early childhood, from about 1 to 8 years, transient synovitis, septic arthritis, Perthes' disease and the juvenile idiopathic arthritides are the predominant causes of hip abnormalities. Most abnormalities present with hip pain and/or limp, with or without fever. An ordered sequence of imaging combined with appropriate laboratory investigations frequently allows rapid differentiation of the diseases that can cause these symptoms (Del Beccaro *et al.* 199, Eggl *et al.* 1999, Kocher *et al.* 1999). Initial imaging with anteroposterior and frog lateral views of the pelvis is preferred as the initial plain films for these patients, showing not only the symptomatic side but also a comparison normal with little increase in radiation. If this investigation provides a diagnosis, therapy is instituted. If these films are normal, ultrasound of the hip joint will allow rapid diagnosis of a hip effusion. If an effusion is present, arthrocentesis will identify a purulent effusion in septic arthritis. If there is no effusion, or the effusion is sterile, and symptoms persist, further imaging by MRI or radionuclide scintigraphy will help in diagnosis. This algorithm can be applied to specific diagnoses as below.

Transient (toxic) synovitis is the most common cause of symptoms in this age group (Do 2000). Initial plain films are usually normal in both. If the clinical and laboratory findings do not allow diagnosis, arthrosonography should be performed as a rapid assessment for joint effusion. If effusion is present, it can be sampled for diagnosis. If the aspirate is sterile, a tentative diagnosis of transient synovitis can be made. If symptoms do not resolve in several days, further investigation is in order (Briggs *et al.* 1990, Hart 1996).

Septic arthritis has clinical findings similar to transient synovitis. Laboratory values are frequently equivocal, and plain films are often normal. Again, arthrosonography will allow rapid diagnosis of joint effusion that can be sampled. Purulent material on aspiration confirms the diagnosis of septic arthritis. Bone scintigraphy may be necessary to confirm or exclude osteomyelitis if bone infection will alter the length of antibiotic therapy (Sundberg *et al.* 1989, Caksen *et al.* 2000, Chen 2001, Hammond and Macnicol 2001). Once the diagnosis is confirmed, plain radiographs will allow monitoring of the affected hip to evaluate postinfectious deformity of the femur and hip.

Perthes' disease has similar clinical findings to transient synovitis and septic arthritis. Plain films of the pelvis may show a small sclerotic femoral head with some fragmentation (Kemp and Boldero 1966, Caffey 1968). If these findings are not present, arthrosonography will show an effusion if present. Aspirates are sterile. However, unlike transient synovitis, symptoms will persist. MRI will show decreased signal on T_1 images due to loss of fat and marrow edema of the ossific nucleus. Since it is at least as sensitive as nuclear scintigraphy in the diagnosis of avascular necrosis, requires a similar degree of sedation or anesthesia as nuclear scintigraphy, and allows evaluation of any deformity of the femoral head and hip joint, MRI is currently preferred over scintigraphy in the diagnosis of suspected Perthes' disease (Oshima *et al.* 1992, Kaniklides *et al.* 1995). If MRI is unavailable, scintigraphy will show decreased perfusion of the affected femoral head. Once a diagnosis of idiopathic avascular necrosis is made, plain radiographs are useful to follow any progressive deformity of the hip. Additional imaging including CT and further MRI should be reserved for surgical planning.

The acute onset of one of the juvenile chronic arthropathies (juvenile rheumatoid arthritis, ankylosing spondylitis, Reiter's syndrome, etc.) involves more than one joint more than half the time, generally the knee or wrist when one joint is involved. The arthritis of Lyme disease usually presents with a typical prodrome and characteristic rash. When these diseases present in atypical fashion involving just the hip joint without prodrome, they mimic any of the above illnesses. Plain films will be normal. Arthrosonography usually shows a joint effusion that is sterile. When symptoms persist, MRI will show evidence of a joint effusion without bony involvement. Nuclear scintigraphy will show increased activity from joint inflammation without bony involvement. In these atypical instances, final diagnosis rests with further laboratory investigation.

Neoplasms involving bone are uncommon in the first eight years of life. Leukemia and neuroblastoma do occur, frequently exhibit bone involvement, and are a cause of hip pain. The radiographic appearance of these malignancies is varied and fairly nonspecific, seen as metaphyseal lucent bands, localized areas of bone destruction, and/or periosteal reaction (Rogalsky *et al.* 1986, Gallagher *et al.* 1996).

Once identified, further investigation to define the primary lesion is in order.

After the age of about 8 years trauma predominates as the cause of symptoms referable to the hip. Primary neoplasms of bone also become more frequent. Usually plain films will identify the abnormality accurately. Occasionally, further imaging with CT or MRI will be helpful for further evaluation of lesions discovered. It is important to remember that lesions at the knee may cause pain in the hip, and hip abnormalities may cause knee pain. Therefore, if initial imaging of the symptomatic joint is normal, images of the other joint (knee or hip) should be obtained. If symptoms persist after normal plain films, radionuclide scintigraphy or MRI should be considered.

Slipped capital femoral epiphysis is the most common and most insidious of these fractures (Ozonoff 1992). The majority of patients present with a painful limp without history of antecedent trauma. Radiographs of the pelvis are usually diagnostic. Changes on the anteroposterior view are subtle except in more advanced cases, so that a frog leg lateral pelvis should be obtained at the same time. Simultaneous imaging of both hips is mandatory both at diagnosis and during treatment because bilateral slipping occurs in up to 33% of cases (Loder 1995). CT and MRI should be reserved for surgical planning or to confirm the diagnosis if plain films are equivocal (Umans *et al.* 1998).

Avulsed superior and inferior iliac spines, avulsed ischial synchondroses and stress fractures are generally athletic injuries (Sundar and Carty 1994, Mares 1998, Rossi and Dragoni 2001). They are readily diagnosed with anteroposterior and frog lateral pelvis films as well. The appearance of these avulsion fractures can be quite disturbing, mimicking neoplasm. However, biopsy in these lesions should be avoided, since these benign lesions can have a quite malignant appearance at pathology.

Bone neoplasms are quite common in children. The role of imaging is to separate these tumors into those that should be observed or left alone (benign), and those that require immediate intervention (Miller and Hoffer 2001). Fortunately, the majority are benign (Senac *et al.* 1986), usually incidental findings on radiographs obtained for trauma. Fibrous lesions of bone including fibrous cortical defects and nonossifyng fibromas, cartilage lesions of bone including enchondromas and cartilaginous exostoses, and unicameral bone cysts all share sharp demarcations between normal and abnormal bone, usually with sclerotic margins. Their position and typical appearance usually allow confident diagnoses (Kumar *et al.* 1990). Occasionally, especially following trauma, the appearance may be confusing. CT or MRI will help in further identifying these lesions to exclude malignancy.

Osteoid osteoma is the exception in this benign tumor group. This tumor causes characteristic night pain relieved by aspirin or ibuprofen (Frassica *et al.* 1996). The plain film images are usually diagnostic, showing an area of cortical sclerosis with a radiolucent central nidus. CT may be helpful for surgical planning. If the lesion is intracapsular in the femoral neck, the symptoms are more those of the synovitis induced by the lesion (White and Kandel 2000). Plain films show demineralization of the femoral head and neck with a widened joint space from the reactive joint effusion. The typical reactive bone is absent. Under these circumstances, CT will help localize the lesion. If symptoms persist with normal plain films, radionuclide scintigraphy should be performed, and will be strikingly positive if osteoid osteoma is present.

Osteosarcoma and Ewing's tumor are the common malignancies that can affect the pelvis and hip (Yaw 1999). Their presentation is usually one of pain, commonly associated with minor trauma. A palpable mass is present in 30–40% of patients at presentation (Widhe and Widhe 2000). Because of these nonspecific findings, the initial diagnostic imaging will be plain films. Once malignancy is suspected, further evaluation with radionuclide scintigraphy, CT or MRI will be required.

Osteosarcoma is the most common malignant bone tumor in this age group, more frequently occuring in the knee than in the hip or pelvis. These tumors are primarily metaphyseal in location. Plain films show a mixed destructive and productive lesion with osteoid matrix. These tumors require further evaluation, usually with MRI, to show the extent of the lesion and the size of the soft tissue mass. MRI will also show the relationship to contiguous neurovascular structures for surgical planning (Sundaram *et al.* 1987, Saifuddin 2002).

Ewing's tumor is the second most common malignant tumor of bone in this age group, and most common in the hip and pelvis. It is frequent in the flat bones of the pelvis. Plain radiographs show a predominately sclerotic lesion in flat bones with some bony destruction and an associated soft tissue mass. In the long bones, the tumor is more frequently lytic, with associated periosteal reaction.30 Again, MRI will show the extent of the lesion as well as the size of the soft tissue mass, allowing therapy planning (Weber and Sim 2001).

In summary, the imaging algorithm for knee complaints is straightforeward. In the young infant where developmental dysplasia of the hips predominates, ultrasound will be the diagnostic tool of choice. In all other situations, plain films of the pelvis should be the initial modality used. The results of those films will then help direct further work-up.

REFERENCES

Briggs, R.D., Baird, R.S., Gibson, P.H. (1990) 'Transient synovitis of the hip joint.' *Journal of the Royal College of Surgeons of Edinburgh*, **35**, 48–50.
Caffey, J. (1968) 'The early roentgenographic changes in essential coax plana: Their significance in pathogenesis.' *American Journal of Radiology*, **103**, 620–634.
Caksen, H., Ozturk, M.K., Uzum, K., Yuksel, S., Ustunbas, H., Per, H. (2000) 'Septic arthritis in childhood.' *Pediatrics International*, **42**, 534–540.
Chen, C.E., Ko, J.Y., Li, C.C., Wang, C.J. (2001) 'Acute septic arthritis of the hip in children.' *Archives of Orthopaedic and Traumatic Surgery*, **121**, 521–526.
Del Beccaro, M.A., Champoux, A.N., Bockers, T., Mendelman, P.M.. (1992) 'Septic arthritis versus transient synovitis of the hip: the value of screening laboratory tests.' *Annals of Emergency Medicine*, **21**, 1418–1422.
Do, T.T. (2000) 'Transient synovitis as a cause of painful limp in children.' *Current Opinion in Pediatrics*, **12**, 48–51.
Eggl, H., Drekonja, T., Kaiser, B., Dorn, U. (1999) 'Ultrasonography in the diagnosis of transient synovitis of the hip and Legg–Calvé–Perthes disease.' *Journal of Pediatric Orthopaedics, Part B*, **8**, 177–180.
Eich, G.F., Superti-Furga, A., Umbricht, F.S., Willi, U.V. (1999) 'The painful hip: evaluation of criteria for clinical decision making.' *European Journal of Pediatrics*, **158**, 923–928.

Fischer, S.U., Beattie, T.F. (1999) 'The limping child: epidemiology, assessment and outcome.' *Journal of Bone and Joint Surgery, British Volume*, **81**, 1029–1034.

Frassica, F.J., Waltrip, R.L., Sponseller, P.D., Ma, L.D., McCarthy, E.F.(1996) 'Clinicopathologic features and treatment of osteoid osteoma and osteoblastoma in children and adolescents.' *Orthopedic Clinics of North America*, **27**, 559–574.

Gallagher, D.J., Phillips, D.J., Heinrich, S.D. (1996) 'Orthopedic manifestations of acute pediatric leukemia.' *Orthopedic Clinics of North America*, **27**, 635–644.

Grissom, L.E., Harcke, H.T., Kumar, S.J., Bassett, G.S., MacEwen, G.D. (1988) 'Ultrasound evaluation of hip position in the Pavlick harness.' *Journal of Ultrasound in Medicine*, **7**, 1–6.

Hammond, P.J., Macnicol, M.F. (2001) 'Osteomyelitis of the pelvis and proximal femur: diagnostic difficulties.' *Journal of Pediatric Orthopaedics, Part B*, **10**, 113–119.

Harcke, H.T., Grissom, L.E. (1986) 'Sonographic evaluation of the infant hip.' *Seminars in Ultrasound, CT, and MRI*, **7**, 331–338.

Harcke, H.T., Clarke, N.M.., Lee, M.S., Borns, P.F., MacEwen, G.D. (1984) 'Examination of the infant hip with real-time ultrasonography.' *Journal of Ultrasound in Medicine*, **3**, 131–137.

Hart, J.J. (1996) 'Transient synovitis of the hip in children.' *American Family Physician*, **54**, 1587–1591, 1595–1596.

Kaniklides, C., Lonnerholm, T., Moberg, A., Sahlstedt, B. (1995) 'Legg–Calvé–Perthes disease. Comparison of conventional radiography, MR imaging, bone scintigraphy and arthrography.' *Acta Radiologica*, **36**, 434–439.

Kemp, H.S., Boldero, J.L. (1966) 'Radiologic changes in Perthes' disease.' *British Journal of Radiology*, **39**, 744–760.

Kocher, M.S., Zurakowski, D., Kasser, J.R. (1999) 'Differentiating between septic arthritis and transient synovitis of the hip in children: an evidence-based clinical prediction algorithm.' *Journal of Bone and Joint Surgery, American Volume*, **81**, 1662–1670.

Kumar, R., Madewell, J.E., Lindell, M.M., Swischuk, L.E. (1990) 'Fibrous lesions of bones.' *Radiographics*, **10**, 237–256.

Loder, R.T. (1995) 'Slipped capital femoral epiphysis in children.' *Current Opinion in Pediatrics*, **7**, 95–97.

MacEwan, G.D., Bassett, G.S. (1984) 'Current trends in the management of congenital dislocation of the hip.' *International Orthopedics*, **8**, 103–111.

Mandell, G.A., Harcke, H.T., Kumar, S.J. (1990) *Imaging Strategies in Pediatric Orthopedics*. Gaithersburg, MD: Aspen.

Mares, S.C. (1998) 'Hip, pelvic, and thigh injuries and disorders in the adolescent athlete.' *Adolescent Medicine*, **9**, 551–568, vii.

Maroo, S. (1999) 'Diagnosis of hip pain in children.' *Hospital Medicine*, **60**, 788–793.

McBeath, A.A. (1985) 'Some causes of hip pain. Physical diagnosis is the key.' *Postgraduate Medicine*, **77**, 189–192, 194–195, 198.

Miller, S.L., Hoffer, F.A. (2001) 'Malignant and benign bone tumors.' *Radiologic Clinics of North America*, **39**, 673–699.

Oshima, M., Yoshihasi, Y., Ito, K., Asai, H., Fukatsu, H., Sakuma, S. (1992) 'Initial stage of Legg–Calvé–Perthes disease: comparison of three phase bone scintigraphy and SPECT with MR imaging.' *European Journal of Radiology*, **15**, 107–112.

Ozonoff, M.B. (1992) *Pediatric Orthopedic Radiology*. Philadelphia: W.B. Saunders.

Polaneur, P.A., Harcke, H.T., Bowen, J.R. (1990) 'Effective use of ultrasound in the management of congenital dislocation and/or dysplasia of the hip (CDH).' *Clinical Orthopedics and Related Research*, **252**, 176–181.

Rogalsky, R.J., Black, G.B., Reed, M.H.(1986) 'Orthopedic manifestations of leukemia in children.' *Journal of Bone and Joint Surgery, American Volume*, **68**, 494–501.

Rossi, F., Dragoni, S. (2001) 'Acute avulsion fractures of the pelvis in adolescent competitive athletes: prevalence, location and sports distribution of 203 cases collected.' *Skeletal Radiology*, **30**, 127–131.

Saifuddin, A. (2002) 'The accuracy of imaging in the local staging of appendicular osteosarcoma.' *Skeletal Radiology*, **31**, 191–201.

Senac, M.O., Isaacs, H., Gwinn, J.L. (1986) 'Primary lesions of bone in the first decade: retrospective survey of biopsy results.' *Radiology*, **160**, 491–495.

Sundberg, S.B., Savage, J.P., Foster, B.K. (1989) 'Technetium pyrophosphate bone scan in the diagnosis of septic arthritis in childhood.' *Journal of Pediatric Orthopedics*, **9**, 579–585.

Sundar, M., Carty, H. (1994) 'Avulsion fractures of the pelvis in children: a report of 32 fractures and their outcome.' *Skeletal Radiology*, **23**, 85–90.

Sundaram, M., McGuire, M.H., Herbold, D.R. (1987) 'Magnetic resonance imaging of osteosarcoma.' *Skeletal Radiology*, **16**, 23–9.

Umans, H., Leibling ,MS.,. Moy, L., Haramati, N., Macy, N.J., Pritzker, H.A. (1998) 'Slipped capital femoral epiphysis: a physeal lesion diagnosed by MRI, with radiographic and CT correlation.' *Skeletal Radiology*, **27**, 139–144.

Weber, K.L., Sim, F.H. (2001) 'Ewing's sarcoma: presentation and management.' *Journal of Orthopaedic Science*, **6**, 366–371.

White, L.M., Kandel, R. (2000) 'Osteoid-producing tumors of bone.' *Seminars in Musculoskeletal Radiology*, **4**, 25–43.

Widhe, B., Widhe, T. (2000) 'Initial symptoms and clinical features in osteosarcoma and Ewing sarcoma.' *Journal of Bone and Joint Surgery, American Volume*, **82**, 667–674.

Yaw, K.M. (1999) 'Pediatric bone tumors.' *Seminars in Surgical Oncology*, **16**, 173–183.

4
DEVELOPMENTAL DYSPLASIA OF THE HIP

Peter A. DeLuca

Developmental dysplasia of the hip (DDH) remains the musculoskeletal problem of highest concern and frequent anxiety for the pediatric practitioner. A thorough examination of the newborn and infant hip remains the mainstay of early diagnosis and the Pavlik harness the universal form of treatment. Since the disorder may not always be detectable at birth it is felt that the term "developmental" best describes this entity which should be continually sought out on repeated clinical examinations (Aronsson *et al.* 1994). Although cases of DDH can occur in the older child in the face of a normal neonatal clinical examination (Walker 1971), it is felt by some practitioners that many of those hips would have been detected as abnormal by early ultrasonography.

Terminology
The term DDH is meant to encompass the entire spectrum of abnormalities from mild underdevelopment of the newborn hip to the stiff non-reducible teratologic hip dislocation. *Dysplasia* generally refers to a shallow or underdeveloped acetabulum, while *subluxation* refers to a hip that is not totally reduced or centered and demonstrates some degree of instability, excessive mobility or laxity (Fig. 4.1). A hip may be dysplastic but very stable, or lax in the face of acceptable acetabular development. When the femoral head is not contained in the acetabulum, it is *dislocated*.

The *teratologic* hip is dislocated at birth and not reducible. As dislocation occurred in utero, it is generally rigid and remains in a dislocated position on examination. Such hips may be associated with chromosomal abnormalities and neuromuscular conditions such as myelodysplasia and arthrogryposis, but can also occur in the normal infant.

Incidence and risk factors (Table 4.1)
Dysplasia of the hip occurs in approximately 1% of live births, while dislocation is present in 1–2 per 1000 (Chan *et al.* 1999). It is found more commonly in whites and those of European heritage, while it is unusual in blacks (Edelstein 1966). The left hip predominates in 60% of cases, but frequently the contralateral hip demonstrates at least some degree of radiographically confirmed involvement. Girls with DDH far outnumber boys by six to one, and the firstborn female presenting breech represents the highest risk for DDH at 8%. Family history is a very strong risk factor, and essentially all children with DDH share a familial

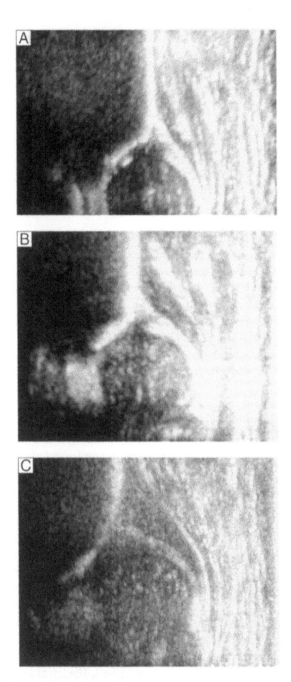

Fig. 4.1. Coronal ultrasound of the neonatal hip.

(A) Normal hip. More than 50% of the femoral head is within the acetabulum.

(B) Mild hip dysplasia and subluxation. Less than 50% of the femoral head is within the acetabulum. Acetabular roof (alpha angle) is steep.

(C) Hip subluxation.

TABLE 4.1
Relative and absolute risks for finding a positive examination result at newborn screening by using the Ortolani and Barlow signs*

Newborn characteristics	Relative risk of positive examination result	Absolute risk of positive examination result per 1000 newborn infants with risk factors
All newborn infants		11.5 (25 using ultrasound)
Boys	1.0	4.1
Girls	4.6	19
Positive family history	1.7	
Boys		6.4
Girls		32
Breech presentation	7.0	
Boys		29
Girls		133

*Adapted by permission from American Academy of Pediatrics (2000).

ligamentous laxity. Risk in subsequent pregnancies is 6% without an affected parent, 12% with a parent with hip dysplasia and 36% with both an affected parent and child (Wynne-Davies 1970).

Other intrauterine associations appear to implicate a restricted environment as an etiologic factor; these include firstborns, preterm birth, oligohydramnios (Hinderaker *et al.* 1994), torticollis coexistence (8–17%) (Walsh and Morrissy 1998, Tien *et al.* 2001), and metatarsus adductus (0–10%) (Jacobs 1996, Chan *et al.* 1999).

Only 40% of infants with clinically detectable hip dysplasia have risk factors. Thus, the clinical examination is more important than dependence upon risk factors. Hips that are found to be unstable on ultrasound and in need of treatment are usually clinically evident (Omeroglu and Koparal 2001).

However, routine screening programs based on clinical examination alone have had varied success in reducing the late presentation of DDH requiring treatment. Chan *et al.* (1999) found that screening done at birth, prior to hospital discharge and again at 6 weeks of age resulted in late presentation in only 2.4% of all the DDH cases in South Australia. Clinical screening reduced the presentation of DDH after age 18 months from 1.2 to 0.2 per 1000 in another series (Ref???). Yet in a series from the UK, clinical screening before 3 months of age failed to detect 70% of the cases eventually requiring surgery (Godward and Dezateux 1998).

Pathology
Instability of the hip may initially be the result of some combination of maternal hormonal laxity, genetic (familial) laxity and intrauterine (and even postnatal) malpositioning. Initially, the acetabulum may be normal with no signs of acetabular dysplasia. The longer the femoral head remains in a subluxated position, the more likely that progressive changes in acetabular anatomy will occur.

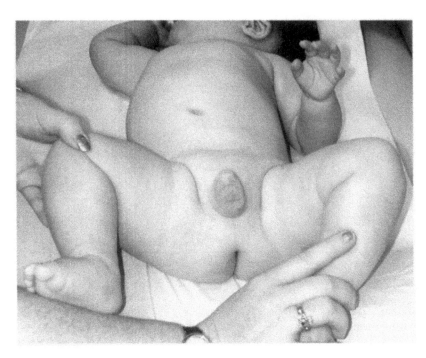

Fig. 4.2. Limitation of hip abduction due to tightening of the hip adductor muscles.

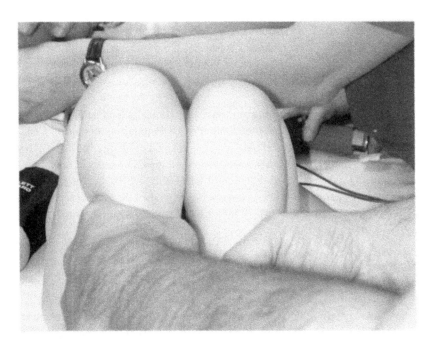

Fig. 4.3. Galleazzi test. The femur has a foreshortened appearance when subluxated or dislocated.

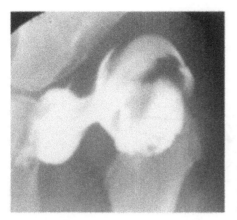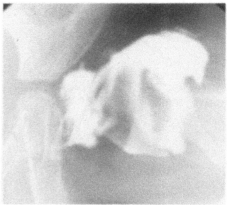

Fig. 4.4. Hip dislocation with secondary acetabular changes as seen by arthrogram. Left: hip dislocated, capsule narrowed. Right: reduction fails as femoral head cannot pass through constriction.

First, the femoral head causes pressure on the labrum or cartilaginous acetabular rim, causing it to thicken and be flattened outward. The underlying bony acetabulum also deforms under such pressure and results in the anterolateral edge being steeper than normal. These findings are very evident on ultrasound with increased echogenicity of the labrum and an increase in the alpha angle (representing the acetabular orientation) (Fig. 4.1C).

With the femoral head proximal and lateral, the hip adductors shorten, resulting in a limitation of hip abduction (Fig. 4.2). The femur assumes a foreshortened position (Galleazzi test) (Fig. 4.3).

If the hip progresses to dislocation, the labrum becomes infolded and thickened under the pressure of the femoral head, gradually closing down the superior and posterior acetabulum (Fig. 4.4). The inferior transverse acetabular ligament drifts upward, closing off the lower opening to the acetabulum. As these two structures close in, they create an obstacle to reduction of the femoral head back into the acetabulum. Also, over time the psoas tendon presses on and can tighten down the hip capsule contributing to a tightening of the "buttonhole". If treatment is begun prior to this occurrence there is a high probability of achieving a successful reduction. The longer the dislocation persists, the more resistant it becomes to reduction.

Presentation and diagnosis
In the *neonatal period* (0–3 months) hip instability allows for the clinical diagnosis.

A reduced hip may be *subluxated* (incompletely dislocated) or even *dislocated* (dislocatable) by the maneuver of adduction, flexion and posterior pressure. Once the force is released, the hip returns to a reduced position. Such a test is the *Barlow maneuver*, and the hip described as a "Barlow positive hip" (Fig. 4.5). These hips may or may not be associated with concurrent acetabular dysplasia (Barlow 1962). The instability demonstrated by these hips is due to inherent collagen laxity in combination with maternal relaxing hormones.

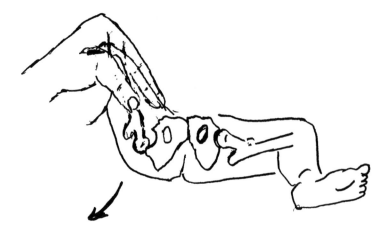

Fig. 4.5. Barlow maneuver.

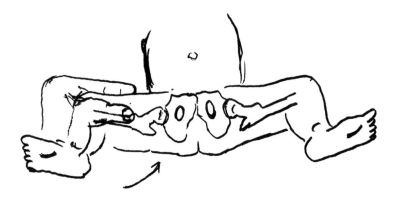

Fig. 4.6. Ortolani maneuver. With the hip in the dislocated position, it is reduced by abduction and lifting forward of the proximal thigh. This results in a feeling of acceleration then deceleration or a "clunk".

As the hormonal influences diminish, stability generally returns. However, acetabular dysplasia may remain and require treatment.

Some dislocated hips can be "reduced" back into the acetabulum by spreading the legs apart (abduction) and lifting the thigh forward (*Ortolani maneuver*) (Ortolani 1976). This elicits a sensation of rapid acceleration and deceleration as the femoral head returns into the socket, and the sensation of a "clunk" (Fig. 4.6). Some examiners have described this feeling as a "click", although that term actually is more applicable to the benign high-pitched noises frequently elicited at abduction. A dislocated hip that reduces is best termed an "Ortolani positive hip". It is usually accompanied by a variable degree of acetabular maldevelopment.

The examiner should be fascile with the Ortolani and Barlow examinations and practice them repeatedly at each well child examination during this period. Special attention should be paid to those children with the above risk factors, but all infants require examination. The Galeazzi or Allis test is useful from this period in those with severe subluxation or dislocation. With the hips flexed up 90°, the observer will note a decrease in height of the involved knee (see Fig. 4.3). When any of the above abnormalities are found, the child should be referred to an orthopedic specialist. The decision for radiographic studies should be made by the treating orthopedist.

In the *infant* older than 3 months, the signs of instability become less distinct, while signs of limitation of motion predominate. The dislocated or subluxated side will develop tightness of the hip adductors and thus abduction will be limited and asymmetric. In cases of bilateral involvement, the asymmetry may be absent (including Galleazzi), and the decrease in typical spread of the hips may be the only sign. However, when present as an isolated finding, limitation of hip abduction is fairly nonspecific, with only 18% of cases positive for DDH (Castelein *et al.* 1992). Family complaints of unusual leg positions or crawling problems should be investigated.

In the *toddler*, restricted motion and asymmetries remain, and a Trendelenburg limp from hip abductor weakness may be evident. In bilateral cases, a waddling gait may be seen. Adolescents have these findings and may also complain of fatigue, instability or hip, thigh or knee pain.

Radiology/ultrasound

Graf (1980, 1984) introduced the morphological approach of hip ultrasonography to evaluate the infant hip. He classified hips based on the degree of femoral head displacement and the degree of acetabular maldevelopment. Modern ultrasound interpretation generally combines the anatomic evaluation popularized by Graf and the assessment of instability (Dynamic Standard Minimum Examination) proposed by Harcke *et al.* (1984). Its use allows for earlier diagnosis and reduces the rate and the duration of treatment of DDH (Anderssen *et al.* 2000). Ultrasound also reduces exposure to radiography (Grissom *et al.* 1988). Both techniques suffer from a high degree of interobserver variability.

Although the screening of all newborn hips with ultrasound persists in many countries, it should be used as an adjunct to the physical examination in the infant aged between 1 and 4–5 months (Aronsson *et al.* 1994). Although very sensitive for abnormalities of the newborn hip, it is poorly specific for DDH requiring treatment (Patel 2001). Routine screening is generally not cost-effective. While the ultrasound evaluation of those infants with abnormal physical findings or risk factors has proven beneficial, screening all newborn infants has not significantly reduced the incidence of late-diagnosis DDH (Rosendahl *et al.* 1996, Lewis *et al.* 1999).

As there is a very high incidence on ultrasound of immature hips that do not require treatment, it is recommended that such screening by ultrasound be deferred until 4–6 weeks. (Clarke 1986, Castelein *et al.* 1992). Hips that show dysplasia but no instability do not benefit from early treatment, as more than 95% of hips that are immature or show mild dysplasia by ultrasound spontaneously normalize (Castelein *et al.* 1992, Rosendahl *et al.* 1996, Wood

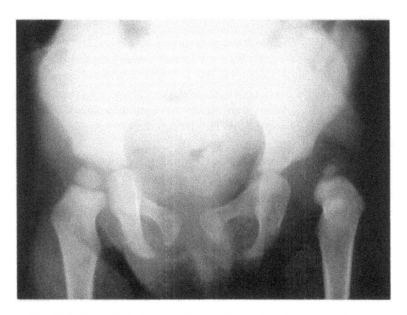

Fig. 4.7. Radiograph of a 2-year-old child with complete dislocation of left hip.

et al. 2000). In the series by Castelein and coworkers, 21% of neonatal hips (144 of 691) had ultrasound abnormalities but normal clinical examinations. After 6 months only four had DDH requiring treatment, and three of these had associated risk factors. As long as the practitioner does not allow the child to slip though the system and miss the follow-up study, the DDH will be readily treated.

After 4–5 months, radiographs replace ultrasound in the evaluation. By this age, the femoral head ossification center has generally appeared, and the acetabular parameters of importance become more readily defined (Fig. 4.7).

Treatment
DYSPLASIA

The treatment of the dysplastic and unstable hip should be differentiated from that of the truly dislocated hip. From the *neonatal period until 7–9 months of age*, the dysplastic or subluxated hip is best managed with the Pavlik harness (Fig. 4.8). This device is designed to maintain hip flexion and limit adduction. In those hips identified as having risk factors, some beneficial increase in hip abduction can be achieved with extra diapering (double or triple) pending ultrasound evaluation at 4–6 weeks. However, once a treatable dysplasia is documented, diapering is inadequate and the Pavlik brace should be fitted. The harness has anterior adjustable straps that are set to keep the hips flexed approximately 100°. Excessive flexion may produce a femoral nerve palsy. The posterior straps allow for a gentle encouragement of abduction. They should be loose enough to allow two to three finger breadths between the knees when they are held flexed and adducted. Thus prevention of any forced abduction helps to minimize the complication of avascular necrosis.

54

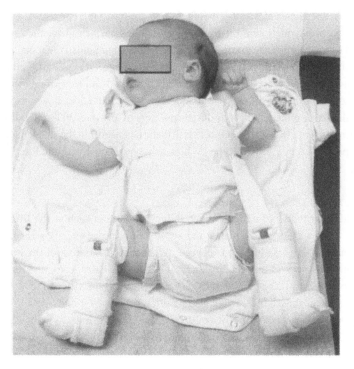

Fig. 4.8. Child in Pavlik harness.

Thus in a *Barlow positive hip*, if the ultrasound at 4–6 weeks is normal, the instability has resolved and the child does not require treatment or radiographic follow-up. However, serial clinical examinations of the hips must continue until walking age.

If the ultrasound demonstrates acetabular pathology or persistent subluxation, treatment with a Pavlik harness is begun, and progress monitored with serial ultrasound studies every four to six weeks. Once the study is normal, the child is weaned from the harness over a period of time. After six months, follow-up is done with anteroposterior radiographs through the growing years. There is a 10% risk of recurrence of deformity that makes follow-up to maturity necessary (Falliner *et al*. 1999).

DISLOCATION
The hip that is Ortolani positive in a child under 2 months of age may also be treated in a Pavlik harness. However, the child is re-examined weekly to assure that the hip has reduced, and then studied by ultrasound to confirm the clinical impression. Once the hip becomes stable, it is managed as described above.

If the hip has not stabilized after three weeks, the harness is discontinued. Continuation of the harness beyond this period increases the risk of worsening the acetabular dysplasia. Approximately 3.6% of cases of DDH, although clinically detected before 3 months of age will still require surgery (Chan *et al*. 1999). The child is taken to surgery for an arthrogram

55

under general anesthesia and a closed reduction, maintained in a spica cast. The hip arthrogram confirms the reduction of the hip or demonstrates obstacles to reduction. A CT scan is obtained following surgery to confirm that the hip has maintained the reduction achieved.

A hip that is dislocated but not reducible (*Ortolani negative dislocation*) may be briefly treated in a Pavlik harness, but if reduction is not achieved and confirmed by ultrasound in two to three weeks, treatment must be abandoned. Ultrasound does have prognostic value, as an initially irreducible hip that has initial coverage of less than 20% will fail Pavlik treatment (Lerman *et al.* 2001). Also, Graf classification is useful in the dislocated hip as over 95% of type III but only 50% of type IV hips achieve success with the Pavlik (Mostert *et al.* 2001).

THE OLDER CHILD
In the child older than 7–9 months, other abduction devices such as the Ilfeld brace may be used to treat acetabular dysplasia and subluxation; however, after 18 months, brace management alone is less likely to succeed. An excessive twisting of the femur, femoral anteversion, may prevent acetabular remodeling. In such cases, proximal femoral derotational osteotomy may be beneficial. If the acetabular dysplasia is judged severe, a rotational osteotomy such as that of Salter may also be offered.

Hip dislocations presenting in children older than 18 months will usually require operative closed or open reduction in conjunction with correction of femoral anteversion and acetabular dysplasia.

Natural history
Persistent acetabular dysplasia alone does not correlate well with later problems, but in conjunction with hip subluxation does increase the risk of degenerative arthritis. Subluxation with abnormal head–acetabular forces leads to early overload of cartilage and pain. Such hips may fare worse than those that remain frankly dislocated. High-riding dislocations from birth, where the femoral head rests within a muscular bed and away from bony contact, may be well tolerated for up to 30–40 years before causing pain. However, such patients may suffer from abnormal waddling gait due to muscle insufficiency, increased lumbar lordosis (sometimes painful) and limitation in hip flexibility. Unilateral persistent dislocations are less well tolerated due to relative leg length inequality and pelvic obliquity.

Missed cases of DDH
Missed cases of DDH continue to occur for a number of reasons. The initial signs of laxity (Ortolani, Barlow) are short lived, and in some instances they may be clinically undetectable, even in the face of dysplasia. Residual dysplasia may be present but the examinations fail to elicit any findings until the subluxation becomes pronounced. (Godward and Dezateux 1998). The examination may be performed in a timely fashion at each well child visit, but the examiner may lack sufficient experience to appreciate the diagnosis. Children may be lost to follow-up, or they may be sidetracked as they are seen for episodic medical maladies.

The best protection for the pediatric practitioner is to maintain complete medical records that document the consistent performance of the hip examination. Attention must be paid

TABLE 4.2
Screening for DDH: American Academy of Pediatrics recommendations*

1. All newborn infants should be clinically screened by a properly trained health professional
2. Routine ultrasound is not recommended
     May reduce late cases, need for surgery
     But, operator dependent
     Availability
     Increases treatment rate
     High interobserver variability
3. Positive Ortolani or Barlow test (unequivocal clunk): refer to orthopedist; no ultrasound, no radiograph
4. Follow-up equivocal findings at 2 weeks with referral or ultrasound at 4–6 weeks
5. Triple diapers are not treatment, but serve as a reminder
6. Risks:
     Ultrasound 4–6 weeks and/or radiograph 4 months
     Girl with family history
     Breech girl>boy, but all
7. Examine hips at each well baby visit

*American Academy of Pediatrics (2000).

to children with associated risk factors, any abnormalities on physical examination and special concerns raised by the family. These measures are delineated in a series of recommendations by the American Academy of Pediatrics (2000), summarized in Table 4.2.

REFERENCES

American Academy of Pediatrics (2000) 'Clinical practice guideline: Early detection of developmental dysplasia of the hip. Committee on Quality Improvement, Subcommittee on Developmental Dysplasia of the Hip. American Academy of Pediatrics.' *Pediatrics*, **105**, 896–905.
Anderssen, S., Silberg, I.E., Soukop, M., Andersen, A.E. (2000) 'Congenital hip dysplasia in Ostfold 1990–96.' *Tidsskrift for den Norske Laegeforening*, **120**, 3530–3533.
Aronsson, D.D., Goldberg, M.J., Kling, T.F., Roy, D.R. (1994) 'Developmental dysplasia of the hip.' *Pediatrics*, **94**, 201–208.
Barlow, T.G. (1962) 'Early diagnosis and treatment of congenital dislocation of the hip.' *Journal of Bone and Joint Surgery, British Volume*, **44**, 292–301.
Castelein, R., Sauter, A., de Vlieger, M., van Linge, B. (1992) 'Natural history of ultrasound hip abnormalities in clinically normal newborns.' *Journal of Pediatric Orthopedics*, **12**, 423–427.
Chan, A., Cundy, P.J., Foster, B.K., Keane, R.J., Byron-Scott, R. (1999) 'Late diagnosis of congenital dislocation of the hip and presence of a screening programme: South Australian population-based study.' *Lancet*, **354**, 1514–1517.
Clarke, N. (1986) 'Sonographic clarification of the problems of neonatal hip instability.' *Journal of Pediatric Orthopedics*, **6**, 527–532.
Edelstein, J. (1966) 'Congenital dislocation of the hip in the Bantu.' *Journal of Bone and Joint Surgery, British Volume*, **48**, 397 *(abstract)*.
Falliner, A., Hahne, H.J., Hassenpflug, J. (1999) 'Sonographic hip screening and early management of developmental dysplasia of the hip.' *Journal of Pediatric Orthopaedics, Part B*, **8**, 112–117.
Godward, S., Dezateux, C. (1998) 'Surgery for congenital dislocation of the hip in the UK as a measure of the outcome of screening.' *Lancet*, **351**, 1149–1152.
Graf, R. (1980) 'The diagnosis of congenital hip-joint dislocation by the ultrasonic compound treatment.' *Archives of Orthopaedics and Trauma Surgery*, **97**, 117–133.
Graf, R. (1984) 'Classification of hip joint dysplasia by means of sonography.' *Archives of Orthopaedics and Trauma Surgery*, **102**, 248–255.

Grissom, L.E., Harcke, H.T., Kumar, S.J., Bassett, G.S., MacEwen, G.D. (1988) 'Ultrasound evaluation of hip position in the Pavlik harness.' *Journal of Ultrasound Medicine*, 7, 1–6.

Harcke, H.T., Clarke, N.M., Lee, M.S., Borns, P.F., MacEwen, G.D. (1984) 'Examination of the infant hip with real-time ultrasonography.' *Journal of Ultrasound Medicine*, 3, 131–137.

Hinderaker, T., Daltveit, A.K., Irgens, L.M., Uden, A., Reikeras, O. (1994) 'The impact of intra-uterine factors on neonatal hip instability: an analysis of 1,059,479 children in Norway.' *Acta Orthopaedica Scandinavica*, 65, 239–242.

Jacobs, J.E. (1996) 'Metatarsus varus and hip dysplasia.' *Clinical Orthopaedics and Related Research*, 16, 203–213.

Lerman, J., Emans, J.B., Millis, M.B., Share, J., Zurakowski, D., Kasser, J.R. (2001) 'Early failure of Pavlik harness treatment for developmental hip dysplasia: clinical and ultrasound predictors.' *Journal of Pediatric Orthopedics*, 21, 348–353.

Lewis, K., Jones, D.A., Powell, N. (1999) 'Ultrasound and neonatal hip screening: the five-year results of a prospective study in high-risk babies.' *Journal of Pediatric Orthopedics*, 19, 760–762.

Mostert, A.K., Tulp, N.J., Castelein, R.M. (2001) 'Results of Pavlik harness treatment for neonatal hip dislocation as related to Graf's sonographic classification.' *Journal of Pediatric Orthopedics*, 21, 306–310.

Omeroglu, H., Koparal, S. (2001) 'The role of clinical examination and risk factors in the diagnosis of developmental dysplasia of the hip: a prospctive study in 188 referred young infants.' *Archives of Orthopaedics and Trauma Surgery*, 121, 7–11.

Ortolani, M. (1976) 'The classic: Congenital hip dysplasia in the light of early and very early diagnosis.' *Clinical Orthopaedics and Related Research*, 119, 5–10.

Patel, H. (2001) 'Preventive health care, 2001 update: Screening and management of developmental dysplasia of the hip in newborns.' *Canadian Medical Association Journal*, 164, 1669–1677.

Rosendahl, K., Markestad, T., Lie, R.T. (1996) 'Developmental dysplasia of the hip. A population-based comparison of ultrasound and clinical findings.' *Acta Paediatrica*, 85, 64–69.

Tien, Y.C., Su, J.Y., Lin, G.T., Lin, S.Y. (2001) 'Ultrasonographic study of the coexistence of muscular torticollis and dysplasia of the hip.' *Journal of Pediatric Orthopedics*, 21, 343–347.

Walker, G. (1971) 'Problems in the early recognition of congenital hip dislocation.' *British Medical Journal*, 3, 147–148.

Walsh, J.J., Morrissy, R.T. (1998) 'Torticollis and hip dislocation.' *Journal of Pediatric Orthopedics*, 18, 219–221.

Wood, M., Conboy, V., Benson, M.K. (2000) 'Does early treatment by abduction splintage improve the development of dysplastic but stable neonatal hips?' *Journal of Pediatric Orthopedics*, 20, 302–305.

Wynne-Davies, R. (1970) 'Acetabular dysplasia and familial joint laxity: two etiological factors in congenital dislocation of the hip: a review of 529 patients and their families.' *Journal of Bone and Joint Surgery, British Volume*, 52, 704–716.

5
THE PAINFUL HIP JOINT

Jeffrey D. Thomson

When the clinician is faced with a child with a painful hip there is a wide spectrum of potential pathological conditions that may have caused either the general complaint of discomfort voiced by the older child, or the irritability or visible limp seen in a toddler. A useful algorithm to remember is the following classic etiologic classification: congenital, traumatic, infectious, metabolic, neoplastic. As a guide to this approach to the diagnosis of the painful hip, a review of presentation of symptoms, important physical examination techniques and diagnostic procedures will be presented. For conditions other than those of neoplastic origin, the reader is directed to the specific conditions covered in detail in the other chapters of this book.

Diagnosis
It is vital to obtain a careful history from the child (if they are old enough to participate) and the parents. With the great increase in laboratory and radiological techniques there is a tendency today in the shortened medical curriculum devoted to the musculoskeletal system to pay less attention to obtaining a detailed complete history (Laurence 1998, Flynn and Widmann 2001). It is important to ascertain the onset of pain and its relationship to time of day. Morning pain if associated with stiffness may herald the onset of rheumatologic problems, whereas night pain only should alert the examiner to the possibility of a neoplasm.

The diagnosis of "growing pains" is often overused and misunderstood. There are three characteristics of growing pains: (a) the pain is usually in the legs; (b) the pain occurs only at night; and (c) the patient has no limp, pain or symptoms during the day (Schaller 1996). One caveat to remember: do not mistake fatigue and tiredness as pain or limp. "Pain" that occurs in the evening when the child is tired (and just before bedtime) can be related to muscle fatigue from overuse.

The presence of any constitutional symptoms such as significant loss of appetite, lethargy, fevers, rash or malaise can be a symptom of a systemic illness such as juvenile rheumatoid arthritis or malignancy and should automatically alert the clinician to obtain appropriate laboratory studies. If the child is systemically ill, obviously an immediate thorough work-up including appropriate laboratory and radiology studies is indicated (Royle 1992).

Physical examination
Obviously the child presenting with hip pain may show a wide range of discomfort from vague symptoms to severe discomfort that limits walking or even passive range of motion.

TABLE 5.1
Common causes of limp by location and age

	0–3 years	4–10 years	>10 years
Spine	Diskitis	Diskitis Spondylolisthesis Tumor	Diskitis Spondylolisthesis Tumor
Hip/femur	Septic arthritis Toxic synovitis Perthes' disease DDH	Toxic synovitis Perthes' disease Septic arthritis	SCFE Acetabular dysplasia Perthes' disease Overuse Snapping hip
Knee/leg	Toddler's fracture Septic arthritis JRA	JRA Diskoid meniscus Lyme disease Leukemia	Meniscus tear Patello-femoral pain Lyme disease Osteochondritis dessicans Stress fracture Osgood–Schlater disease Overuse injuries Bone tumors
Ankle/foot	Foreign body Tight shoes JRA (subtalar joint)	Kohler's disease Sever's disease JRA Bone cyst	Osteochondritis (talus) Sever's disease Tarsal coalition Bone cyst Overuse Accessory navicular

DDH = developmental dysplasia of the hip; JRA = juvenile rheumatoid arthritis; SCFE = slipped capital femoral epiphysis.

One clue to the localization of discomfort is to ask the child to stand on one leg. Often this will indicate the involved side, as the child will unconsciously spare discomfort to a mildly irritable hip. This can be further expanded by having the child perform repetitive maneuvers such as "duck squatting" or ascending and descending a flight of stairs. In this way vague inconsistent discomfort can often be accentuated at the time of the physical examination. These techniques can be most helpful in the diagnosis of the early stages of Legg–Calvé–Perthes disease (Perthes' disease).

With even mild pain the child will often show an antalgic gait characterized by reduced stance phase on the involved side. If there is associated weakness of the musculature of the affected hip a Trendelenburg sign may be present in which the contralateral pelvis will drop during stance phase on the involved limb. Pain associated with non-traumatic hip dislocation is not seen in the young child so careful examination of a child's gait pattern is essential to any physical examination. Lastly, a child who complains of vague discomfort in the lower extremity and who refuses to walk but will crawl may have other problems in the leg, ankle or foot. One must be aware of the condition of the so-called "toddler's fracture" (a non-displaced tibia fracture in a child under the age of 3 years in which the initial X-ray is often negative) (John *et al.* 1997).

Pain secondary to traumatic or infectious processes invariably results in a loss of range of motion of the hip. This is most evident with irritation or actual loss of range of internal rotation of the hip. Remember that with internal rotation the volume of the intracapsular space of the hip joint is reduced as the Y ligament of Bigalow and the iliopsoas tendon constrict the anterior aspect of the hip joint capsule. Passive rotation of the lower extremity with the child in a supine and relaxed position will elicit discomfort in a hip joint in the early stages of toxic synovitis, as well as Perthes' disease or early slipped capital femoral epiphysis.

Pelvic pain may radiate to the hip and thigh region and can often be elicited by the flexion, abduction and external rotation maneuver (the so-called FABER sign). Pain from an inflamed iliopsoas tendon, or retropsoas abscess causing hip joint pain will be exacerbated by hyperextending the affected thigh (Gaenslen's sign).

Imaging studies

Radiographic examination of the child with a painful hip is mandatory and it is vital that the radiographs always include not only the joint above and below the area of tenderness. The radiology request should always specify an anteroposterior (AP) as well as a lateral view of the entire *pelvis* because isolated views of only one hip joint can be deceptive. This is especially true in the adolescent with a slipped epiphysis who may present with a vague complaint of distal thigh or knee pain. Radiographs are easily obtained and are both sensitive and specific for a wide variety of disorders (Myers and Thompson 1997). An AP radiograph of both lower extremities from hips to ankles can be useful in young children who limp or refuse to walk and in whom the locus of injury cannot be clearly identified (Table 5.1).

Ultrasound is useful in evaluating the hip for effusion if the initial radiograph was normal. Ultrasound-guided hip aspiration in the radiology suite can be performed thus decreasing the patient's exposure to X-rays, and if the aspiration is positive for pus then antibiotics can be started sooner than if one had to wait to go to the operating room for hip aspiration (Fig. 5.1).

If the site of tenderness or the source of limp cannot be identified, a three-phase technetium-99m bone scan is very useful. The technicium accumulates at the site of increased blood flow and osteoblastic activity in osteomyelitis, stress fractures, occult fractures, neoplasm and metastases (Flynn and Widmann 2001). Bone scans have a high sensitivity and specificity in suspected early bone infections. Bone scans have been proven to be especially helpful in localizing infections and bone tumors in the pelvis and spinal column. It is very important to note that bone scans are not affected by arthrocentesis or by bone aspiration. Computerized tomography (CT) and magnetic resonance imaging (MRI) are useful if the particular area in question can be exactly localized.

Laboratory studies

Laboratory studies are indicated in a child with non-traumatic limp who has signs and symptoms of fever, malaise, night pain, vague or localized tenderness and especially if the pain has not resolved after a few weeks of observation. Appropriate screening tests include not only a complete blood count with differential white blood cell count (WBC), but also

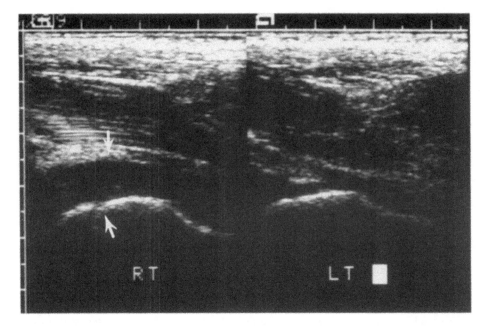

Fig. 5.1. Ultrasound of the right hip of an infant who presented with an acute onset pyarthrosis, compared to the uninvolved left hip (on the right side of the illustration). Note the increased capsular distention on the right side directly above the convex outline of the femoral neck and head. The small irregularity in the left side of the convex white line represents the lateral border of the physeal plate (lower arrow) with the lateral border of the femoral head directly to the far left of the illustration. These findings usually predate a positive bone scan by at least several days.

the erythrocyte sedimentation rate (ESR), C-reactive protein, antinuclear antibodies (ANA), rheumatoid factor (RF) and Lyme screen.

The ESR is an excellent screening lab test that is usually elevated in conditions such as juvenile rheumatoid arthritis, osteomyelitis and septic arthritis. If these studies are positive and the physical examination cannot isolate the location of the pain then a bone scan is an excellent test that will have a high probability of being able to locate the area of inflammation. The reader is referred to the decision matrix presented in Table 5.1 for evaluating a child with hip pain.

Differential diagnosis
Children under 5 years of age with hip pain can be the most difficult to evaluate because of difficulty in communication and anxiety. The following are common clinical problems faced when evaluating a child under age 5 with limp or refusal to walk.

SEPTIC ARTHRITIS VS TOXIC SYNOVITIS
The differential diagnosis of septic arthritis and toxic synovitis can be difficult. In general, children with septic arthritis will be more "ill", with a higher fever and a higher WBC and

TABLE 5.1
Decision matrix for evaluating a child with hip pain

	Physical exam (+)	Physical exam (−)
Labs (+)	Aspirate hip	Bone scan
Labs (−)	Ultrasound hip	Observe

Physical exam (+) implies there is a significantly decreased range of motion of the hip with pain. Physical exam (−) means there is full range of motion without pain.

Labs are white blood cell count (WBC) and erythrocyte sedimentation rate (ESR). They are positive if WBC >14,000 and ESR >30.

ESR, but most importantly their hip range of motion will be significantly reduced to less than 30% of normal. Typically, any attempts to move a septic joint will result in significant pain for the child. In toxic synovitis, however, the joint range of motion is better than with septic arthritis, with pain mostly at the extremes of normal motion. Also, children with septic arthritis will typically refuse to walk or move their hip, whereas children with toxic synovitis will walk with a significant limp. An ultrasound of the hip can be useful to identify not only the presence but also the size of an effusion. A positive ultrasound is commonly noted before a bone scan becomes positive.

Kocher *et al.* (1999) have published a clinical prediction algorithm to help differentiate between septic arthritis and toxic synovitis that uses four independent clinical predictors: history of fever, non-weight-bearing, ESR ≥40mm per hour, and serum WBC >12,000 cells/mm³. When all four were present they found a 99.6% probability of septic arthritis versus toxic synovitis; with three predictors present the probability was 93.1%; with two, 40.0%; and with only one, 3.0%.

Neonates with suspected hip infections are a particularly challenging clinical problem and deserve special comment. It is vital to check both hips in neonates with a suspected septic hip, and ultrasound may be the most reliable method. Bone scans have a high false-negative rate in neonates so one should not be misled by a negative bone scan in a neonate with suspected osteomyelitis or septic joint. There is a high incidence of bilateral hip involvement in septic arthritis in neonates, so both hips should be checked with ultrasound and aspirated if there is an effusion.

TODDLER'S FRACTURE VS TOXIC SYNOVITIS
It can be difficult to distinguish between a toddler's fracture and toxic synovitis. Children with a toddler's fracture will typically crawl but refuse to stand or walk. If they crawl this is a good sign that the hip, femur and knee are not involved, so one should focus on the tibia, ankle and foot. One important suggestion is to examine the child in the mother's lap, which will hopefully put the child at ease. By carefully palpating along the anterior tibia one can often localize a tender spot that is usually in the lower one-third of the tibia. If the X-ray is negative (and the child is otherwise healthy), observation is the recommended treatment. The child typically will refuse to weight-bear for five to seven days, then they

will slowly start to put the foot down over the next five to seven days, and finally, usually by the second or third week, they are walking well. If the X-ray reveals a fracture line, casting is essential to protect the affected bone. The concept of a "toddler's fracture" has been expanded to include other fractures of the tibia (compression, impaction and stress) as well as tarsal foot and metatarsal fractures (John *et al.* 1997). All of these can present with the same clinical manifestations as the classic toddler's fracture and eventually resolve without treatment.

DISKITIS

Diskitis typically presents in children aged between 1 and 5 years as a pain with walking and sometimes refusal to walk. The hip, knee and ankle range of motion will be relatively normal unless the involved disk is at the lumbosacral junction. The child characteristically moves with a rigid spine, resisting efforts to bend over. They will pick up objects from the floor but they will not bend their spine and instead bend at the hips and knees. The L2–L3 and L3–L4 disk spaces are the most commonly involved, but radiographs early in the disease process can be normal. Disk space narrowing and end-plate erosion can be seen radiographically after two weeks, but a bone scan or MRI can provide an earlier diagnosis. *Staphylococcus aureus* is the most common cause, and disk space aspiration or biopsy is usually not necessary. Blood cultures are usually positive, and treatment with short-term intravenous antibiotics followed by oral antibiotics is usually effective (Ring *et al.* 1995).

JUVENILE RHEUMATOID ARTHRITIS

Juvenile rheumatoid arthritis (JRA) can present with a limp that classically affects the knee joint, but the subtalar joint of the foot or the hip joint can be involved and be the source of pain and limp. The joint effusion can be subtle, but careful physical examination will usually elicit a difference in the range of motion of the affected joints. Many children are seronegative so ANA and RF tests may be negative, but if the limp and joint swelling have been present for more than six weeks it is likely to be JRA.

SLIPPED CAPITAL FEMORAL EPIPHYSIS

Children with long-standing hip pathology will exhibit pain on active or passive motion of the hip joint; however, the condition will be self-evident from the obvious signs of the underlying disease process such as spastic cerebral palsy. In cases with slipped capital femoral epiphysis (SCFE) it is important to remember that in up to 50% of cases bilateral involvement may occur, and the unaffected hip must be followed carefully. SCFE classically presents in the overweight adolescent as hip pain with a mild limp. However, it can also present with groin, thigh or knee pain. This is why it is always necessary not only to examine the joint above and below the site of pain, but also to obtain appropriate radiographs of the regions above as well as below the site of pain. The patient's limp can be very subtle and easily overlooked, especially in adolescents who may tend to be less verbal and less willing to undergo a physical examination. One especially needs to be mindful of the adolescent presenting with knee pain who actually has an SCFE but because of the phenomenon of referred pain via branches of the obturator and femoral nerves complains of knee pain. Again,

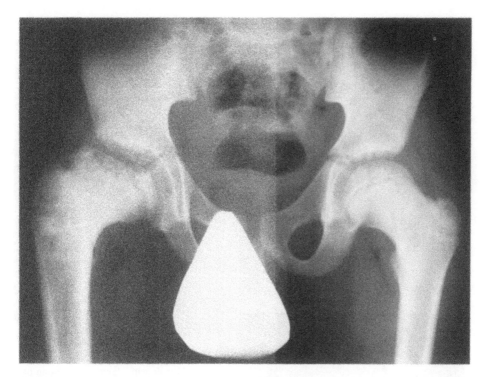

Fig. 5.2. Anteroposterior view of the pelvis of a 7-year-old patient with advanced Perthes' disease of the right hip. Mild pain led over several months to severe limp and loss of range of motion as the femoral capital nucleus underwent collapse. A high index of suspicion would have led to an earlier radiograph and institution of containment treatment to prevent femoral head collapse.

a simple check of the patient's hip internal and external range of motion will reveal the true source of the pain.

PERTHES' (SMITH–CALVÉ–PERTHES) DISEASE
Children between the ages of 5 to 10 may have Perthes' disease, which usually presents with a relatively painless limp. With time the patient will develop hip and thigh pain as well as thigh and calf atrophy. Loss of hip abduction and internal rotation are common and very reliable signs that one should obtain a radiograph of the hips. Radiographs may initially appear as normal but with time a subchondral lucency and eventually collapse and fragmentation of the femoral head develops (Fig. 5.2). Some patients with Perthes' disease will present with an acute painful limp. Careful examination of the child's hip internal and external range of motion should demonstrate asymmetry between the involved and uninvolved sides, with loss of hip internal rotation being the most sensitive finding.

NEOPLASMS
Neoplasms of the femur and pelvis may often present with vague ill-defined pain and

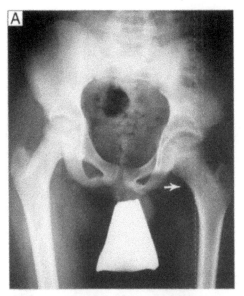

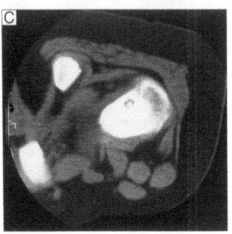

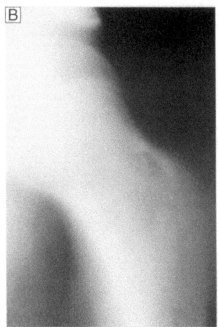

Fig. 5.3. (A) Anteroposterior radiograph of an 8-year-old male with chronic unremitting pain in his left femur. Note the small area of radio lucency immediately medial to the greater trochanter physis.

(B) On tomographic examination the nidus is readily visible beneath the lateral cortex of the base of the femoral neck.

(C) Computer assisted tomogram showing the central nidus as well as the well-defined border of the lesion. This would be an ideal candidate for radio frequency ablation of the lesion.

discomfort, frequently characterized by night pain. Osteoid osteomas are painful and are often found in the proximal femur (Fig. 5.3). On plain X-rays there is a small lucency (nidus) surrounded by a sclerotic border. Treatment frequently required surgical resection, which was often complicated by difficulty in identifying the exact location of the lesion, and the resultant bone resection could leave the femur prone to pathologic fracture during the healing phase. Recently, Rosenthal *et al.* (1998) have reported on the successful ablation of these lesions by means of percutaneous radio frequency coagulation of the tumor with results superior to that of conventional surgical excision.

Osteochondromas are benign lesions that usually occur in the metaphyseal regions of long bones. Recent evidence suggests that these lesions may have a molecular basis for their

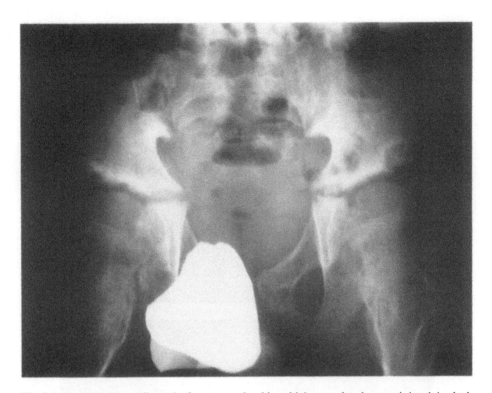

Fig. 5.4. Anteroposterior radiograph of a young male with multiple osteochondromatosis involving both femora. Note the lesions in the base of the neck of both femora. He presented with hip pain and limp characterized by limitation of hip extension as well as reduced arc of hip rotation.

origin, hence being neoplastic and not the result of ectopic portions of the physis in long bones (Porter and Simpson 1999). There is an autosomal dominant form resulting in multiple exostoses which may involve the proximal femoral metaphyseal areas. In such cases mild pain with exertion and abnormal hip motion may be noted (Fig. 5.4). In rare cases surgical resection may be advocated to improve hip motion and reduce symptoms of mechanical impingement.

Unicameral bone cysts and aneurysmal bone cysts may occur in the proximal femur and first be noted either on incidental radiographs or present as pathological fracture (Fig. 5.5). MRI has been shown to be valuable in differentiating aneurysmal bone cysts by the appearance of a double density fluid level within the lesion (Sullivan *et al.* 1999). Unicameral bone cysts are more commonly encountered, and current treatment recommendations have suggested filling the cavity with demineralized bone matrix leading to successful healing of the medullary defect (Killian *et al.* 1998).

Plain radiographs of the hip are always indicated in the presence of persistent pain and occasionally may identify early stress fracture either from extreme overuse or following previous surgery (Canale *et al.* 1997) (Fig. 5.6)

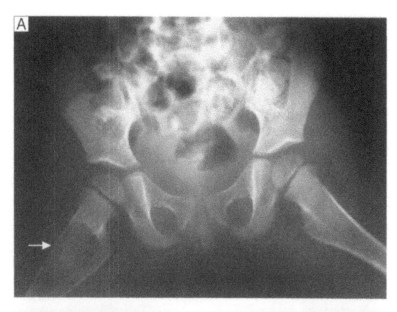

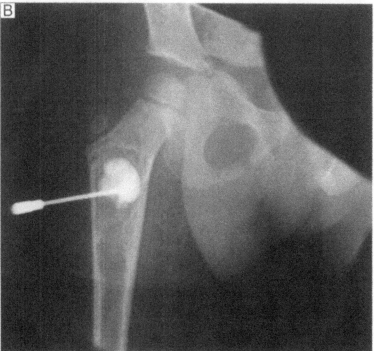

Fig. 5.5. (A) Frog view of the pelvis of a child with a painful right hip due to a large unicameral bone cyst. Note the thin cortical margin which will lead to a pathologic fracture.

(B) Intraoperative radiograph at the time of injection of renographin, demonstrating the partial healing of the defect following introduction of demineralized bone matrix.

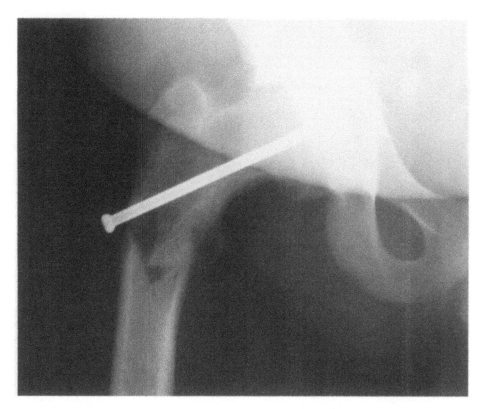

Fig. 5.6. Anteroposterior radiograph of a young male who had undergone uneventful *in situ* pinning of a mild slipped capital femoral epiphysis several months before the onset of pain in the affected hip. A stress fracture developed at the point of entry of the screw, which acted as a stress riser.

Chondroblastoma is a benign neoplasm that can occasionally present in the proximal femur with pain often referred to the region of the knee. Radiographs demonstrate a lytic lesion with focal calcifications and smooth margins (Fig. 5.7). Excisional curettage and bone grafting are recommended for this lesion (Schuppers 1998).

Fibrous dysplasia of bone may affect the femur and result in not only pain but also significant deformity of the proximal femur (Fig. 5.8). The etiology of this disorder is related to a mutation of the *GNAS1 1* gene. Chapurlat *et al.* (1997) have reported beneficial effects of the intravenous administration of pamidronate providing pain relief and improvement in the bone structure.

Ewing's sarcoma commonly presents as a painful lesion not uncommonly noted in the long bones and the pelvis. The radiological appearance is that of an aggressive lesion with periosteal elevation sometimes referred to as an "onion skin" appearance (Fig. 5.9). The diagnosis and to some extent the prognosis of this tumor have been aided by recent advances in genetic research (Dagher *et al.* 2001), and the combination of chemotherapy followed by surgical resection and radiation has resulted in improved survival for many patients.

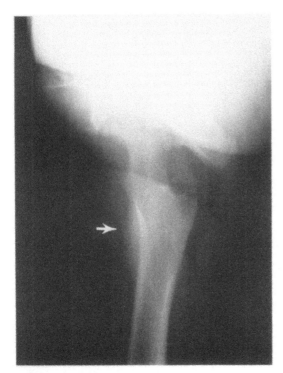

Fig. 5.7. Lateral radiograph of a young patient presenting with a painful hip due to an osteochondroma best visualized at the inferomedial border of the intertrochanteric region.

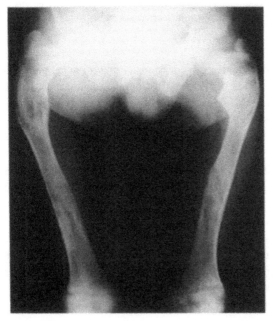

Fig. 5.8. Anteroposterior radiograph of the pelvis of a patient with polyostotic fibrous dysplasia. Note the involvement of both femora with varus deformation of the intertrochanteric region. This patient presented with a bilateral painful Trendelenberg gait. Pain from the lesions and the Trendelenberg gait pattern were caused by the relative weakness of the abductor muscles due to the severe varus deformity.

70

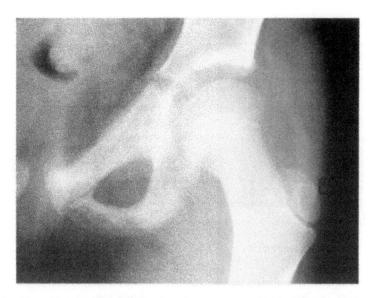

Fig. 5.9. Anteroposterior view of the left hip of a patient presenting with hip pain due to Ewing's sarcoma involving the inferior acetabulum, and the ischial and pubic rami.

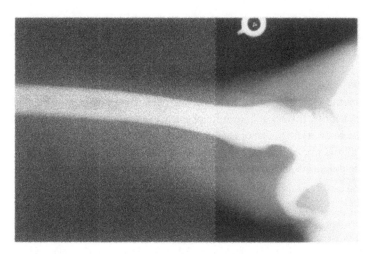

Fig. 5.10. Lateral radiograph of a patient presenting with hip and thigh pain due to extensive involvement of the entire femur with osteogenic sarcoma.

The last major malignant tumor commonly presenting with pain is osteosarcoma, which can frequently present in the proximal femur or pelvis (Fig. 5.10). Current treatment regimens include intravenous chemotherapy preceding surgical resection and further chemotherapy, with survival rates now approaching 80% (Grimer *et al.* 1999).

TABLE 5.3
Differential diagnosis

Trauma	**Developmental**
Fracture	Perthes' (Legg–Calvé–Perthes) disease
Stress fracture	Slipped capital femoral epiphysis
Toddler's fracture	Osteochondritis dessicans
Contusion	Spondylolisthesis
Sprain	**Neurologic**
Infection	Cerebral palsy
Cellulitis	Charcot–Marie–Tooth disease
Osteomyelitis	Friedreich's ataxia
Septic arthritis	**Tumor**
Diskitis	Benign
Post-streptococcal reactive arthritis	Osteoid osteoma
Inflammatory	Bone cyst
Toxic synovitis	Fibrous dysplasia
Juvenile rheumatoid arthritis	Osteochondromas
	Chondroblastoma
Congenital	Malignant
Developmental dysplasia of the hip	Osteosarcoma
Congenital short femur	Ewing's sarcoma
Tarsal coalition	Leukemia
Diskoid meniscus	Lymphoma

The range of conditions involved in the differential diagnosis of hip pain is summarized in Table 5.3.

Conclusion

In summary, the evaluation of the child with hip pain can be challenging but with an orderly approach to taking a history and a careful physical examination one can usually differentiate between the basic etiologic factors of congenital, traumatic, infectious or neoplastic origin. This then allows one to order the most valuable radiological and laboratory examinations to make the diagnosis and start appropriate treatment.

REFERENCES

Canale, S.T., Casillas, M., Banta, J.V. (1997) 'Displaced femoral neck fractures at the bone–screw interface after in situ fixation of slipped capital femoral epiphysis.' *Journal of Pediatric Orthopedics*, **17**, 212–215.

Chapurlat, R.D., Delamans, P.D., Liers, D., Meunier, P.J. (1997) 'Long term effects of intravenous pamidronate in fibrous dysplasia of bone.' *Journal of Bone and Mineral Research*, **12**, 1746–1752.

Dagher, R., Sorbara, L., Kumar, S., Long, L., Bernstein, D., Mackall, C., Raffeld, M., Tsokos, M, Helman, L. (2001) 'Molecular confirmation of Ewing sarcoma.' *Journal of Pediatric Hematology and Oncology*, **23**, 221–224.

Flynn, J.M., Widmann, R.F. (2001) 'The limping child: Evaluation and diagnosis.' *Journal of the American Academy of Orthopaedic Surgeons*, **9**, 89–98.

Grimer, R.J., Carter, S.R., Tillman, R.M., Spooner, D., Mangham, D.C., Kabukcuoglu, Y. (1999) 'Osteosarcoma of the pelvis.' *Journal of Bone and Joint Surgery, British Volume*, **81**, 796–802.

John, S.D., Moorthy, C.S., Swischuk, L.E. (1997) 'Expanding the concept of the toddler's fracture.' *Radiographics*, **17**, 367–376.

Killian, J.T., Wilkinson, L., White, S, Brassard, M. (1998) 'Treatment of unicameral bone cyst with demineralized bone matrix.' *Journal of Pediatric Orthopedics*, **18**, 621–624.

Kocher, M.S., Zurakowski, D., Kasser, J.R. (1999) 'Differentiating between septic arthritis and transient synovitis of the hip in children: An evidence-based clinical prediction algorithm.' *Journal of Bone and Joint Surgery, American Volume*, **81**, 1662–1670.

Laurence, L.L. (1998) 'The limping child.' *Emergency Medicine Clinics of North America*, **16**, 911–929.

Myers, M.T., Thompson, G.H. (1997) 'Imaging the child with limp.' *Pediatric Clinics of North America*, **44**, 637–658.

Porter, D.E., Simpson, A.H. (1999) 'The neoplastic pathogenesis of solitary and multiple osteochondromas.' *Journal of Pathology*, **188**, 119–125.

Ring, D., Johnston, C.E., Wenger, D.R. (1995) 'Pyogenic infectious spondylitis in children: the convergence of discitis and vertebral osteomyelitis.' *Journal of Pediatric Orthopedics*, **15**, 652–660.

Royle, S.G. (1992) 'Investigation of the irritable hip.' *Journal of Pediatric Orthopedics*, **12**, 396–397.

Rosenthal, D.I., Hornicek, F.J., Wolfe, M.W., Jennings, L.C., Gebhardt, M.C., Mankin, H.J. (1998) 'Percutaneous radiofrequency coagulation of osteoid osteoma compared with operative treatment.' *Journal of Bone and Joint Surgery, American Volume*, **80**, 815–821.

Schaller, J.G. (1996) 'Pain syndromes.' *In:* Nelson, W.E. (Ed.) *Textbook of Pediatrics*. Philadelphia: W.B. Saunders, p. 686.

Schuppers, H.A., van der Eijken, J.W. (1998) 'Chondroblastoma during the growing age.' *Journal of Pediatric Orthopaedics, Part B*, **7**, 293–297.

Sullivan, R.J., Meyer, J.S., Dormans, J.P., Davidson, R.S. (1999) 'Diagnosing aneurysmal and unicameral bone cysts with magnetic resonance imaging.' *Clinical Orthopaedics and Related Research*, **366**, 186–190.

6
SLIPPED CAPITAL FEMORAL EPIPHYSIS

Kristan A. Pierz

Slipped capital femoral epiphysis (SCFE) is one of the most common disorders of the pediatric hip and is characterized by displacement of the proximal femoral metaphysis with respect to the capital epiphysis. Because the slippage occurs through the growing physeal plate, this condition can only occur prior to skeletal maturity. The epiphysis, attached by the ligamentum teres, remains in the acetabulum as the femoral neck displaces, resulting in pain and varying degrees of deformity. Most commonly, the femoral neck displaces anteriorly and laterally, resulting in an apparent decreased angle between the femoral head and neck, or varus deformity. The displacement may be in other directions, but this occurs much less frequently (Segal *et al.* 1996, Shanker *et al.* 2000). Early diagnosis of SCFE is critical since a delay in treatment can result in further progression of the slip and compromise a patient's outcome.

Etiology
Multiple theories have been proposed regarding the etiology of SCFE, and it is unlikely that only one single factor causes the disorder. Instead, biomechanical and biochemical factors, acting together during puberty, are probably responsible for producing SCFE (Weiner 1996).

Biomechanically, an increase in shear stress across the physis can put a hip at risk for SCFE. Obesity, which results in increased shear stress, is seen in the majority of patients with SCFE. Loder (1996a) noted that the weight of 63.2% of 1630 children with SCFE was at or above the 90th percentile. Obesity has also been associated with reduced femoral anteversion, which, along with a decreased femoral shaft neck angle, has been implicated in increasing shear stresses and the risk of SCFE (Pritchett *et al.* 1989, Williams *et al.* 1999, Kordelle *et al.* 2001, Loder *et al.* 2001). Normally, the femoral neck projects anterior to the femoral shaft in the sagittal plane, referred to as anteversion, whereas the femoral neck shaft angle describes alignment in the coronal plane (Fig. 6.1). Kordelle *et al.* observed 30 SCFEs in 22 patients that demonstrated reduced femoral anteversion of 7.0° (compared with 12.7° in the normal hip) and a reduced femoral shaft neck angle of 134.2° (vs. 141.0° in normal hips). After comparing radiographs of 50 normal adolescents with those of 50 patients with SCFE, Pritchett *et al.* found the angle between a line drawn along the femoral neck and a line perpendicular to the growth plate to be 23° in the normal population, between 10° and 20° in those with unilateral slips, and less than 10° for those with bilateral slips. Aronson and Tursky (1996) postulated a torsional basis for slips, reporting that shear in two planes (coronal and sagittal) results in a spiral deformity through the epiphyseal cartilage columns.

74

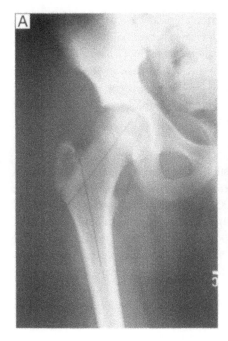
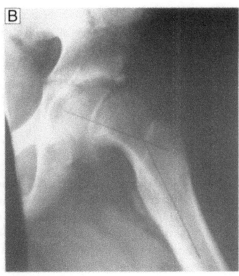

Fig. 6.1. (A) Anteroposterior, and (B) lateral radiographs of the hip, demonstrating the femoral neck shaft angle and anteversion, respectively.

Within the physis, slips tend to occur through the zone of chondrocyte hypertrophy. Core biopsy specimens of physes from patients with SCFE revealed that the cartilage matrix within the zone of hypertrophy contained only scattered fine collagen fibrils in a homogenous ground substance, whereas the resting zone's matrix contained large, densely packed collagen fibrils (Mickelson *et al.* 1977). During puberty, the entire growth plate is weakened, and alterations in the hormonal balance of thyroid hormone, growth hormone, testosterone and estrogen may increase the susceptibility of the physis to mechanical risk factors (Weiner 1996). The finding that estrogen tends to reduce physeal width and increase physeal strength, whereas testosterone tends to decrease physeal strength, may help explain the male predominance of SCFE and the rare occurrence of SCFE in postmenarchal girls (Loder *et al.* 2001).

Biochemically, hormonal changes occur normally during puberty, and most patients with SCFE lack a demonstrable endocrinopathy, although many have a delayed bone age when compared to chronological age (Loder *et al.* 2001). Endocrine disorders such as primary or secondary hypothyroidism, panhypopituitarism, hypogonadal conditions and renal osteodystrophy can increase a patient's risk of SCFE, and such conditions should be considered, especially in patients who present with SCFE before age 10 or after age 16 years (Kehl 2001, Mann 1996). In particular, growth hormone treatment has been associated with an increased risk of SCFE, and children with growth hormone deficiency or Turner syndrome are more likely to develop SCFE, before or during growth hormone replacement, than those with idiopathic short stature (Blethen and Rundle 1996). GnRH-agonist treatment has also been considered a risk factor for the occurrence of SCFE (Kempers *et al.* 2001).

Additionally, radiation therapy for the treatment of malignancy has been implicated as a risk factor for SCFE. Unlike patients with idiopathic slips, patients with radiation-therapy associated SCFE are usually young (10.4 ± 3.2 years) and thin (median weight in the 10th percentile), and a negative linear relationship exists between the age at presentation of the SCFE and the amount of radiation therapy received (Loder *et al.* 1998). Finally, attempts to link specific human leukocyte antigen phenotypes with SCFE have been inconclusive (Gunal and Ates 1997, Wong-Chung *et al.* 2000).

Prevalence

The true prevalence of SCFE is not known, and estimates vary based on geography. In eastern Japan the prevalence has been reported as 0.2 per 100,000 (Ninomiya *et al.* 1976), whereas the USA has a reported prevalence of 2.13 per 100,000 in the southwest and as high as 10.08 per 100,000 in the northeast (Kelsey *et al.* 1970). In an international, multicenter study of 1630 children (1993 SCFEs), Loder (Loder 1996a) found the relative racial frequency of SCFE compared to the white population to be 4.5 for the Polynesian, 2.2 for the black, 1.05 for the Amerindian (native and Hispanic), 0.5 for the Indonesian-Malay, and 0.1 for the Indo-Mediterranean children.

Since the early 20th century, the male predominance of SCFE has decreased to its current estimate of 60% (Loder 1996a, Loder *et al.* 2001). The average age of presentation is 13.5 years for boys and 11.5 years for girls (Kehl 2001). The range of ages (12–16 years for boys and 10–13 years for girls) was similar across races in Loder's international study (Loder 1996b). This same study also noted a seasonal variation of onset and presentation of SCFE: for children living north of 40°N latitude, onset was greatest in mid-July (±2.4 months), and presentation was greatest in early September (±2.5 months).

Presentation

Since SCFEs are characterized by either a sudden or a gradual displacement of the femoral neck from the epiphysis, it is not surprising that the onset of symptoms may be either abrupt or insidious over many months. Slips may occur acutely after high-energy trauma or gradually over time. Traditionally, slips have been classified as acute, acute-on-chronic, or chronic. Acute slips are those that have a sudden onset of symptoms for less than three weeks, whereas chronic slips are characterized by a more gradual onset of symptoms for more than three weeks. Those with acute-on-chronic slips may report a prodrome of symptoms for greater than three weeks followed by a more recent sudden exacerbation.

A more recent classification system, which also has prognostic implications, is based on the patient's ability to bear weight (Loder *et al.* 1993). According to this system, slips are considered stable if the patient is able to bear weight on the affected limb, with or without crutches. Unstable slips, however, result in such severe pain that the patient is unable to bear weight, even with crutches, on the affected limb. The unstable slips are associated with a high rate (up to 47%) of developing avascular necrosis, whereas stable slips, which are more common, have a more favorable outcome.

Patients with stable or chronic slips frequently demonstrate a mildly antalgic gait with external rotation of the affected side. Depending on the severity of displacement, the affected limb may appear shortened. Flexion of the hip results in varying degrees of obligatory external rotation depending on the severity of the slip. For unilateral cases, hip rotation, best documented with the patient lying in the prone position, will be asymmetric. Attempts to internally rotate the affected hip often cause increased pain, and the arc of passive internal hip rotation is decreased compared to the unaffected side.

Typically, pain is experienced in the hip or groin. It is not uncommon, however, for patients to experience referred pain to the medial thigh or knee due to the sensory distribution of the obturator nerve (Kehl 2001). In fact, some patients complain only of knee pain, thus making it critical to have a high index of suspicion and to examine the hips as part of the routine knee evaluation. Focusing only on the knee can result in a higher rate of unnecessary knee radiographs, misdiagnoses, and increased severity of slips due to delays in diagnosis (Matava *et al.* 1999). Any asymmetry of hip motion warrants radiographic evaluation of the pelvis.

Imaging studies
Any patient suspected of having an SCFE should be screened with standard orthogonal radiographs. Additionally, any obese adolescent with vague knee pain warrants a screening radiograph of the pelvis, especially if there is any asymmetry in hip rotation, due to the prevalence of SCFEs in this population. The anteroposterior (AP) and frog lateral views of the pelvis allow for evaluation of both hips simultaneously. If only one hip is affected, the other hip provides a reference for comparison. If, however, the patient has bilateral SCFEs and only one side is symptomatic, imaging both sides simultaneously decreases the chance of missing the diagnosis on the asymptomatic side. The technique for obtaining the frog lateral view of the pelvis requires that the patient be able to externally rotate and abduct his or her hips. In acute, unstable cases, this maneuver should be avoided because it can potentially increase the amount of physeal displacement. For these patients, a cross-table, or shoot-through, lateral image should be obtained. Although this image better elucidates the amount of posterior displacement, it can be difficult to obtain in obese patients.

Most SCFEs can be identified on the AP radiograph (Fig. 6.2A). However, for patients who present very early and before any measurable slipping (frequently referred to as pre-slip), radiographic changes may be very subtle. Any widening or irregularity of the physis should be viewed as suspicious for an SCFE. Additionally, the height of the epiphysis may appear decreased compared to the contralateral side. With increasing amounts of slippage, the radiographic changes become more obvious. As the epiphysis becomes posteriorly displaced with respect to the femoral neck, the superimposed structures create a crescent-shaped density that may become apparent just distal to the physis. This radiographic finding is referred to as the metaphyseal blanch sign of Steel (1986). Another radiographic entity that can assist in making the diagnosis is a line drawn along the superior edge of the femoral neck. This line, referred to as Klein's line, normally intersects the lateral corner of the femoral head as it is extended proximally (Klein *et al.* 1952). With increasing slippage, the amount of epiphysis intersected by the projected line decreases.

The lateral view is useful for identifying subtle slips and can be used to quantify the amount of posterior displacement of the epiphysis (Fig. 6.2B). In chronic cases, the anterior

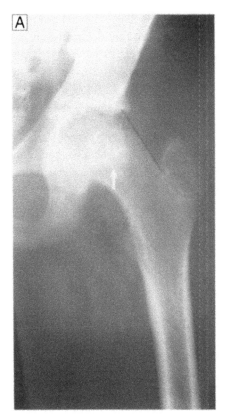

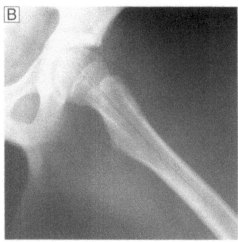

Fig. 6.2. (A) Anteroposterior, and (B) lateral radiographs of a patient with a slipped capital femoral epiphysis (SCFE). The blanch sign of Steel (arrow) and Klein's line are indicated on the AP view, and the slip angle is demonstrated on the lateral view. Descriptions of these findings are given in the text.

femoral neck may show evidence of metaphyseal remodeling with blunting of this edge. Additionally, periosteal new bone formation may be detected at the epiphyseal–metaphyseal junction. The severity of the slip can be graded based on the percentage of epiphyseal displacement with respect to metaphyseal width of the femoral neck. Slippage is considered mild if displacement is less than one-third of the femoral neck width; moderate if displacement is between one-third and one-half of the width; and severe if displacement is greater than one-half of the width of the femoral neck (Jacobs 1972). Southwick (1967) recommended measuring the angle between the femoral head and the femoral shaft. A head–shaft angle, or slip angle, of 30° or less is considered mild; 30–50° is moderate; and greater than 50° is severe (Boyer *et al.* 1981).

The diagnosis of SCFE can usually be made from plain radiographs alone. Other imaging studies, however, may be used in the evaluation of an affected child. Computed tomography (CT) offers three-dimensional evaluation of the deformity and can be useful for assessing physeal plate closure and possible slip progression (Magid *et al.* 1988) (Fig. 6.3). Magnetic resonance imaging (MRI) allows for early detection of osteonecrosis and chondrolyis, and it can be useful in identifying preslips before standard radiographic changes occur (Umans *et al.* 1998). Bone scans can identify ischemia and help predict which patients are at

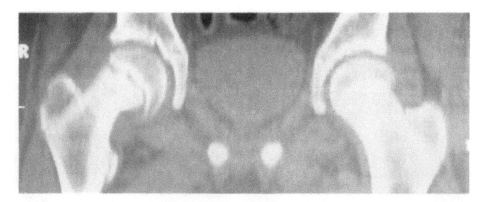

Fig. 6.3. CT image demonstrating a slipped capital femoral epiphysis.

increased risk for avascular necrosis of the femoral head (Rhoad *et al.* 1999). Ultrasonography not only reveals the presence or absence of a slip, but also can quantify the amount of physeal step-off and identify a hip joint effusion (Castriota-Scanderbeg and Orsi 1993). The presence of an effusion suggests an acute, unstable slip, whereas metaphyseal remodeling is a sign of chronicity (Kallio *et al.* 1993).

Treatment
As with most conditions, the first goal of treatment of any patient with an SCFE is *primum non nocere* (first, do no harm). Because prognosis correlates with slip severity, treatment should be aimed at preventing further slippage by stabilizing the physis and promoting premature physeal closure. Correction of the deformity remains controversial and is usually reserved for more severe cases. Any patient suspected of having an SCFE should be made non-weight-bearing (bedrest for unstable cases, wheelchair or crutches for stable cases) and referred immediately to an orthopedist. For patients who are able to ambulate on their own, it is reasonable to obtain radiographs before referral. If a patient presents with an acute, unstable slip (unable to bear weight), referral should not be delayed. Such a patient requires an efficient clinical and radiographic evaluation that can usually best be provided in a hospital setting. Once the diagnosis of SCFE has been confirmed, the recommended treatment is almost always surgical. In a recent study investigating the quality of evaluation and management of 142 children requiring timely orthopedic surgery before admission to a tertiary pediatric facility, Skaggs *et al.* (2002) found that 32% experienced problems or delays in medical care prior to their transfer. Although this population included patients with a variety of diagnoses, including open fractures, infections and compartment syndromes, six of the patients had missed SCFEs, and five of these had not been made non-weight-bearing prior to their transfer.

Although a variety of treatments have been used to treat slips, *in situ* stabilization with single or multiple screws is currently the most frequently used technique (Morrissy 1990, Aronson and Carlson 1992) (Fig. 6.4). Often, patients are referred to pediatric orthopedists

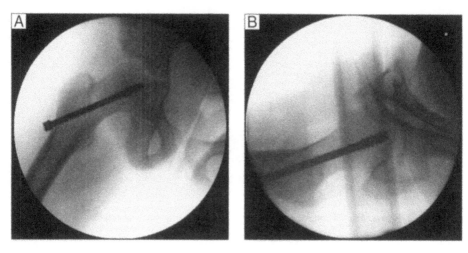

Fig. 6.4. Intraoperative fluoroscopy of (A) anteroposterior and (B) lateral images of *in situ* screw fixation of a stable SCFE.

at tertiary care facilities; however, the development of intraoperative fluoroscopy has made it possible for most orthopedists to safely perform this procedure. The technique involves placing a guide pin through a tiny skin incision and advancing it under fluoroscopic guidance up the femoral neck and into the femoral head, crossing perpendicular to the physis. After measuring with a depth gauge, the appropriate length 7.3 mm or 7.0 mm screw can then be placed over the guide pin. A radiolucent table and AP and lateral images are required for this percutaneous technique so as to decrease the risk of improper screw placement. Ideally, the screw should be targeted into the center of the epiphysis (Aronson and Carlson 1992). As the femoral head slips more posterior with respect to the metaphysis, the screw's starting point will need to be more anterior to allow centralized placement within the epiphysis without exiting out the back of the femoral neck. The main blood supply to the femoral head enters the posterosuperior quadrant via the lateral epiphyseal branches of the medial femoral circumflex artery (Brodetti 1960). Screws that enter the femoral head's posterosuperior quadrant may damage the terminal branches, whereas screws that inadvertently exit the femoral neck posteriorly may compromise the circumflex vessel. Either scenario can increase the risk of avascular necrosis (Fig. 6.5). Screws that are too long and penetrate the articular cartilage can increase the risk of chondrolysis (loss of cartilage thickness, increased hip pain, and decreased range of motion). As the number of screws increases, so too does the potential for improper screw placement. Karol *et al.* (1992) evaluated single-screw fixation versus double-screw fixation in a bovine model. They concluded that the small gains in stiffness from the second screw did not offset the risk of complications and, therefore, recommended single-screw fixation for the treatment of SCFEs. Blanco *et al.* (1992) noted that patients treated with single-pin fixation experienced fewer complications than those treated with multiple pins, yet the time to physeal closure was similar.

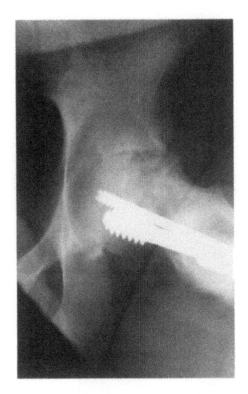

Fig. 6.5. Example of improper hardware placement. Note the screw exiting the posterior aspect of the femoral neck.

Treatment of unstable or acute slips is similar to, though more controversial than, that of stable slips. The risk of osteonecrosis is higher in patients with unstable slips (seen in 14 of 30 unstable hips vs none of 25 stable hips among the 54 patients studied by Loder *et al.* 1993). Most believe, however, that the poor outcome is due to damage done at the time of injury rather than the result of treatment (Herman *et al.* 1996, Rhoad *et al.* 1999, Maeda *et al.* 2001). There are conflicting views as to what measures to take to minimize the damage caused by kinking of the posterior vessels by the displaced femoral head. Peterson *et al.* (1997) advocate immediate reduction (<24 hours) and pinning; Aronson and Loder (1996) recommend preoperative bedrest until the synovitis and effusion improve, followed by *in situ* screw fixation; Casey *et al.* (1972) suggest preoperative traction. Although single-screw fixation may be adequate for most slips, the risk of further progression in acute cases may warrant multiple screw techniques (Sanders *et al.* 2002) (Fig. 6.6). To avoid the risk of osteonecrosis associated with screw placement in the superolateral corner, it is recommended that the first screw be directed into the center of the femoral head. Subsequent screws can be placed inferior to this.

Additional treatment options exist, but these are used much less frequently and are mentioned here mostly for historical purposes. Spica cast immobilization has been used to successfully treat some slips, and it offers the advantage of simultaneously immobilizing the contralateral hip (Betz *et al.* 1990). The cast, however, cannot actually stabilize the physis.

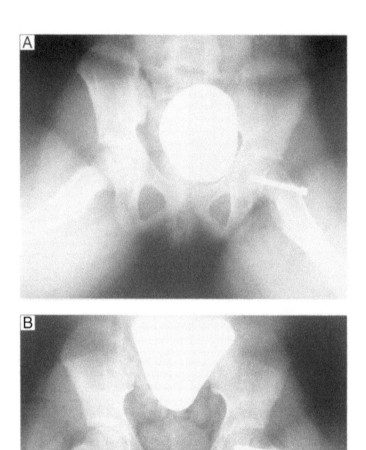

Fig. 6.6. (A) Example of single-screw fixation in a patient with an unstable SCFE. (B) A second screw was added due to persistent symptoms and concern for further progression.

Because spica cast treatment has been associated with further slip progression, chondrolysis, cast pressure sores and family inconvenience, this technique is no longer recommended (Meir *et al.* 1992). Open bone graft epiphysiodesis is accomplished by creating a tunnel up the femoral neck and across the physis, followed by placing multiple corticocancellous strips of iliac crest bone graft within the tunnel. Although this technique can result in successful physeal fusion and stability without the potential for hardware failure, the increased surgical exposure, operative time, blood loss and risk of graft resorption or fracture limit its indications (Ward and Wood 1990). Finally, a variety of corrective osteotomies have been developed to reorient the displaced femoral head. Osteotomies through the physis (Dunn and Angel 1978), the base of the neck (Kramer *et al.* 1976, Barmada *et al.* 1978), and intertrochanteric regions (Southwick 1967, Ito *et al.* 2001) have all been attempted. Such osteotomies, which are beyond the scope of this chapter, are usually reserved for severe slips and are rarely indicated for initial treatment. Due to the technically demanding nature of these procedures, only experienced specialists should be performing them.

Treatment of a patient with an SCFE requires urgent stabilization of the actual slip, but caregivers must also be cognizant of potentially coexisting medical conditions. Because most patients with SCFE do not have a demonstrable endocrinopathy, it is probably not cost-effective to screen all patients with SCFE for such disorders. Nevertheless, certain patients do warrant further investigation. Since idiopathic SCFE is associated with puberty, it is not surprising that it occurs most frequently in boys between 10 and 16 years of age (average, 13.5 years) and in girls between 10 and 14 years (average, 11.5 years) (Kehl 2001). Presentation outside these age ranges should alert the physician to a potential endocrinopathy. Burrow *et al.* (2001) demonstrated that height may be used as a screening tool. They found that the sensitivity and negative predictive value of detecting an endocrinopathy in patients with SCFE and short stature (defined as 10th percentile or less for height) were 90.2% and 98.6%, respectively. They therefore recommend screening patients for endocrinopathies if they are on or below the 10th percentile for height at the time of presentation with SCFE. Thyroid-stimulating hormone and free thyroxine are their recommended screening tests. For patients with a known endocrine deficiency and a unilateral slip, Wells *et al.* (1993) recommend prophylactic pinning of the uninvolved hip, having found simultaneous or subsequent bilateral involvement in 100% of 131 such cases that they reviewed. Prophylactic pinning of the uninvolved hip in such high-risk patients is generally accepted (Fig. 6.7). Additionally, patients with poor access to medical care who may be unable to obtain follow-up treatment to monitor the uninvolved hip may benefit from prophylactic pinning. More recently, however, the practice of prophylactically pinning the unaffected contralateral hip in any patient with a unilateral SCFE has gained some support. Proponents for this practice accept the minimal risks associated with *in situ* pin fixation of the unaffected hip in the same surgical setting rather than the risk of potential secondary slippage requiring further surgery (Seller *et al.* 2001). Such prophylactic surgery, however, remains controversial.

Prognosis
The natural history of the untreated SCFE remains somewhat unpredictable. Certainly, some patients may go undetected if their symptoms are mild. Once the physis has closed, further slippage does not occur, but residual malalignment may result in early degenerative joint disease. In a study of 200 adult patients who were thought to have primary degenerative joint disease, Murray (1964) found 40% with a tilt deformity that he considered compatible with an old SCFE. Stulberg *et al.* (1975) reported a similar deformity in 40% of patients undergoing a total hip arthroplasty who previously had no known history of hip disease. They also concluded that this deformity, referred to as the pistol grip deformity, was compatible with an old SCFE. As for patients who had a known SCFE, yet still went untreated, long-term follow-up suggests that the risk of degenerative arthritis increases

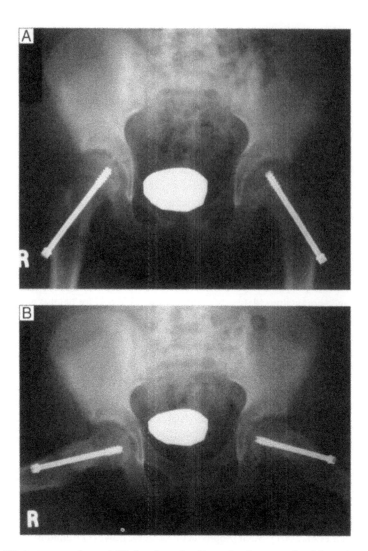

Fig. 6.7. (A) Anteroposterior and (B) frog lateral radiographs demonstrating bilateral *in situ* screw fixation in a 10-year-old patient with a left unilateral SCFE. Because of her young age, thyroid function tests were obtained: these confirmed hypothyroidism and prompted the surgeon to prophylactically pin the asymptomatic side.

with increasing displacement, whereas those with chronic slips with minimal displacement have a favorable outcome (Carney and Weinstein 1996). Unfortunately, even very mild slips, if left untreated, can progress, making surgical stabilization the current standard of care.

For patients whose slips are stabilized with screw fixation, osteonecrosis and chondrolyis, with subsequent degenerative joint disease, are the most dreaded complications. Fortunately, modern techniques using fluoroscopic guidance and proper screw placement have made these complications quite rare in patients with stable SCFEs (Loder *et al.* 1993, 2001). Patients presenting with unstable slips, however, have a much higher complication rate, approaching 47%, regardless of the degree of displacement, attempts at reduction, or the number of screws used (Loder *et al.* 1993, Kennedy *et al.* 2001). These patients should be counseled about such risks at the time of initial presentation and treatment. Nevertheless, in situ screw fixation seems to provide the best long-term function with a low risk of complications in most cases of SCFE (Dobbs and Weinstein 2001). Even for those with severe slips who initially lose hip motion, soft-tissue stretching and bone resorption in the anterolateral femoral neck may occur and result in improved motion and gait (Siegel *et al.* 1991). Because such remodeling occurs gradually over time, some authors advocate waiting at least two years before considering a realignment osteotomy (Siegel *et al.* 1991, Wong-Chung and Strong 1991).

Conclusion

SCFE remains one of the most common disorders affecting the pediatric hip. Fortunately, the majority of slips can be successfully stabilized with minimally invasive surgical techniques that produce reliably favorable outcomes. In order to ensure the best results, early recognition of the problem and prompt referral to an orthopedic surgeon are of utmost importance. This chapter provides an overview of the common features associated with SCFE and offers the reader an explanation of current treatment strategies. For further study, the reader is referred to Kehl (2001) and Loder *et al.* (2001).

REFERENCES

Aronson, D.D., Carlson, W.E. (1992) 'Slipped capital femoral epiphysis: a prospective study of fixation with a single screw.' *Journal of Bone and Joint Surgery, American Volume*, **74**, 810–819.

Aronson, D.D., Loder, R.T. (1996) 'Treatment of the unstable (acute) slipped capital femoral epiphysis.' *Clinical Orthopaedics and Related Research*, **322**, 99–110.

Aronson, J., Tursky, E. (1996) 'The torsional basis for slipped capital femoral epiphysis.' *Clinical Orthopaedics and Related Research*, **322**, 37–42.

Barmada, R., Bruch, R.F., Gimbel, J.S., Ray, R.D. (1978) 'Base of the neck extracapsular osteotomy for correction of deformity in slipped capital femoral epiphysis.' *Clinical Orthopaedics and Related Research*, **132**, 98–101.

Betz, R.R., Steel, H.H., Emper, W.D., Huss, G.K., Clancy, M. (1990) 'Treatment of slipped capital femoral epiphysis. Spica-cast immobilization.' *Journal of Bone and Joint Surgery, American Volume*, **72**, 587–600.

Blanco, J.S., Taylor, B., Johnston, C.E. (1992) 'Comparison of single pin versus multiple pin fixation in treatment of slipped capital femoral epiphysis.' *Journal of Pediatric Orthopedics*, **12**, 384–389.

Blethen, S.L., Rundle, A.C. (1996) 'Slipped capital femoral epiphysis in children treated with growth hormone. A summary of the National Cooperative Growth Study experience.' *Hormone Research*, **46**, 113–116.

Boyer, D.W., Mickelson, M.R., Ponseti, I.V. (1981) 'Slipped capital femoral epiphyis: long-term follow-up of one hundred and twenty-one patients.' *Journal of Bone and Joint Surgery, American Volume*, **63**, 85–95.

Brodetti, A. (1960) 'The blood supply of the femoral neck and head in relation to the damaging effects of nails and screws.' *Journal of Bone and Joint Surgery, British Volume*, **42**, 794–801.

Burrow, S.R., Alman, B., Wright, J.G. (2001) 'Short stature as a screening test for endocrinopathy in slipped capital femoral epiphysis.' *Journal of Bone and Joint Surgery, British Volume*, **83**, 263–268.

Carney, B.T., Weinstein, S.L. (1996) 'Natural history of untreated chronic slipped capital femoral epiphysis.' *Clinical Orthopaedics and Related Research*, **322**, 43–47.

Casey, B.H., Hamilton, H.W., Bobechko, W.P. (1972) 'Reduction of acutely slipped upper femoral epiphysis.' *Journal of Bone and Joint Surgery, British Volume*, **54**, 607–614.

Castriota-Scanderbeg, A., Orsi, E. (1993) 'Slipped capital femoral epiphysis: ultrasonographic findings.' *Skeletal Radiology*, **22**, 191–193.

Dobbs, M.B., Weinstein, S.L. (2001) 'Natural history and long-term outcomes of slipped capital femoral epiphysis.' *Instructional Course Lectures*, **50**, 571–575.

Dunn, D.M., Angel, J.C. (1978) 'Replacement of the femoral head by open operation in severe adolescent slipping of the upper femoral epiphysis.' *Journal of Bone and Joint Surgery, British Volume*, **60**, 394–403.

Gunal, I., Ates, E. (1997) 'The HLA phenotype in slipped capital femoral epiphysis.' *Journal of Pediatric Orthopedics*, **17**, 655–656.

Herman, M.J., Dormans, J.P., Davidson, R.S., Drummond, D.S., Gregg, J.R. (1996) 'Screw fixation of grade III slipped capital femoral epiphysis.' *Clinical Orthopaedics and Related Research*, **322**, 77–85.

Ito, H., Minami, A., Suzuki, K., Matsuno, T. (2001) 'Three-dimensionally corrective external fixator system for proximal femoral osteotomy.' *Journal of Pediatric Orthopedics*, **21**, 652–656.

Jacobs, B. (1972) 'Diagnosis and natural history of slipped capital femoral epiphysis.' *Instructional Course Lectures*, **21**, 167–173.

Kallio, P.E., Paterson, D.C., Foster, B.K., Lequesne, G.W. (1993) 'Classification in slipped capital femoral epiphysis: sonographic assessment of stability and remodeling.' *Clinical Orthopaedics and Related Research*, **294**, 196–203.

Karol, L.A., Doane, R.M., Cornicelli, S.F., Zak, P.A., Haut, R.C., Manoli, A. (1992) 'Single versus double screw fixation for treatment for slipped capital femoral epiphysis: a biomechanical analysis.' *Journal of Pediatric Orthopedics*, **12**, 741–745.

Kehl, D.K. (2001) 'Slipped capital femoral epiphysis.' *In:* Morrissy, R.T., Weinstein, S.L. (Eds.) *Lovell and Winter's Pediatric Orthopaedics, 5th Edn.* Philadelphia: Lippincott, Williams & Wilkins, pp. 999–1034.

Kelsey, J.L., Keggi, K.J., Southwick, W.O. (1970) 'The incidence and distribution of slipped capital femoral epiphysis in Connecticut and southwestern United States.' *Journal of Bone and Joint Surgery, American Volume*, **52**, 1203–1216.

Kempers, M.J., Noordam, C., Rouwe, C.W., Otten, B.J. (2001) 'Can GnRH-agonist treatment cause slipped capital femoral epiphysis?' *Journal of Pediatric Endocrinology and Metabolism*, **14**, 729–734.

Kennedy, J.G., Hresko, M.T., Kasser, J.R., Shrock K.B., Zurakowski, D., Waters, P.M., Millis, M.B. (2001) 'Osteonecrosis of the femoral head associated with slipped capital femoral epiphysis.' *Journal of Pediatric Orthopedics*, **21**, 189–193.

Klein A., Joplin, R.J., Reidy, J.A., Hanelin, J. (1952) 'Slipped capital femoral epiphysis: early diagnosis and treatment facilitated by "normal" roentgenograms.' *Journal of Bone and Joint Surgery, American Volume*, **34**, 233–239.

Kordelle, J., Millis, M., Jolesz, F.A., Kikinis, R., Richolt, J.A. (2001) 'Three-dimensional analysis of the proximal femur in patients with slipped capital femoral epiphysis based on computed tomography.' *Journal of Pediatric Orthopedics*, **21**, 179–182.

Kramer, W.G., Craig, W.A., Noel, S. (1976) 'Compensating osteotomy at the base of the femoral neck for slipped capital femoral epiphysis.' *Journal of Bone and Joint Surgery, American Volume*, **58**, 796–800.

Loder, R.T. (1996a) 'The demographics of slipped capital femoral epiphysis. An international multicenter study.' *Clinical Orthopaedics and Related Research*, **322**, 8–27.

Loder, R.T. (1996b) 'A worldwide study on the seasonal variation of slipped capital femoral epiphysis.' *Clinical Orthopaedics and Related Research*, **322**, 28–36.

Loder, R.T., Richards, B.S., Shapiro, P.S., Reznick, L.R., Aronsson, D.D. (1993) 'Acute slipped capital femoral epiphysis: The importance of physeal stability.' *Journal of Bone and Joint Surgery, American Volume*, **75**, 1134–1140.

Loder, R.T., Hensinger, R.N., Alburger, P.D., Aronsson, D.D., Beaty, J.H., Roy, D.R., Stanton, R.P., Turker, R. (1998) 'Slipped capital femoral epiphysis associated with radiation therapy.' *Journal of Pediatric Orthopedics*, **18**, 630–636.

Loder, R.T., Aronsson, D.D., Dobbs, M.B., Weinstein, S.L. (2001) 'Slipped capital femoral epiphysis.' *Instructional Course Lectures*, **50**, 555–570.

Maeda, S., Kita, A., Funayama, K., Kokubun, S. (2001) 'Vascular supply to slipped capital femoral epiphysis.' *Journal of Pediatric Orthopedics*, **21**, 664–667.

Magid, D., Fishman, E.K., Sponseller, P.D., Griffin, P.P. (1988) '2D and 3D computed tomography of the pediatric hip.' *Radiographics*, **8**, 901–933.

Mann, D.C. (1996) 'Endocrine disorders and orthopedic problems in children.' *Current Opinion in Pediatrics*, **8**, 68–70.

Matava, M.J., Patton, C.M., Luhmann, S., Gordon, J.E., Schoenecker, P.L. (1999) 'Knee pain as the initial symptom of slipped capital femoral epiphysis: an analysis of initial presentation and treatment.' *Journal of Pediatric Orthopedics*, **19**, 455–460.

Meir, M.C., Meyer, L.C., Ferguson, R.L. (1992) 'Treatment of slipped capital femoral epiphysis with a spica cast.' *Journal of Bone and Joint Surgery, American Volume*, **74**, 1522–1529.

Mickelson, M.R., Ponseti, I.V., Cooper, R.R., Maynard, J.A. (1977) 'The ultrastructure of the growth plate in slipped capital femoral epiphysis.' *Journal of Bone and Joint Surgery, American Volume*, **59**, 1076–1081.

Morrissy, R.T. (1990) 'Slipped capital femoral epiphysis technique of percutaneous in situ fixation.' *Journal of Pediatric Orthopedics*, **10**, 347–350.

Murray, R.O. (1964) 'The aetiology of primary osteoarthritis of the hip.' *British Journal of Radiology*, **38**, 810–824.

Ninomiya, S., Nagasaka, Y., Tagawa, H. (1976) 'Slipped capital femoral epiphysis. A study of 68 cases in the eastern half area of Japan.' *Clinical Orthopaedics and Related Research*, **119**, 172–176.

Peterson, M.D., Weiner, D.S., Green, N.E., Terry, C.L. (1997) 'Acute slipped capital femoral epiphysis: the value and safety of urgent manipulative reduction.' *Journal of Pediatric Orthopedics*, **17**, 648–654.

Pritchett, J.W., Perdue, K.D., Dona, G.A. (1989) 'The neck shaft–plate shaft angle in slipped capital femoral epiphysis.' *Orthopaedic Review*, **18**, 1187–1192.

Rhoad, R.C., Davidson, R.S., Heyman, S., Dormans, J.P., Drummond, D.S. (1999) 'Pretreatment bone scan in SCFE: a predictor of ischemia and avascular necrosis.' *Journal of Pediatric Orthopedics*, **19**, 164–168.

Sanders, J.O., Smith W.J., Stanley, E.A., Bueche, M.J., Karol, L.A., Chambers, H.G. (2002) 'Progressive slippage after pinning for slipped capital femoral epiphysis.' *Journal of Pediatric Orthopedics*, **22**, 239–243.

Segal, L.S., Weitzel, P.P., Davidson, R.S. (1996) 'Valgus slipped capital femoral epiphysis: fact or fiction?' *Clinical Orthopaedics*, **322**, 91–98.

Seller, K., Raab, P., Wild, A., Krauspe, R. (2001) 'Risk–benefit analysis of prophylactic pinning in slipped capital femoral epiphysis.' *Journal of Pediatric Orthopaedics, Part B*, **10**, 192–196.

Shanker, V.S., Hashemi-Nejad, A., Catterall, A., Jackson, A. (2000) 'Slipped capital femoral epiphysis: is the displacement always posterior?' *Journal of Pediatric Orthopaedics, Part B*, **9**, 119–121.

Siegel, D.B., Kasser, J.R., Sponseller, P, Gelberman, R.H. (1991) 'Slipped capital femoral epiphysis: a quantitative analysis of motion, gait, and femoral remodeling after in situ fixation.' *Journal of Bone and Joint Surgery, American Volume*, **73**, 659–666.

Skaggs, D.L., Roy, A.K., Vitale, M.G., Pfiefer, C., Baird, G., Femino, D., Kay, R.M. (2002) 'Quality of evaluation and management of children requiring timely orthopaedic surgery before admission to a tertiary pediatric facility.' *Journal of Pediatric Orthopedics*, **22**, 265–267.

Southwick, W.O. (1967) 'Osteotomy through the lesser trochanter for slipped capital femoral epiphysis.' *Journal of Bone and Joint Surgery, American Volume*, **49**, 807–835.

Steel, H.H. (1986) 'The metaphyseal blanch sign of slipped capital femoral epiphysis.' *Journal of Bone and Joint Surgery, American Volume*, **68**, 920–922.

Stulberg, S.D., Cordell, L.D., Harris, W.H., Ramsey, P.L, MacEwen, G.D. (1975) 'Unrecognized childhood hip disease: a major cause of idiopathic osteonecrosis of the hip.' *In:* The Hip Society (Ed.) *The Hip: Proceedings of the Third Open Scientific Meeting of the Hip Society*. St Louis: C.V. Mosby, pp. 212–230.

Umans, H., Liebling, M.S., Moy, L., Haramati, N., Macy, N.J., Pritzker, H.A. (1998) 'Slipped capital femoral epiphysis: a physeal lesion diagnosed by MRI, with radiographic and CT correlation.' *Skeletal Radiology*, **27**, 139–144.

Ward, W.T., Wood, K. (1990) 'Open bone graft epiphyseodesis for slipped capital femoral epiphysis.' *Journal of Pediatric Orthopedics*, **10**, 14–20.

Weiner, D. (1996) 'Pathogenesis of slipped capital femoral epiphysis: current concepts.' *Journal of Pediatric Orthopaedics, Part B*, **5**, 67–73.

Wells, D., King, J.D., Roe, T.F., Kaufman, F.R. (1993) 'Review of slipped capital femoral epiphysis associated with endocrine disease.' *Journal of Pediatric Orthopedics*, **13**, 610–614.

Williams, J.L, Vani, J.N., Eick, J.D., Petersen, E.C., Schmidt, T.L. (1999) 'Shear strength of the physis varies with anatomic location and is a function of modulus, inclination, and thickness.' *Journal of Orthopaedic Research*, **17**, 212–222.

Wong-Chung, J., Strong, M.L. (1991) 'Physeal remodeling after internal fixation of slipped capital femoral epiphyses.' *Journal of Pediatric Orthopedics*, **11**, 2–5.

Wong-Chung, J., Al-Aali, Y., Farid, I., Al-Aradi, A. (2000) 'A common HLA phenotype in slipped capital femoral epiphysis.' *International Orthopaedics*, **24**, 158–159.

7
PERTHES' DISEASE

J. Mark H. Paterson

About 90 years ago, descriptions of a curious condition affecting children's hips began to appear in the medical literature. They noted a self-limiting process in which the femoral head went through successive stages of degeneration and varying degrees of collapse, followed by regeneration and healing, albeit not necessarily with complete restitution of the original shape.

In recognition of the contributions made by three physicians at that time, the condition became known as Legg–Calvé–Perthes disease, although nowadays this is commonly shortened to Perthes' disease, particularly in Europe. No-one seemed sure about the aetiology, but it seemed to be a different condition to the hip joint tuberculosis prevalent at the time. Whatever the cause, it was widely believed that prolonged relief from weight bearing was important to prevent osteoarthritic changes in the hip. This led to many children spending months or even years in traction in bed, or in various types of caliper and other so-called weight-relieving devices.

In the 1930s, the concept of containment of the damaged femoral head became popular. It was thought that if the hip were maintained in abduction, more of the femoral head would be contained within the acetabulum, which could then act as a mould to help maintain the spherical shape of the femoral head. There followed a succession of operative and non-operative treatment regimes designed to improve containment. Claims were made for the relative advantages of either femoral or pelvic osteotomies to achieve this containment, while others promoted orthotic devices designed to maintain the affected hip in a contained position.

As arguments raged over the correct management, one basic and extremely important observation was frequently ignored or forgotten, the fact that many children with Perthes' disease had an excellent outcome without being subjected to any specific treatment.

We still do not know precisely what causes Perthes' disease, so treatment of the condition remains largely empirical. If we are to attempt to provide a rational management programme, it is important to have a full understanding of the pathology and natural history of the condition. Specific interventions can clearly only be recommended if they are likely to result in a better outcome than that expected from the untreated disease.

In the following sections, we will firstly consider what we do know about Perthes' disease from a pathological, clinical and radiological viewpoint. We will then look at the various outcomes from Perthes' disease, treated and untreated. Finally, we will put all this information together to produce a logical plan of management for this condition.

The cause of Perthes' disease: what do we know?

A ligature wound tightly around the femoral neck of a dog produces infarction of the femoral head and pathological features that superficially resemble those seen in Perthes' disease (Freeman and England 1969). There is general agreement that the underlying patho-physiological process in Perthes' disease is that of bone infarction. However, a single episode of acute ischaemia does not produce the prolonged features of bone death, collapse and subsequent repair that characterize the hip in Perthes' disease. It appears that multiple episodes of ischaemia are necessary to produce these features, and that even then the process of Perthes' disease will not be initiated unless these ischaemic episodes lead to structural collapse in the femoral head. (This will be developed further in the section on pathology.)

What causes the ischaemia that leads to these changes? Over the years, the following observations about Perthes' disease have been made, some of which may be relevant:

• Angiographic studies have demonstrated obstruction of superior capsular arteries of the femoral head in some patients during the early stages of the disease (Theron 1980).

• Disruption of normal venous drainage of the affected hip has been demonstrated, though whether this is a cause rather than a result of Perthes' disease is unclear (Heikkinen *et al.* 1980).

• More recently, coagulation abnormalities have been demonstrated in children suffering from Perthes' disease. In one study, deficiencies in proteins C and S were found in the majority of children with Perthes' disease, leading to a tendency to thrombophilia or hypofibrinolysis (Glueck *et al.* 1997), although a subsequent study by McDougall *et al.* (1998) did not provide support for this finding.

• Children who develop Perthes' disease tend to be shorter than average and have a delayed bone age (Fisher 1972).

• In the UK, epidemiological studies have demonstrated a particularly high prevalence of the condition in socially deprived urban areas, suggesting a possible nutritional influence (Hall *et al.* 1983).

• There appears to be an unusually high proportion of children with hyperactivity syndrome or attention deficit disorder (ADD) amongst those suffering from Perthes' disease. It is possible that hyperactivity may have some role in the onset of Perthes' disease, perhaps because of a higher incidence of trauma (Loder *et al.* 1993).

• Perthes' disease can present initially as an acute synovitis in much the same way as a common transient synovitis (the "irritable hip" associated with a viraemia). Although it has been suggested that a proportion of children with a transient synovitis can go on to develop Perthes' disease, there is little evidence to show that such an inflammatory episode is actually the cause of Perthes' disease.

It has become fashionable to talk of the 'predisposed' or 'susceptible' child who may have some of the characteristics listed above, and whose femoral head is unable to tolerate the effects of minor repeated ischaemic episodes which in 'normal' children would not lead to structural damage. Support for the concept of a more generalized predisposition comes from the observation that isotope bone scans performed on the contralateral hip in unilateral Perthes' disease can show avascular changes which subsequently recover without development of Perthes' disease in that hip.

Pathology

It seems likely that the capital epiphysis of the growing femoral head is subject to frequent threats to its vascular integrity from which it is usually able to recover. In susceptible children, however, the key event that pushes the ischaemic femoral head over the brink into the full condition of Perthes' disease is the trabecular fracture.

It is thought that repeated ischaemic events in the susceptible child will lead to bone death and structural collapse of the bony trabeculae in at least part of the femoral head. These trabecular fractures lead to a variable degree of flattening of the epiphysis. This process will be much more apparent in the older child, where more of the cartilaginous epiphysis has converted to bone. In the early stages, there is also an overgrowth of articular cartilage that leads to an enlarged head or coxa magna; this is of importance in consideration of the containment concept of treatment. This is the initial period and it lasts about 6–12 months.

Once the infarct becomes established, repair processes come into play. As revascularization occurs, avascular but intact trabeculae are replaced by the process of 'creeping substitution' characterized by sequential bone resorption and new bone formation. Loose, crushed necrotic bone is replaced by fibrocartilage. Islands of new bone formation start to appear within the enlarged volume of articular cartilage and bone starts to be laid down again at the outer margins of any part of the bony nucleus that has remained viable. These scattered areas of bone produce a radiographic appearance of fragmentation. At the same time, there is disruption of the growth plate. Unossified cartilage columns extend into the metaphysis forming metaphyseal cysts. Severe distortions of the growth plate lead to partial arrests of growth and these will influence the final shape of the head and neck. This is the period of fragmentation and it may last up to 24–30 months. During this time, the femoral head is large, soft and deformable, and vulnerable to distortion.

Healing is completed by coalescence of all separate areas of ossification within the cartilage of the head. The head hardens again, effectively frozen in the shape adopted during the earlier phases of the disease. This final stage of the disease process may last for several years. Further remodelling can occur, the extent of this process being dependent to a great extent on the age of the child and the number of years left for growth.

Throughout the disease process, there may be secondary changes in the acetabulum in response to changes in the shape and size of the femoral head. The resulting shape of the femoral head and the acetabulum, and their relationship to each other, will determine the long-term outcome of the disease, as will be shown below.

Clinical features

The onset of the condition occurs between the ages of 2 and 12 years, with most cases occurring between 4 and 9 years of age. It is much more common in boys. The '80% rule' is useful: 80% of children with Perthes' disease are boys, 80% have unilateral involvement, and 80% have an onset at between 4 and 9 years of age. The incidence is in the region of 1 in 10,000 children, although this varies between different ethnic and possibly also social groupings. There is a low incidence in black children, and, as noted above, a high incidence in socially deprived families living on inner-city estates.

The most common presentation is of a limp, with pain felt in hip, thigh or knee. The onset can be quite insidious, with rather vague and intermittent symptoms during the early months. For this reason, the disease process is frequently well advanced by the time the diagnosis is made. The limp and pain are usually aggravated by physical activity and are more pronounced later in the day. The pain may be localized to the groin or lateral hip region, or may be referred to the thigh or knee. Often there is an accompanying history of trauma, but the relevance of this is unclear; there is an understandable tendency for parents to try to relate the onset of symptoms to a particular event. The truth is that minor trauma is very common in children, and particularly so in those hyperactive children who seem to make up a large proportion of cases of Perthes' disease.

The clinical signs include a limp that may be either antalgic or Trendelenburg in type, or a combination of the two. In the former, there is a shortened stance phase as the child attempts to reduce the time spent bearing weight on the affected limb. In the latter, abductor muscle dysfunction on the affected side leads to a dropped pelvis and a leaning of the upper body over the affected side. There may be some wasting of the gluteal and quadriceps musculature. Muscle spasm will be manifest as a reduction in the range of hip movement, particularly that of abduction and internal rotation, though this reduction in range is very variable.

As the condition progresses, these clinical findings will change. Episodes of pain, limp and restriction of movement become more frequent and pronounced as collapse of the femoral head occurs. Progress thereafter is dictated largely by the nature and extent of the ensuing femoral head deformity. If the head remains spherical or ovoid, the hip will continue to act as a ball-and-socket joint, and rotational movements will return as the head heals. If the head becomes flattened, congruency with the acetabulum will be lost, and the joint will fail to act as a ball-and-socket articulation. Instead, it adopts the configuration of a 'roller bearing' type joint that allows flexion and extension but no rotation. Furthermore, if the flattened head has extruded significantly from the confines of the acetabulum, attempts at abduction will result in 'hinging' of the flattened head on the lateral lip of the acetabulum. Thus, movement at the hip will remain restricted even after healing has occurred.

Diagnostic imaging

The early radiographic findings in Perthes' disease are subtle and nonspecific. They include mild apparent widening of the medial joint space due to a combination of cartilage hypertrophy and synovitis (including swelling of the ligamentum teres). In about one-third of cases, a lateral radiograph will demonstrate a thin lucent line just under the surface of the bony epiphysis. This is the subchondral fracture line. These early signs are followed by a loss of height and increased density of the femoral head. This increased density is due to a combination of trabecular collapse and the accumulation of new bone on the trabeculae in the head (Fig. 7.1).

Isotope bone scanning will detect the avascular changes and help to determine the extent of epiphysis involved in the process. MRI is probably as good if not better than bone scanning in mapping the extent of involvement of the epiphysis. However, it is debatable if either of these investigations help to inform management decisions, and serial radiography remains the mainstay of imaging investigation in Perthes' disease.

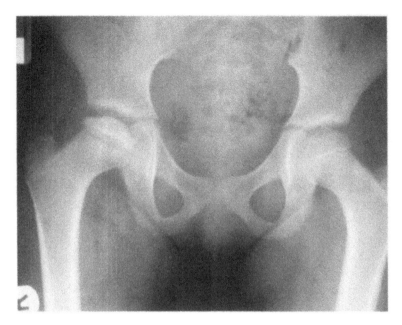

Fig. 7.1. Early changes in the right hip in Perthes' disease: flattening and sclerosis.

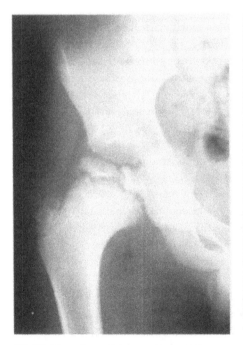

Fig. 7.2. More advanced changes: fragmentation and metaphyseal cysts.

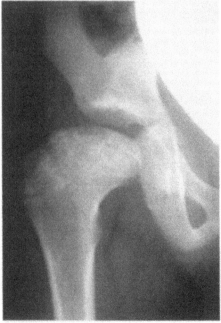

Fig. 7.3. The hip recovers: re-ossification of the epiphysis.

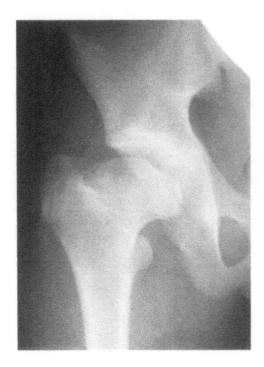

Fig. 7.4. The final outcome: a flattened head with growth disturbance resulting in a high trochanter.

The fragmentation phase is characterized radiologically by areas of radiolucency appearing within the otherwise sclerotic head. The appearance of calcification in the lateral part of the epiphysis is evidence of extrusion of the soft, flattened head from under the cover of the acetabulum. Changes are frequently seen also in the metaphysis where unossified cartilage cell rests appear as cysts (Fig. 7.2).

The healing phase is heralded on radiographs by the reappearance of bone in the sub-chondral region. This often starts in the periphery, with the centre of the head and the anterior segment being the last areas to re-ossify (Fig. 7.3).

Further remodelling over time means that the final appearance of the hip may only become apparent at skeletal maturity. Radiographs made at that time may show hips that appear to be virtually normal; at the other end of the spectrum, marked residual flattening of the femoral head may have persisted. Furthermore, damage to the growth plate may lead to decreased growth in the femoral neck, and relative overgrowth of the greater trochanter (Fig. 7.4).

Differential diagnosis

The radiological appearance of Perthes' disease can be mimicked by other conditions. In the first place, any condition such as sickle cell disease, thalassaemia or leukaemia that can cause avascular change in the femoral head may look superficially like Perthes' disease. It is sometimes difficult to distinguish the late sequelae of septic arthritis or developmental displacement of the hip from Perthes' disease. Gaucher's disease and lymphoma should

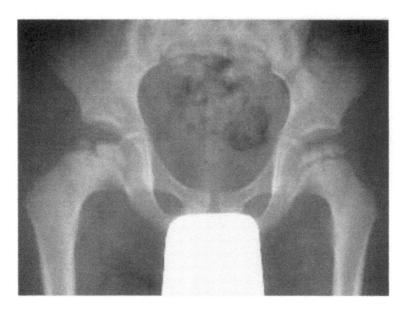

Fig. 7.5. Bilateral Perthes' disease can be differentiated from multiple epiphyseal dysplasia by the asymmetry of changes and absence of changes in other joints.

also be considered. A careful history and examination should enable these conditions to be ruled out. Certain skeletal dysplasias feature abnormal ossification of cartilage and may give rise to radiological appearances similar to those seen in Perthes' disease. The commonest of these is multiple epiphyseal dysplasia. Here, the changes in the hips are symmetrical. This should help to differentiate the condition from bilateral Perthes' disease, where hip involvement tends to be sequential rather than simultaneous (Fig. 7.5). Finally, children with hypothyroidism sometimes develop appearances of fragmentation of the bony femoral head, leading to flattening deformity of the head.

Prognostic factors—who do we treat?

Catterall (1971) showed that 57% of untreated cases of Perthes' disease had a good long-term outcome. In order to manage this condition in a rational way, we need to be able to identify which patients are likely to do well if left alone, and which patients may be helped by intervention. In other words, we need to know the risk factors for a poor prognosis and target active treatment accordingly.

There are three main factors influencing outcome in Perthes' disease: the extent of involvement of the femoral head, the age at onset of disease, and the gender of the patient. To these must be added a series of clinical and radiological warning signs that all is not well with the affected hip.

DEGREE OF FEMORAL HEAD INVOLVEMENT

There is a strong correlation between the extent of femoral head involvement and final outcome.

94

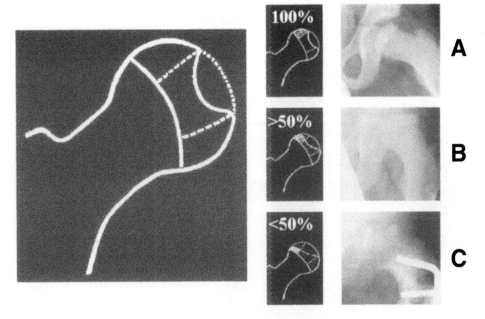

Fig. 7.6. The lateral pillar classification (Herring). The lateral third of the head is designated the lateral pillar. In group A the height of the lateral pillar is maintained, whereas in groups B and C there is progressive loss of pillar height.

The extent of involvement can be classified using either of two widely used systems, the Catterall (Catterall 1971) and the Herring or lateral pillar (Herring *et al.* 1992) classifications. The Catterall classification has been more widely used in the past, but some have found it difficult to apply, and interobserver error is high. The more recently described lateral pillar classification has the advantage of simplicity and its power as a predictive indicator of outcome has been demonstrated. This latter system is illustrated in Fig. 7.6.

Preservation of the height of the lateral pillar indicates a less severe degree of involvement and is associated with a relatively good outcome.

AGE AT ONSET
In general terms, the younger the age at onset the better the outcome.

GENDER
Boys have a better prognosis than girls do, although this distinction is blurred at the more severe end of the spectrum of head involvement. In mild disease the sex ratio is about 14:1 in favour of males, whereas this difference decreases dramatically to about 3:1 in severe involvement.

CLINICAL AND RADIOGRAPHIC RISK FACTORS
In addition to the degree of head involvement, Catterall (1971) listed a series of radiographic

TABLE 7.1
Catterall's 'head at risk' signs*

Clinical	Radiographic
• Progressive loss of movement	• Gage's sign
• Adduction contracture	• Lateral calcification
• Flexion with abduction	• Lateral subluxation
• Overweight child	• Metaphyseal cysts
	• Horizontal growth plate

*Catterall (1971).

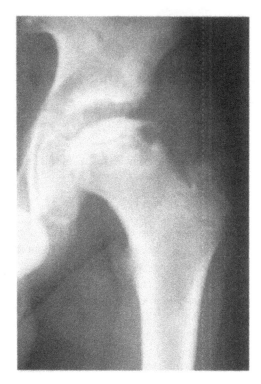

Fig. 7.7. An 'at risk' hip. There are metaphyseal cysts and a positive Gage's sign (lateral defect of ossification at the level of the physis, indicative of the presence of articular cartilage unconstrained by the acetabulum).

and clinical features that were thought to signify impending femoral head deformity (Table 7.1). It has been shown that the presence of two or more signs has an adverse effect on the outcome in untreated cases. This is the concept of the so-called 'head at risk' (Fig. 7.7).

From this, it seems likely that a young boy with partial head involvement and without 'at risk' signs would be one of those who would have a good outcome without specific treatment. Conversely, the older child with whole-head involvement and signs of lateral extrusion and flattening is destined for a poor outcome without treatment.

We now need to look at what that treatment might involve, and the principles guiding it.

Management

We have seen that Perthes' disease is a self-limiting pathological process characterized by changes that at a cellular level are entirely reversible. Provided the mechanical environment for healing is favourable, there is every chance that the hip will recover a normal or near-normal shape and function.

How then can we optimize the conditions in which the affected hip is operating? We can be guided by the following two principles:

• *Reduction of forces acting through the hip.* Weight relief and maintenance of abduction will reduce the degree of collapse of the trabeculae of the femoral head, and give a better chance of maintenance of femoral head sphericity and height. Reduction of force per unit area of weight-bearing surface may also be achieved surgically by providing an extension to the roof of the acetabulum in cases where the softened head is extruding laterally.

• *Restoration and maintenance of movement.* Free concentric movement of the hip will help to provide a congruous joint in the long term. In the early stages of Perthes' disease, before significant head deformity has occurred, restoration and maintenance of movement may best be achieved by containment of the femoral head within the acetabulum. On the other hand, if in the later stages of the disease there has been flattening of the head with hinge abduction, movement may best be restored by surgery to improve joint congruity rather than by femoral head containment.

Thus, these principles remain valid throughout the disease process although the means by which they are achieved will differ depending on the stage of the disease.

NON-OPERATIVE TREATMENT

The majority of children with Perthes' disease will escape surgery. Their experience of the disease will be characterized by long periods of frustrating restrictions on their sporting activities, interspersed with episodes of painful limp requiring the use of crutches and therapy to regain movement range. The paediatrician or surgeon has an important role in explaining the nature of the disease process to children and their carers, who have to learn to appreciate that there is a sequence of events in the healing process that cannot be bypassed or hurried.

The forces acting through the hip can be reduced by relief of weight bearing and by the encouragement of abduction. The former may mean asking the child to use a crutch, or at least to avoid playing sports and running. It would seem logical to ensure that the child avoids activities involving repetitive high-impact forces on the hip such as trampolining. Specific exercises to target hip abduction and swimming may also be recommended. Use of weight-relieving calipers is no longer popular. One problem with keeping the affected limb off the ground is that it tends to encourage adduction rather than abduction.

The episodes of pain, limp and spasm may need to be treated with simple analgesic or non-steroidal anti-inflammatory medication. Short periods of bed rest may be necessary. Use of home traction may reduce spasm. If traction is used, it should allow the hip to be kept in flexion. In this position, the joint is at its greatest volume and less prone to problems arising from high intra-articular pressures.

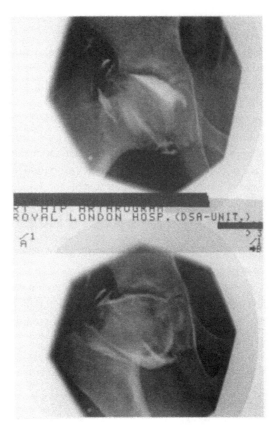

Fig. 7.8. The hinging phenomenon. Arthrography demonstrates that in the neutral position of the hip there is medial pooling of contrast and point contact between the lateral lip of the acetabulum and the femoral head. When the hip is adducted, the joint becomes congruous.

Abduction of the hip in the early stages will improve containment and reduce the risk of lateral extrusion of a deforming and enlarged femoral head. This may be achieved by abduction casts and orthoses, or by surgery in the form of either femoral or pelvic osteotomy.

Signs that such measures are indicated include increasingly painful stiffness of the joint, with limitation particularly of abduction. Application of 'broomstick casts' (bilateral long leg cylinder casts separated by an adjustable bar) will enable an abduction range to be regained in a gradual manner over a period of a few weeks, while allowing flexion movement of the hips. A variety of ambulatory abduction braces have been used over the years in an attempt to maintain this abduction while retaining independent mobility. Their success has been questioned in recent years, and patient compliance is often dubious. Recently, some surgeons have used botulinum toxin as a myoneural blocking agent to reduce spasm in the adductors and allow a greater range of abduction.

Examination under anaesthetic combined with arthrography is an important part of the management of the child with Perthes' disease who is starting to run into problems. The arthrogram enables one to appreciate the true size and shape of the femoral head, which with the cartilaginous overgrowth may well be larger and less well contained within the acetabulum than had been apparent on plain radiographs. Using image intensifier (fluoroscopy) screening, it is possible not only to determine the range of available hip movement but also to see if a position of improved containment can be achieved by abducting the hip. If this is the case, there may be an indication for an osteotomy on either the femoral or pelvic side of the joint that will place the femoral head and acetabulum in this improved relationship. Finally, it is possible with screening to check if the hip moves concentrically within its socket. An enlarged, poorly contained head will lose ability to rotate within the acetabulum, and attempts to abduct the hip will result in the head hinging on the lateral margin of the acetabulum (Fig. 7.8). This hinge phenomenon is an important factor affecting progress in the later stages of Perthes' disease, and may require surgical intervention.

OPERATIVE TREATMENT

Proximal femoral varus osteotomy
By reducing the angle that the femoral neck makes with the shaft, the femoral head may be centralized better within the acetabulum (Fig. 7.9). The operation involves removing a wedge of bone from the proximal femur and securing the divided bone with one of a variety of implants (Fig. 7.9B). Although technically straightforward, the procedure has the disadvantages of (a) incurring an obvious lateral thigh scar, (b) requiring subsequent removal of implant at a second surgery, and (c) contributing to overall shortening of the lower limb. This last feature does not reliably correct spontaneously, particularly in the older child. Most authors are agreed that the results of varus osteotomy after the age of 9–10 years are no better than those of the untreated disease. However, in the younger child whose femoral head is at risk but can still be contained, varus osteotomy offers a 'one-off' alternative to months of wearing abduction braces.

Innominate (Salter) osteotomy
Containment may also be achieved by redirecting the acetabulum to provide better cover of exposed aspects of the involved femoral head. In a young child, division of the pelvic bone above the acetabulum allows the section of pelvis below the osteotomy to be rotated downwards, outwards and forwards to achieve this aim. The bone is held in this corrected position by bone graft cut from the same side of the pelvis and secured with Kirschner wires (Fig. 7.9C). This procedure has the advantages of (a) leaving a scar that is usually cosmetically more acceptable than that of a varus osteotomy of the femur, and (b) involving no additional shortening of the limb.

Acetabular augmentation (shelf) procedures
The femoral head that cannot be contained is by definition extending beyond the confines of the acetabulum. If the head has escaped beyond the stage where a containment procedure is possible, some benefit may be gained from extending the roof of the acetabulum anterolaterally to increase the area of weight-bearing surface. This can be achieved by a shelf procedure (Fig. 7.10). The force per unit area on the softened head is thereby decreased.

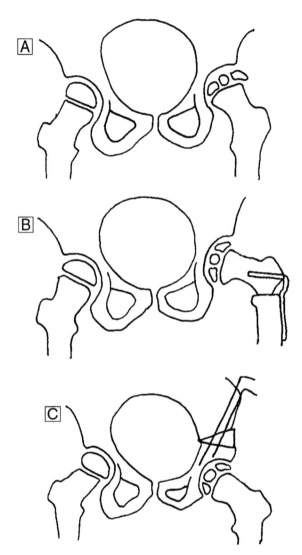

Fig. 7.9. Diagram showing how an uncovered femoral head (A) may be contained either by femoral varus osteotomy (B) or by Salter's pelvic osteotomy (C).

In addition, the shelf discourages the development of hinging. In the latter stages of the disease, a shelf procedure can provide cover for the exposed part of the femoral head following a valgus osteotomy (see below).

Proximal femoral valgus osteotomy
At first glance it may appear confusing that a valgus osteotomy as well as a varus osteotomy may have a role in the management of Perthes' disease. However, this procedure is

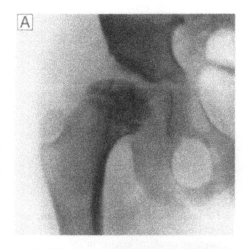

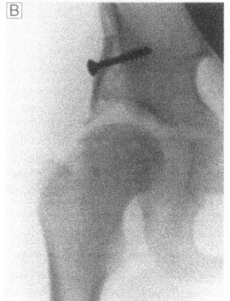

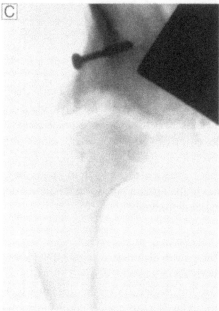

Fig. 7.10. Uncovering of the femoral head (A) treated by an acetabular shelf procedure (B) with good final result (C).

indicated in the healing stages of the disease process when there is established deformity of the head, and attempted abduction of the hip results in the hinging phenomenon. In this situation, arthrography often shows that the head and acetabulum are congruous with the hip in adduction and sometimes with a little flexion (see Fig. 7.8). In those circumstances, removing a laterally based wedge of bone from the proximal femur places the lower limb in a neutral position whilst the hip remains, in effect, adducted and congruous (Fig. 7.11). The level of patient satisfaction following this procedure is generally very high. Not only do the children regain comfortable abduction but also the osteotomy effectively lengthens

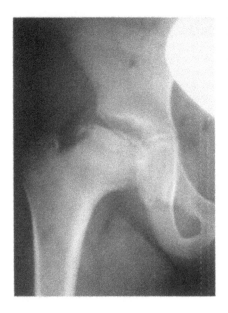

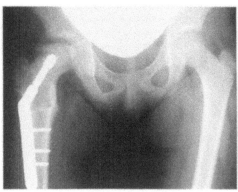

Fig. 7.11. Treatment for hinging. An abduction osteotomy has restored congruity to the hip in the neutral range, increased comfortable range of abduction, and restored limb length.

them a little and improves the biomechanics of the proximal femur, giving them an improved gait. The procedure inevitably leaves part of the femoral head uncovered. There is no consensus over the appropriate action here, but some surgeons will fashion a shelf to cover the exposed anterolateral aspect of the femoral head. It should be emphasized that this is a salvage procedure designed for the late case with established deformity. In the author's experience, results from valgus osteotomy are not so good when it is performed earlier in the disease process at a time when the femoral head is still somewhat plastic and easily deformable.

Other salvage procedures

The growth disturbance at the capital femoral physis may lead to a shortened neck, particularly on its superior aspect. This will give rise to a relatively high greater trochanter (see Fig. 7.4). Because this is the area into which some of the hip abductors insert, these muscles are acting at a mechanical disadvantage and an abductor lurch or Trendelenburg gait may develop. As well as being cosmetically unattractive, such a gait and stance are tiring. The trochanter can be transferred down the shaft of the femur to improve the mechanical advantage and thereby improve the gait.

Where there is significant residual incongruity between femoral head and acetabulum, it may be possible to alter the relationship between the two by osteotomies on either side of the joint. For example, in certain circumstances a rotational osteotomy of the femoral head and neck would bring a more congruent pair of surfaces into the main weight-bearing area of the joint.

Occasionally the central section of the head fails to heal completely. The resulting osteochondritic lesion is visible on radiographs as a persistent lucent area. The osteochondral

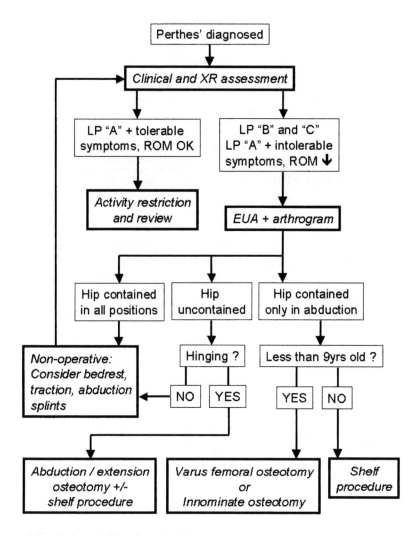

LP = Lateral pillar classification

Fig. 7.12. Algorithm for management of Perthes' disease.

fragment may be unstable and in time become a loose body within the joint. Arthroscopy or open arthrotomy may be required to remove loose fragments and to debride any resulting cavity.

PLAN OF TREATMENT
The algorithm (Fig. 7.12) shows a suggested plan of management for this condition based on the observations above. It will be noted that active treatment is targeted at the middle age range and in those cases where the femoral head is deemed to be at risk.

TABLE 7.2
The Stulberg classification for outcome from Perthes' disease*

Class I	Normal hip
Class II	Spherical head, minor abnormalities of neck or acetabulum
Class III	Non-spherical head but not flat, acetabular abnormalities
Class IV	Flattened head with acetabular abnormalities
Class V	Flattened head but normal acetabulum

Classes I and II (spherically congruent) → Good prognosis
Classes III and IV (aspherically congruent) → Late-onset osteoarthritis
Class V (aspherically incongruent) → Early-onset osteoarthritis

*Stulberg *et al.* (1981).

Outcomes

Although the avascular femoral head regains its blood supply, we have seen that this may not occur before there has been irreversible deformity of the femoral head. This deformity, and the loss of congruity between the head and the acetabulum, leads to abnormal uneven wear in the joint, giving rise to premature degenerative osteoarthritic changes and a painful, dysfunctional hip joint. Thus, it is the extent of the femoral head deformity that dictates the final outcome.

The Stulberg classification concerns the radiographic appearance of the hip at maturity (Table 7.2). It describes the shape of the femoral head and its relationship to the acetabulum. It has been shown to correlate well with secondary osteoarthritic changes (Stulberg *et al.* 1981). Stulberg class I and II hips do not develop arthritis in the long term. Class III and IV hips develop arthritis in late adult life. Class V hips, in which there is 'aspherical incongruency' due to a flattened femoral head articulating with an unaltered acetabulum, are characterized by severe arthritis before the age of 50 years.

Children presenting before the age of 6 years without 'at risk' signs are likely to end up with Stulberg class I or II hips regardless of whether or not they have received any specific treatment. Conversely, children who present after the age of 9 years with whole-head disease are more likely to develop Stulberg IV and V hips, again irrespective of treatment given. It is likely that active intervention in the form of operative treatment will have its greatest effect on the intermediate group of children between 6 and 9 years, in whom judicious intervention may well bring the affected hip back into a Stulberg I or II category (Coates *et al.* 1990).

In a long-term follow-up study, McAndrew and Weinstein (1984) studied patients at an average follow-up of 48 years. They found that 40% of affected hips had become sufficiently painful to require total hip arthroplasty, mostly between the ages of 40 and 60 years. This correlates well with the oft-repeated statement that the prognosis is good for about 60% of all affected hips.

Those involved with adolescents and young adults who have recovered from Perthes' disease are often uncertain how to advise them with regard to safe activity levels and appropriate careers. Radiographs of the hip at skeletal maturity and estimation of the Stulberg class are helpful in this situation. Stulberg I or II hips are probably capable of supporting

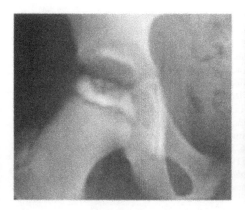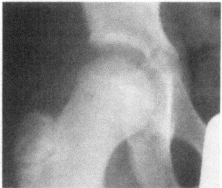

Fig. 7.13. Untreated hip in patient with Perthes' disease. Many cases will have an excellent long-term outcome without surgical intervention.

their owner through a normal range of physical activities in both work and recreational life for at least the first 30 years of adult life. Those with Stulberg III or worse hips should probably be discouraged if possible from following a career involving manual labour.

Conclusion

Perthes' disease is a self-limiting condition that may nevertheless give rise to long-term sequelae. At the very least, it will involve a period of several years of disruption of normal activity, discomfort and disability. At worst, it will lead to early degenerative change in the affected hip, limiting the range and nature of physical activities available to the patient and resulting ultimately in total hip arthroplasty. Supportive symptomatic treatment is applicable to all cases during the disease process. In certain cases, which can usually be identified through a combination of radiographic and clinical features, more active surgical intervention can favourably influence the long-term outcome. However, many cases will do well in the long term without operative surgery (Fig. 7.13).

REFERENCES

Catterall, A. (1971) 'The natural history of Perthes' disease.' *Journal of Bone and Joint Surgery, British Volume*, **53**, 37–53.

Coates, C.J., Paterson, J.M., Woods, K.R., Catterall, A., Fixsen, J.A. (1990) 'Femoral osteotomy in Perthes' disease. Results at maturity.' *Journal of Bone and Joint Surgery, British Volume*, **72**, 581–585.

Fisher, R.L. (1972) 'An epidemiological study of Legg–Perthes disease.' *Journal of Bone and Joint Surgery, American Volume*, **54**, 769–778.

Freeman, M.A.R., England, J.P.S. (1969) 'Experimental infarction of the immature canine femoral head.' *Proceedings of the Royal Society of Medicine*, **62**, 431–433.

Glueck, C.J., Brandt, G., Gruppo, R., Crawford, A., Roy, D., Tracy, T., Stroop, D., Wang, P., Becker, A. (1997) 'Resistance to activated protein C and Legg–Perthes disease.' *Clinical Orthopaedics and Related Research*, **338**, 139–152.

Hall, A.J., Barker, D.J., Dangerfield, P.H., Taylor, J.F. (1983) 'Perthes' disease of the hip in Liverpool.' *British Medical Journal*, **287**, 1757–1759.

Heikkinen, E., Lanning, P., Suramo, I., Puranen, J. (1980) 'The venous drainage of the femoral neck as a prognostic sign in Perthes' disease.' *Acta Orthopaedica Scandinavica*, **51**, 501–503.

Herring, J.A., Neustadt, J.B., Williams, J.J., Early, J.S., Browne, R.H. (1992) 'The lateral pillar classification of Legg–Calvé–Perthes disease.' *Journal of Pediatric Orthopedics*, **12**, 143–150.

Hresko, M.T., McDougall, P.A., Gorlin, J.B., Vamvakas, E.C., Kasser, J.R., Neufeld, E.J. (2002) 'Prospective reevaluation of the association between thrombotic diathesis and Legg–Perthes disease.' *Journal of Bone and Joint Surgery, American Volume*, **84**, 1613–1618.

Loder, R.T., Schwartz, E.M., Hensinger, R.N. (1993) 'Behavioral characteristics of children with Legg–Calvé–Perthes disease.' *Journal of Pediatric Orthopedics*, **13**, 598–601.

McAndrew, M.P., Weinstein, S.L. (1984) 'A long-term follow-up of Legg–Calvé–Perthes disease.' *Journal of Bone and Joint Surgery, American Volume*, **66**, 860–869.

Stulberg, S.D., Cooperman, D.R., Wallensten, R. (1981) The natural history of Legg–Calvé–Perthes disease.' *Journal of Bone and Joint Surgery, American Volume*, **63**, 1095–1108.

Theron, J. (1980) 'Angiography in Legg–Calvé–Perthes disease.' *Radiology*, **135**, 81–92.

8
EPIPHYSEAL DYSPLASIAS

Jayesh Trivedi

The bone dysplasias or osteochondrodysplasias are a spectrum of disorders with a variety of causes. They are characterized by an intrinsic abnormality in the growth and remodeling of cartilage and bone (Sillence *et al.* 1979). Most are heritable. The reported incidence is 1 in 3000 to 1 in 5000 births (Andersen 1989, Erik and Hauge 1989). The skull, spine and extremities are usually affected in various proportions.

Terminology
Bone dysplasias typically cause shortening of the involved bones resulting in short stature. This has led to the use of the term 'dwarfism' in these patients. In *proportionate dwarfism* there is a symmetric decrease in the both the truncal and limb lengths. *Disproportionate dwarfism* may be either of the short limb or the short trunk variety according to whether the limbs or the trunk are more extensively involved. The short-limbed dwarfism is further divided by the region of limb involved as *rhizomelic* (proximal), mesomelic (middle) and *acromelic* (distal).

Classification
Dysplasias are classified according to the region of long bone involvement into epiphyseal, physeal, metaphyseal or diaphyseal (Rubin 1964) (Table 8.1).

This chapter deals with the more common form of physeal and epiphyseal dysplasias and the importance of orthopaedic input in the management of these disorders.

Achondroplasia
Achondroplasia is the most common form of dysplasia with a reported incidence of 1 in 30,000 births (Dietz and Mathews 1996). The condition has been described from early times. Evidence reported in Marc Armand Ruffer's *Studies in the Palaeopathology of Egypt* suggests that achondroplastic dwarfs were recognized 5000 years ago (see Warkany 1964). The ancient Egyptians revered them as the gods Bes and Ka. The emperors of Rome introduced dwarfs to the gladiatorial circus, and the custom of having dwarfs at royal courts was continued into the 18th century.

Achondroplasia is caused by abnormal endochondral bone formation (Ponseti 1970, Rimoin *et al.* 1970, Maynard *et al.* 1981). There is a quantitative defect in the proliferative zone of the physis, such that endochondral bone growth is more affected than appositional growth. Periosteal and intramembranous ossification is normal. Anatomically, achondroplasia is classified as a physeal dysplasia.

TABLE 8.1
Classification of bone dysplasias*

Epiphyseal dysplasia
  Epiphyseal hypoplasia
    Failure of articular cartilage: spondyloepiphyseal dysplasia
    Failure of ossification of centre: multiple epiphyseal dysplasia
  Epiphyseal hyperplasia
    Excess of articular cartilage: dysplasia epiphysealis hemimelia
Physeal dysplasia
  Cartilage hypoplasia
    Failure of proliferating cartilage: achondroplasia
    Failure of hypertrophic layer of cartilage: metaphyseal dysostosis
  Cartilage hyperplasia
    Excess of proliferating cartilage: Marfan syndrome
    Excess of hypertrophic cartilage: enchondromatosis
Metaphyseal dysplasia
  Metaphyseal hypoplasia
    Failure to form primary spongiosa: hypophosphatasia
    Failure to absorb primary spongiosa: osteopetrosis
    Failure to absorb secondary spongiosa: craniometaphyseal dysplasia
  Metaphyseal hyperplasia
    Excessive spongiosa: multiple exostosis
Diaphyseal dysplasia
  Diaphyseal hypoplasia
    Failure of periosteal bone formation: osteogenesis imperfecta
    Failure of endosteal bone formation: idiopathic osteoporosis
  Diaphyseal hyperplasia
    Excessive periosteal bone formation: Engelmann's disease
    Excessive endosteal bone formation: hyperphosphatasemia

*Rubin (1964).

INHERITANCE
The genetic basis of achondroplasia is well established. The responsible gene is transmitted as an autosomal dominant trait, but 80% of cases are the result of a spontaneous mutation. Most parents of an affected individual are normal, and the risk of a second affected child is negligible.

AETIOLOGY
Achondroplasia is due to a point mutation in the gene—located on the short arm of chromosome 4—that codes for fibroblast growth factor receptor-3 (FGFR3) (Shiang *et al.* 1994). Fibroblast growth factor is normally expressed in physeal cartilage and the central nervous system. FGFR3 is thought to limit endochondral bone formation in the proliferative zone of the epiphyses. The mutation is thought to increase this inhibition, thereby further limiting endochondral bone formation and thus leading to the short stature.

CLINICAL FEATURES
Patients have a normal trunk length and short limbs. Limb involvement is rhizomelic with proximal segments more affected than middle and distal ones. Patients have an enlarged

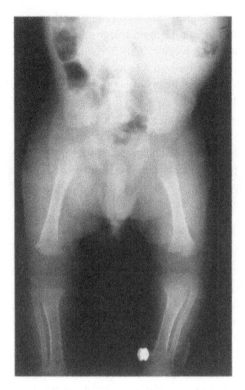

Fig. 8.1. Anteroposterior roentgenogram of the pelvis and lower extremities of a 10-month-old child with achondroplasia. Note the extremely broad flattened acetabular roof and the nearly 'squared' appearance of the ilia. The sacroiliac notch is short. The long bones are not only short but also demonstrate early metaphyseal flaring, and the tibiae already show early bowing.

neurocranium, frontal bossing, button noses, hypoplastic maxillae and flattened nasal bridges, and trident hands with an inability to extend the ring and middle fingers. The development of musculature in extremities is normal and this together with excessive skin and adipose tissue, gives the appearance of shortened, broad extremities. The shortened upper extremities often cause difficulty in dressing and personal care.

DEVELOPMENTAL MILESTONES
Motor milestones are often delayed. Speech and language is however normal, as is sexual development. Patients have a normal intelligence. Sitting height is normal but standing height is below the third percentile for both sexes (Horton *et al.* 1978).

ORTHOPAEDIC MANIFESTATIONS
Ligamentous laxity, abnormalities of spine and skull development and deformities of the upper and lower limbs may all lead to an orthopaedic consultation in the achondroplastic patient.

THE HIP AND PELVIS
Congenital hip dysplasia is usually not encountered. The acetabulum is deep medially and the roof is horizontal giving generous cover to the femoral heads (Fig. 8.1). This may be

due to the fact that the triradiate cartilage, being of identical cellular disposition as the neuro-epiphyseal growth plate, grows at half the rate of the cartilaginous anlage of the acetabular roof (Langer *et al.* 1967, Bailey 1970, Stelling 1973, Kopits 1976). The lumbar lordosis, which develops at ambulation, is associated with a forward rotation of the pelvis. This results in hip flexion contractures. There is a marked ligament laxity and this may be associated with an external rotation deformity of the lower extremities. Osteoarthritis of the hip or the knee has been infrequently reported in patients with achondroplasia over the age of 40, and lower limb symptoms in these patients are usually due to spinal stenosis.

Radiologically, the pelvis is broad and short, with the ilium having a square appearance. The greater sciatic notches are small and deep and the acetabular roofs are horizontal. The greater trochanter is often overgrown with respect to the femoral head and neck. The femoral necks are short, although coxa vara is not seen (Langer *et al.* 1967).

THE SPINE

The growth of the foramen magnum is severely impaired leading to a reduction in the transverse diameter of the foramen magnum (Hecht *et al.* 1985, 1989). Narrowing of the foramen may result in sleep apnoea, cyanotic spells, feeding problems and even sudden death, especially in the first two years of life (Hecht *et al.* 1985, 1989; Nelson *et al.* 1988). A baseline MRI should be performed in these patients to evaluate the extent of the foramen magnum stenosis. Severe symptoms may require foramen magnum decompression, although pro-phylactic surgery is not recommended.

Spinal involvement is common, leading to disabling symptoms. The spinal canal, especially in the lumbar spine, is narrowed secondary to short pedicles, reduced interpedicular distance, thickened laminae and excessive lumbar lordosis (Lutter *et al.* 1977). This leads to spinal stenosis by the third decade of life in most patients (Fig. 8.2). Symptoms include back pain, leg pain, neurogenic claudication and diminished walking distance (Kahanovitz *et al.* 1982). MRI will delineate the extent of neural compression and is a mandatory pre-operative tool. Treatment of stenotic symptoms is usually by a wide decompression through a posterior approach.

Thoracolumbar kyphosis is the most common spinal deformity in these patients (Herring and Winter 1983). The deformity is common before the age of 1 year and is due to ligament laxity and hypotonia in infancy. Spontaneous resolution may occur when ambulation begins. Treatment is usually non-operative as the kyphosis may resolve with growth. The child must be observed until ambulation. If wedging of the apical vertebra persists after independent ambulation, an extension-type orthosis may be considered. Indications for surgery include kyphosis greater than 30° at 5 years of age and neurological symptoms.

DEFORMITY

Genu varum in these patients is secondary to bowing of the tibia and the more rapid growth of the fibula compared to the tibia (Bailey 1970, Kopits 1976). Bracing is not effective due to the short thighs and lax ligaments. Surgery may be required to correct these deformities and usually involves osteotomies of the tibia and the fibula. Surgery is not indicated until after the age of 4 years.

110

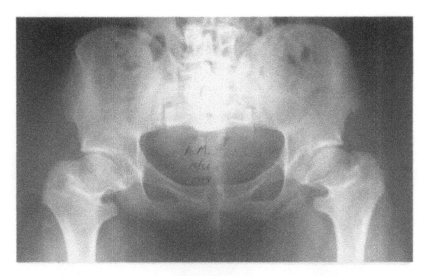

Fig. 8.2. Anteroposterior roentgenogram of the pelvis of a male, aged 19 years 8 months, with achondroplasia. Note the short femoral necks and the relative overgrowth of the greater trochanter. The interpedicular space of the lumbar spine is greatly reduced, leading to lumbar spinal stenosis.

LIMB LENGTHENING IN ACHONDROPLASIA
Hitherto a controversial issue, the concept of lengthening extremities and thereby restoring some height to these individuals is now gaining popularity. The advantages include an improved self-image and better function in the lengthened extremities. The latter has not been conclusively proven. The risks include the possibility of producing angular deformities during lengthening, joint stiffness, and the long period of distraction that is required. Furthermore, any lengthening in the lower extremities in these patients must be accompanied by a concomitant lengthening of the humeri. Failure to do so would jeopardize the ability to facilitate personal care. This would mean six segments of lengthening, which is a major undertaking. The total time required for such a procedure may be in excess of two years. Despite this, several authors have reported good success with limb lengthening in achondroplastic patients (Ganel *et al.* 1979, Aldegheri *et al.* 1988, Bell *et al.* 1992). The concept of restoring length to the extremities is exciting and in the properly selected patient extremely gratifying.

Pseudoachondroplasia
This dysplasia is inherited as an autosomal dominant trait and is clinically similar to achondroplasia. The normal shape and size of the head, the normal facial features, the much greater degree of ligament laxity and the greater severity of lower limb deformities help differentiate it from achondroplasia.

HIP MANIFESTATIONS
Angular deformities of the lower limbs are common. There is rhizomelic shortening of the

111

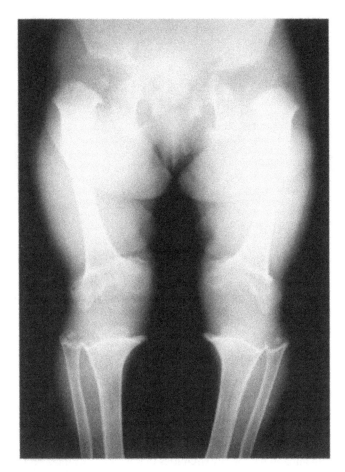

Fig. 8.3. Anteroposterior roentgenogram of the pelvis of a 7-year-old female with pseudoachondroplasia. The ossification of the capital femoral epiphysis is delayed, and there is flaring of the metaphyses. Early genu varum is noted, due to delayed ossification of the distal femoral condyles.

long bones, flaring of the metaphyses and delayed ossification of the epiphyses (Fig. 8.3). The epiphyses of weight-bearing joints are affected, resulting in a deformation of the articular surfaces. This leads to premature osteoarthritis. The hip being a weight-bearing joint is affected. Early deformation of the femoral head leads to a 'sagging rope sign' on the X-rays. This may occur before adolescence. As ossification progresses the changes may mimic Perthes' disease of the hip. The acetabulum poorly contains the large flattened femoral head, and subluxation may develop. Hinge abduction or even a windswept deformity of the femora may occur. Premature osteoarthritis leads to hip pain in early adulthood.

OTHER ORTHOPAEDIC IMPLICATIONS
The upper cervical spine and weight-bearing joints are affected most. Odontoid hypoplasia

and ligamentous laxity lead to instability of the atlantoaxial joint. Myelopathy may develop secondary to this. Stress lateral radiographs of the cervical spine are recommended in these patients until skeletal maturity. Symptomatic instability requires surgical stabilization of the atlantoaxial joint.

Multiple epiphyseal dysplasia (MED)

This common bone dysplasia is characterized by irregular, delayed ossification of several epiphyses. It is usually inherited as an autosomal dominant trait, though autosomal recessive transmission is known (McKusick 1992). A mild form (Ribbing type) and a severe form (Fairbank type) are recognized (Fairbank 1947, Spranger 1976).

CLINICAL FEATURES

Short-limbed, disproportionate dwarfism develops but may not manifest until adolescence. The face and head are normal. Patients usually present with pain in the weight-bearing joints, gait abnormalities or angular deformities of the lower limbs. Joint deformities in these patients result from growth factors and mechanical factors. There is abnormal growth and maturation of cartilage and bone. The delayed ossification leaves the growing epiphyseal cartilage unsupported, predisposing it to progressive deformation with loading forces. Asymmetric physeal growth leads to angular deformities. The joint involvement is symmetrical, mostly affecting the hip joints. The gait is waddling. The more severe cases may become manifest in early childhood. The prognosis is related to the severity of epiphyseal changes. In the severe form the patients may be affected by crippling arthritis before the age of 50 years, being unable to walk or stand. Digits of the hands and feet are shortened. Spine involvement is minimal.

THE HIP AND PELVIS

The epiphyseal centres of ossification are delayed in appearance. After ossification begins, the epiphyses are often found to be small, irregular and fragmented. Multiple sites are affected, predominantly the epiphyses of the femora, tibiae and distal forearms. Hip arthrography may demonstrate a mushroom-shaped femoral head with varying degrees of extrusion or flattening. Coxa vara, subluxation and hinge abduction are common, all leading to premature osteoarthritis. The femoral necks are broad and short. The deformation of the femoral epiphyses is bilateral and often symmetrical (Fig. 8.4). Avascular necrosis of the femoral head may also occur (MacKenzie *et al.* 1989). This usually occurs unilaterally. Sequential X-rays may demonstrate increased density of the femoral head, followed by re-sorption and then re-ossification. Subchondral fracture lines, collapse and extrusion may occur. The radiological appearances are similar to those in Perthes' disease (Griffiths and Witherow 1977, Crossan *et al.* 1983). Table 8.2 outlines the differences between Perthes' disease and MED.

A skeletal survey is indicated in patients suspected of having bilateral Perthes' disease, in order to rule out MED. After physeal closure, the articular surface of the involved joints is deformed, and signs of degenerative arthropathy appear in the third or fourth decade of life.

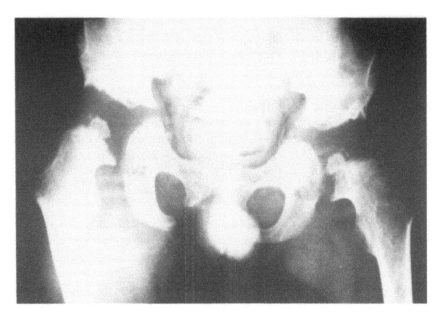

Fig. 8.4. Anteroposterior roentgenogram of the pelvis of a male, aged 7 years 4 months, with multiple epiphyseal dysplasia. There is early coxa vara deformity of the left hip. The capital femoral epiphyses are delayed in development, with irregular ossification. Note also the irregular contour of the acetabulae.

TABLE 8.2
Multiple epiphyseal dysplasia *vs* Perthes' disease

Multiple epiphyseal dysplasia	Perthes' disease
Bilateral and symmetric involvement	Involvement is asymmetric
Acetabulum may be primarily affected	Acetabulum not affected primarily
Metaphyseal cysts not common	Metaphyseal cysts common

SURGICAL TREATMENT

The goals of treatment include correction of deformity and relief of pain. In childhood it is important to evaluate thyroid function in these patients as hypothyroidism may manifest similarly. Corrective osteotomies at the hip and knee may help correct deformity and restore a functional arc of movement in affected joints (Fig. 8.5). In adulthood, total joint arthroplasty forms the main basis of surgical treatment.

Spondyloepiphyseal dysplasia

Spondyloepiphyseal dysplasia is characterized by multiple epiphyseal and vertebral involvement resulting in a short-trunked, short-limbed, disproportionate dwarfism (Spranger and Langer 1970, Davies and Hall 1982). Two forms are recognized, spondyloepiphyseal dysplasia congenita and spondyloepiphyseal dysplasia tarda.

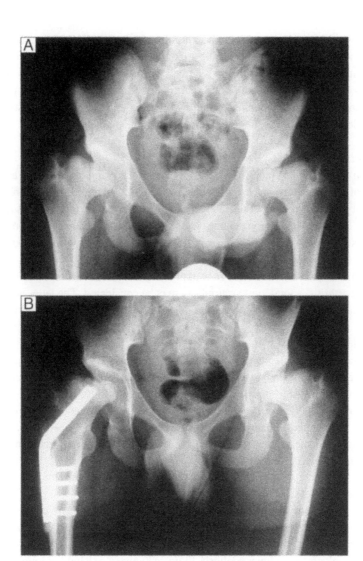

Fig. 8.5. Anteroposterior radiographs of an adolescent male with multiple epiphyseal dysplasia.

(A) There is bilateral coxa vara with deformation of femoral heads bilaterally that is symmetric (in contrast to Perthes' disease where involvement is usually asymmetric).

(B) Corrective osteotomy of the right hip provides a more functional arc of movement.

SPONDYLOEPIPHYSEAL DYSPLASIA CONGENITA

This form is inherited as an autosomal dominant trait, although spontaneous mutation is known (Kaibara *et al.* 1983). The proliferative zone of the epiphyses is primarily affected.

Clinical features

The infant is short at birth. Platyspondyly may be present, with a flat facies and wide-set eyes. Talipes equinovarus may is common. Lumbar lordosis with flexion contractures of the hips may be present even at birth. The proximal and middle segments of the limbs are affected, with the hands and feet being relatively normal. Coxa vara (reduced neck–shaft angle) and genu valgum develop by 3 or 4 years of age. Thoracic scoliosis becomes evident in adolescence. Odontoid hypoplasia resulting in atlantoaxial instability is also common. There is a delay in the ossification of all the lower-limb epiphyses.

The hip and pelvis
Ossification of the femoral epiphysis is delayed. Coxa vara is common, leading to a functional weakness of the abductor muscles. In patients with very severe coxa vara there may be a discontinuity between the femoral head and neck with a proximal migration of the greater trochanter. This leads to a Trendelenburg gait. The associated ligament laxity may lead to dislocations. When the neck–shaft angle is 100° or less, a corrective valgus-extension osteotomy is recommended. Premature degeneration of the hip joint is common. Symptoms include stiffness, pain and difficulty in walking. In young adults with severe clinical and radiological arthritis, a total joint arthroplasty may be considered. The latter is often technically demanding in the setting of angular deformities involving the entire lower limb.

Orthopaedic considerations
Atlanto-axial instability secondary to odontoid hypoplasia is common and may lead to cervical myelopathy. Flexion–extension radiographs of the cervical spine are recommended until skeletal maturity for assessment of the cervical instability. Indications for surgery include neurological signs of instability or MRI evidence of cord compression.

Scoliosis and kyphosis are both common. Severe kyphosis may develop by adolescence and may lead to paraplegia. Screening spinal radiographs should be performed in all patients for detection of these deformities.

SPONDYLOEPIPHYSEAL DYSPLASIA TARDA
Clinical manifestations of this disorder may be delayed until 10 years of age. The spine and the larger joints are primarily affected (Kaibara *et al*. 1983). It is inherited as an X-linked disorder.

Spinal involvement includes scoliosis, thoracic kyphosis and lumbar lordosis. Patients may have back pain and stiffness. Hip involvement is typical. This is again in the form of coxa vara and premature osteoarthritis. Hip pain develops in adolescence. All these symptoms warrant early referral to the orthopaedic surgeon. The osteoarthritis of the hip means that many patients require a total joint arthroplasty in young adulthood.

Summary
The bone dysplasias are a diverse group of disorders. The protean clinical manifestations neccesitate cooperation between the treating paediatrician, a geneticist and an orthopaedic surgeon. Without this multidisciplinary approach the overall care of the patient may be compromised. Appropriate care includes accurate genetic counselling and the recognition and prompt treatment of the medical and musculoskeletal abnormalities.

REFERENCES

Aldegheri, R., Trivella, G., Renzi-Brivio, L., Tessari, G., Agostini, S., Lavini, F. (1988) 'Lengthening of the lower limbs in achondroplastic patients. A comparative study of four techniques.' *Journal of Bone and Joint Surgery, British Volume*, **70**, 69–73.

Andersen, P.E. (1989) 'Prevalence of lethal osteochondrodysplasias in Denmark.' *American Journal of Medical Genetics*, **32**, 484–489.

Bailey, J.A. (1970) 'Orthopaedic aspects of achondroplasia.' *Journal of Bone and Joint Surgery, American Volume*, **52**, 1285–1301.

Bell, D.F., Boyer, M.I., Armstrong, P.F. (1992) 'The use of the Ilizarov technique in the correction of limb deformities associated with skeletal dysplasia.' *Journal of Pediatric Orthopedics*, **12**, 283–290.

Crossan, J.F., Wynne-Davies, R., Fulford ,G.E. (1983) 'Bilateral failure of the capital femoral epiphysis: bilateral Perthes' disease, multiple epiphyseal dysplasia, pseudoachondroplasia, and spondyloepiphyseal dysplasia congenita and tarda.' *Journal of Pediatric Orthopedics*, **3**, 297–301.

Dietz, F.R., Mathews, K.D. (1996) 'Update on the genetic bases of disorders with orthopaedic manifestations.' *Journal of Bone and Joint Surgery, American Volume*, **78**, 1583–1598.

Erik, P., Hauge, M. (1989) 'Congenital generalized bone dysplasias: a clinical, radiological and epidemiological survey.' *Journal of Medical Genetics*, **27**, 37.

Fairbank, T. (1947) 'Dysplasia epiphysialis multiplex.' *British Journal of Surgery*, **34**, 225–232.

Ganel, A., Horoszowski, H., Kamhin, M., Farine, I. (1979) 'Leg lengthening in achondroplastic children.' *Clinical Orthopaedics and Related Research*, **144**, 194–197.

Griffiths, H.E., Witherow, P.J. (1977) 'Perthes' disease and multiple epiphyseal dysplasia.' *Postgraduate Medical Journal*, **53**, 464–472.

Hecht, J.T., Nelson, F.W., Butler, I.J., Horton, W.A., Scott, C.I., Wassman, E.R., Mehringer, C.M., Rimoin, D.L., Pauli, R.M. (1985) 'Computerized tomography of the foramen magnum: Achondroplastic values compared to normal standards.' *American Journal of Medical Genetics*, **20**, 355–360.

Hecht, J.T., Horton, W.A., Reid, C.S., Pyeritz, R.E., Chakraborty, R. (1989) 'Growth of the foramen magnum in achondroplasia.' *American Journal of Medical Genetics*, **32**, 528–535.

Herring, J.A., Winter, R.B. (1983) 'Kyphosis in an achondroplastic dwarf.' *Journal of Pediatric Orthopedics*, **3**, 250–252.

Horton, W.A., Rotter, J.I., Rimoin, D.L., Scott, C.I., Hall, J.G. (1978) 'Standard growth curves for achondroplasia.' *Journal of Pediatrics*, **93**, 435–438.

Kahanovitz, N., Rimoin, D.L., Sillence, D.O. (1982) 'The clinical spectrum of lumbar spine disease in achondroplasia.' *Spine*, **7**, 137–140.

Kaibara, N., Takagishi, K., Katsuki, I., Eguchi, M., Masumi, S., Nishio, A. (1983) 'Spondyloepiphyseal dysplasia tarda with progressive arthropathy.' *Skeletal Radiology*, **10**, 13–16.

Kopits, S.E. (1976) 'Orthopedic complications of dwarfism.' *Clinical Orthopaedics and Related Research*, **114**, 153–179.

Langer, L.O., Baumann, P.A., Gorlin, R.J. (1967) 'Achondroplasia.' *American Journal of Roentgenology, Radium Therapy and Nuclear Medicine*, **100**, 12–26.

Lutter, L.D., Lonstein, J.E., Winter, R.B., Langer, L.O. (1977) 'Anatomy of the achondroplastic lumbar canal.' *Clinical Orthopaedics and Related Research*, **126**, 139–142.

MacKenzie, W.G., Bassett, G.S., Mandell, G.A., Scott, C.I. (1989) 'Avascular necrosis of the hip in multiple epiphyseal dysplasia.' *Journal of Pediatric Orthopedics*, **9**, 666–671.

Maynard, J.A., Ippolito, E.G., Ponseti, I.V., Mickelson, M.R. (1981) 'Histochemistry and ultrastructure of the growth plate in achondroplasia.' *Journal of Bone and Joint Surgery, American Volume*, **63**, 969–979.

McKusick, V.A. (1992) *Mendelian Inheritance in Man. Catalogue of Autosomal Dominant, Autosomal Recessive, and X-linked Phenotypes. 10th Edn.* Baltimore: Johns Hopkins University Press.

Nelson, F.W., Hecht, J.T., Horton, W.A., Butler, I.J. (1988) 'Neurologic basis of respiratory complications in achondroplasia.' *Annals of Neurology*, **24**, 89–93.

Ponsetti, I.V. (1970) 'Skeletal growth in achondroplasia.' *Journal of Bone and Joint Surgery, American Volume*, **52**, 701–716.

Rimoin, D.L., Hughes, G.N., Kaufman, R.L., Rosenthal, R.E., McAlister, W.H., Silberberg, R. (1970) 'Endochondral ossification in achondroplastic dwarfism.' *New England Journal of Medicine*, **283**, 728–735.

Rubin, P. (1964) *Dynamic Classification of Bone Dysplasias.* Chicago: Year Book Medical.

Shiang, R., Thompson, L.M., Zhu, Y.Z., Church, D.M., Fielder, T.J., Bocian, M., Winokur, S.T., Wasmuth,

J.J. (1994) 'Mutations in the transmembrane domain of FGFR3 cause the most common genetic form of dwarfism, achondroplasia.' *Cell*, **78**, 335–342.

Sillence, D.O., Horton, W.A., Rimoin, D.L. (1979) 'Morphologic studies in skeletal dysplasias.' *American Journal of Pathology*, **96**, 813–870.

Spranger, J. (1976) 'The epiphyseal dysplasias.' *Clinical Orthopaedics and Related Research*, **114**, 46–59.

Spranger, J.W., Langer, L.O. (1970) 'Spondyloepiphyseal dysplasia congenita.' *Radiology*, **94**, 313–322.

Stelling, F.H. (1973) 'The hip in heritable conditions of connective tissue.' *Clinical Orthopaedics and Related Research*, **90**, 33–49.

Warkany, J. (1964) *Congenital Malformations: Notes and Comments.* Chicago: Year Book Medical.

Wynne-Davies, R., Hall, C. (1982) 'Two clinical variants of spondylo-epiphyseal dysplasia congenita.' *Journal of Bone and Joint Surgery, British Volume*, **64**, 435–441.

9
TRAUMA

Kristan A. Pierz

Injuries to the pediatric hip may be due to high-energy trauma, such as motor vehicle accidents, or low-energy trauma, such as mishaps during an athletic event. Usually, an isolated incident occurs that results in localized pain; however, repetitive trauma can also produce injuries to the hip region. The etiology, prevalence, treatment and prognosis vary depending on the specific injury. This chapter provides an overview of pediatric hip trauma by addressing injuries to both the pelvic and femoral components of the hip joint.

Before considering the diagnosis and treatment of pediatric hip trauma, one must first have an understanding of the anatomy of the developing hip (see Chapter 1). The child's pelvis consists of three primary centers of ossification, the ilium, ischium, and pubis, which come together within the acetabulum as the triradiate cartilage. On the femoral side, the single proximal femoral physis gives rise to the medial subcapital physis and the lateral greater trochanteric physis during the first few years of life. The subcapital physis is responsible for proximal longitudinal growth (approximately 13% of the total femoral length), whereas the greater trochanter apophysis affects the shape of the proximal femur, especially before the age of 12 years (Raney *et al.* 1993). These physes remain open until after the onset of puberty, at which time the secondary ossification centers, including the iliac crest, ischial apophysis, anterior inferior iliac spine, anterior superior iliac spine, pubic tubercle, ischial spine and secondary acetabular centers of ossification, begin to appear (Fig. 9.1). The appearance of such normal ossification centers on radiographs may easily be misinterpreted as avulsion fractures by those inexperienced at reviewing such films. Additionally, injuries to the cartilage within these growth centers can result in future growth arrest (Canale and Bourland 1977, Ponseti 1978). Also of concern is the blood supply to the proximal femur that can be jeopardized by initial trauma or subsequent treatment, thus putting the femoral head at risk for avascular necrosis. The lateral femoral circumflex artery supplies the metaphysis and greater trochanter, whereas the medial femoral circumflex artery gives rise to the lateral epiphyseal vessels which penetrate the capsule to supply the femoral head (Chung 1976). After approximately 18 months of age and until its closure at skeletal maturity, the physis acts as a barrier between these two networks.

High-energy trauma: pelvic fractures
Any patient involved in a high-energy trauma, such as a large fall or a motor vehicle accident, must be assumed to have a pelvic or proximal femur fracture until proven otherwise. This is true for adults as well as children. Patients sustaining severe multiple trauma should be triaged to a tertiary care facility capable of providing efficient and comprehensive

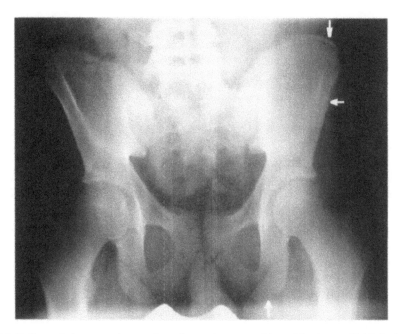

Fig. 9.1. Radiograph demonstrating apophyseal growth centers of the pelvis. Arrows highlight the iliac crest, anterior superior iliac spine and ischial apophyses.

emergency care. Appropriate evaluation and management of the patient's airway, breathing and circulation must be the first priority. Only after stabilizing the patient's overall condition can one focus on specific injuries, such as fractures. Quinby (1966) reported an 18% mortality rate in children with pelvic fractures, emphasizing the importance of recognizing and treating all associated injuries. Other injuries commonly associated with pelvic trauma include closed head or cervical spine injuries in 40–75% of patients, additional fractures in 20–40%, intra-abdominal injuries in 10–20%, and urethral or bladder injuries in 5–10% (Watts 1976, Price *et al.* 2001).

Once a patient has been stabilized and the initial history and physical examination have been performed, evaluation of the patient with a presumed pelvic or hip injury should include a standard anteroposterior radiograph of the pelvis. Orthogonal views of the femur are indicated if any deformity or crepitus is noted in the thigh or if the pelvis film reveals proximal femoral injury. Additional pelvic inlet and outlet views (beam angled 40° caudally and 40° cephalad, respectively) as well as 45° oblique views can be obtained to further assess pelvic fracture displacement and stability (Figs. 9.2, 9.3). Computed tomography (CT) scans offer even more detail than standard radiographs.

Fractures of the pelvis can be categorized according to the *Key and Conwell classification system* (Key and Conwell 1951):

 I. Marginal fractures or avulsions without a break in the continuity of the pelvic ring
  (stable pattern)

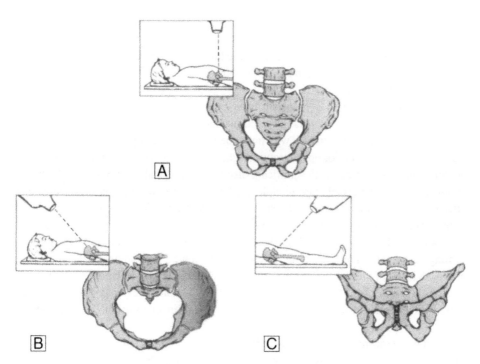

Fig. 9.2. (A) Standard anteroposterior view of the pelvis. (B) 45° external oblique view demonstrating the posterior pelvic column and anterior acetabular wall. (C) 45° internal oblique view demonstrating the anterior pelvic column and posterior acetabular wall. (Reproduced by permission from Swiontkowski 1994.)

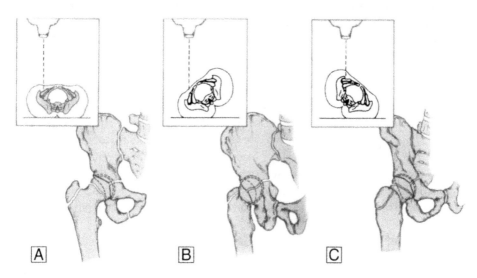

Fig. 9.3. (A) Standard anteroposterior radiograph of the pelvis. (B) 40° caudally angled, or inlet, view demonstrating posterior ring injuries. (C) 40° cephalad, or outlet, view demonstrating anterior ring injuries. (Reproduced by permission from Swiontkowski 1994.)

121

II. Single breaks of the pelvic ring, involving the rami or symphysis separation (stable pattern)

III. Double breaks in the pelvic ring, including bilateral rami fractures (straddle injuries), anterior and posterior ring disruptions, vertical displacement injuries, and multiple fractures (unstable pattern)

IV. Any of the above with an associated acetabular fracture.

Treatment depends on the stability and displacement of the fracture. Most children with pelvic fractures can be treated with initial bed rest followed by protected weight bearing. Surgery is indicated for open fractures, when loose fragments are trapped within the hip joint, and for fractures with significant displacement (Canale and Beaty 1996). When fractures involve the acetabulum in children, four types can occur: small fragments that often occur with a hip dislocation; linear fractures without displacement that are generally stable; linear fractures with hip joint instability; and fractures secondary to central fracture–dislocation of the hip (Watts 1976). Patients who sustain a crush injury to their triradiate cartilage, especially if they are under 10 years of age, have a poor prognosis due to the risk of growth arrest of the physes and subsequent acetabular dysplasia and progressive hip subluxation (Bucholz et al. 1982, Canale and Beaty 1996). Unfortunately, physeal injuries may initially go undetected and be recognized only after significant dysplasia has developed.

High-energy trauma: proximal femur fractures

Like most pelvic fractures, proximal femur fractures are usually caused by high-energy trauma. Representing approximately 1% of all pediatric fractures, proximal femur fractures are associated with other significant injuries in 30% of cases (Price et al. 2001). Child abuse should be suspected as a potential mechanism, especially in young children. Proximal femur fractures may also occur after only minimal trauma in patients with pathologic lesions (e.g. unicameral or aneurysmal bone cysts, fibrous dysplasia, or Langerhans histiocytosis) or disorders of bone metabolism (e.g. osteogenesis imperfecta or rickets). Slipped capital femoral epiphysis is a condition of the adolescent hip that can occur with or without any preceding trauma and is discussed in detail in Chapter 6.

As with pelvic fractures, patients with proximal femur fractures should be triaged to an appropriate trauma center where efficient emergency care can be provided. Most fractures will be detected on a standard anteroposterior pelvis radiograph, and anteroposterior and lateral radiographs of the affected femur are useful for quantifying the extent and amount of displacement of the fracture. Unlike most pelvic fractures, however, most proximal femoral fractures require urgent surgical stabilization, usually within 12 hours of the time of injury. Delay in fracture reduction and stabilization may result in avascular necrosis due to jeopardized blood flow to the femoral head via kinked or tamponaded epiphyseal vessels (Swiontkowski and Winquist 1986).

Fractures of the proximal femur can be categorized according to the *Delbet classification system* (Fig. 9.4):

I. Transphyseal separation, with or without dislocation of the femoral head from the acetabulum

II. Transcervical (femoral neck) fractures

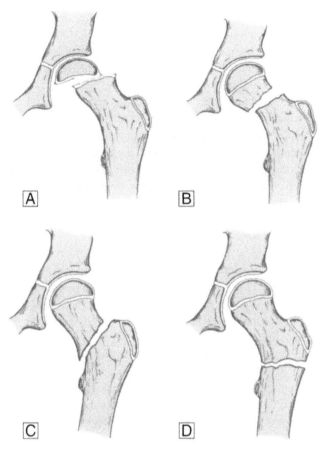

Fig. 9.4. The Delbet classification of pediatric proximal femur fractures. (A) Type I: transepiphyseal. (B) Type II: transcervical. (C) Type III: cervicotrochanteric. (D) Type IV: intertrochanteric. See text for descriptions. (Reproduced by permission from Swiontkowski 1994.)

III. Cervicotrochanteric (base of the femoral neck) fractures
IV. Intertrochanteric fractures.

 Type I (transphyseal) fractures are usually treated with closed or open reduction, internal fixation and spica casting, with most having poor results due to avascular necrosis, premature physeal closure, coxa vara or nonunion (Ingram and Bachynski 1953, Canale and Beaty 1996). In children under 2 years of age, remodeling may restore the anatomic configuration of the proximal femur if the transphyseal separation has only minimal displacement (Canale and Beaty 1996). Type II (transcervical) fractures, the most common of the four types, are also usually treated with closed or open reduction, internal fixation and spica casting. The avascular necrosis rate approaches 43% and may be influenced by the amount of initial displacement (Canale and Bourland 1977, Canale and Beaty 1996). Type III (cervicotrochanteric) fractures are treated like type II fractures and have a similar complication rate if they are displaced (Canale and Beaty 1996). Nondisplaced type III fractures have a more favorable prognosis and may be successfully treated with spica casting alone, provided they are followed carefully to detect and manage any subsequent displacement (Oveson et al. 1989). Type IV (intertrochanteric) fractures are less common and have far fewer complications than the other three types (Canale and Bourland 1977, Oveson et al. 1989). These can usually be managed by traction followed by abduction spica casting, although some may require a formal reduction and possible internal fixation (Canale and Beaty 1996).

Clearly, a complete description of all of the injury patterns and potential complications associated with high-energy fractures is beyond the scope of this chapter. If avascular necrosis is suspected, one can obtain an MRI or bone scan to assess epiphyseal viability. MRI or CT can also provide information regarding premature physeal closure if fractures involve the growth plates. Patients with these high-energy injuries should be managed by pediatric orthopedic specialists and followed for at least two years since alterations in growth may affect long-term sequelae.

Low-energy trauma: contusions, apophyseal injuries, and labral tears

With an increasing number of children and adolescents participating in sports, injuries about the hip and pelvis, although still relatively rare, are increasing in frequency (Canale and Beaty 1996). Since many patients who experience these injuries never present to medical professionals, it is difficult to estimate the prevalence of such problems. Fortunately, most of these injuries require limited intervention and have an excellent prognosis with minimal long-term sequelae. Nevertheless, children complaining of hip pain, even with known antecedent trauma, should have the following considered in their differential diagnosis: slipped capital femoral epiphysis, Perthes' disease, congenital subluxation of the hip, toxic synovitis, systemic neoplasia and infectious process (Waters and Millis 1988). Screening radiographs of the pelvis should be obtained to avoid missing such diagnoses. These conditions are covered elsewhere in this book; the remainder of this section will focus on hip injuries frequently seen in young athletes.

As with other conditions, clinicians seeing patients complaining of hip pain should conduct a careful history and physical examination prior to obtaining radiographs or additional studies. The history can help differentiate between acute traumatic events and overuse-type injuries. Additionally, prodromal pain or other systemic complaints may alert the clinician to nontraumatic conditions of the hip, such as those mentioned above. During the physical examination, observation may reveal an abnormal gait or areas of ecchymosis, abrasions, swelling or atrophy. Palpation of soft tissues and bony prominences should be performed, and the neurovascular status should be documented. Additionally, palpation may reveal hernias or other abdominal wall abnormalities (Taylor et al. 1991). Active and passive motion, including hip flexion, extension, abduction, adduction, and internal and external rotation, should then be documented and compared with the uninvolved hip. Manual resistance can be used to detect weakness. Finally, any crepitus, locking or catching should be noted, as these may indicate intra-articular injury or synovitis. Plain orthogonal radiographs of the hip or pelvis should then be obtained. Studies such as MRI, CT, ultrasound, or bone scans are not routinely necessary but can offer additional information in diagnostic dilemmas.

Contusions and musculotendinous sprains are the most common injuries to occur about the hip (Waters and Millis 1988). Occasionally, a contusion to the piriformis muscle can result in compression of the sciatic nerve, causing buttock and posterior thigh pain. If the injury is anterior and results in compression of the lateral femoral cutaneous nerve, pain and numbness, known as meralgia paresthetica, may occur (Adkins and Figler 2000). When soft tissues move over bony prominences (such as the gluteal muscles and iliotibial band passing over the greater trochanter, or the iliopsoas passing anterior to the femoral head and neck), bursae may form to prevent excessive friction. Overuse injuries or direct trauma to these sites may produce inflammation, or bursitis, which can cause pain and, occasionally, a snapping sensation (Adkins and Figler 2000). For most contusions and sprains, patients usually describe an area of focal tenderness, and radiographs are unremarkable. Additional imaging is rarely necessary; however, an MRI, if obtained, may reveal local soft tissue edema. These injuries can usually be treated conservatively with rest, anti-inflammatory medications and ice massage until the patient is pain free. Once pain free, the athlete may return to sports; however, a stretching program is recommended to prevent future injuries. If a deep muscle contusion or hematoma does not completely heal, scarring and myositis ossificans may occur, resulting in pain during contraction of the affected muscle that may be remedied only by surgical excision (Bowyer and Hollister 1984).

Unlike those fractures that occur during high-energy collision events, a subset of pelvic fractures can occur due to an acute or repetitive over-pull of a muscle at its point of origin or insertion or by a direct contusion of an apophysis, the so-called "hip-pointer" (Lombardo *et al.* 1983). Additionally, repetitive microtrauma and muscle–tendon imbalance can cause apophysitis about the hip (Peck 1995). Attachment of the sartorius to the anterior superior iliac spine, the direct head of the rectus femoris to the anterior inferior iliac spine, the hamstrings and adductors to the ischial tuberosity, and the iliopsoas to the lesser trochanter places these apophyses at risk during maximal muscle exertion (see Fig. 9.1). Hip extension and knee flexion, as performed in kicking sports, may result in avulsion of the anterior inferior iliac spine or anterior superior iliac spine, whereas gymnasts and sprinters are more likely to avulse their ischial apophyses (Canale and Beaty 1996) (Fig. 9.5). Iliac apophyseal injuries are usually due to repetitive stress, direct contusion, or forceful twisting of the torso, as during a baseball swing (Lambert and Fligner 1993).

Occurring most commonly between the ages of 14 and 25 years (before fusion of the secondary centers of ossification to the pelvis), apophyseal injuries are usually associated with point tenderness, localized edema, and pain with stretching of the attached muscle (Canale and Beaty 1996). Plain radiographs can usually confirm the diagnosis, although ultrasound may be useful for detecting avulsions prior to ossification of the apophyses (Lazovic *et al.* 1996). Such injuries may be classified as Key and Conwell type I injuries (marginal fractures or avulsions without a break in the continuity of the pelvic ring) and do not result in an unstable pelvis. After reviewing the literature, Canale and Beaty summarized that, of 91 reported avulsion fractures, 38% were ischial avulsions, 32% were avulsions of the anterior superior iliac spine, 18% were avulsions of the anterior inferior iliac spine, 9% were avulsions of the lesser trochanter of the femur, and 3% were iliac crest avulsions. Additionally, a German study reviewed 22 patients with apophyseal fractures and found a similar

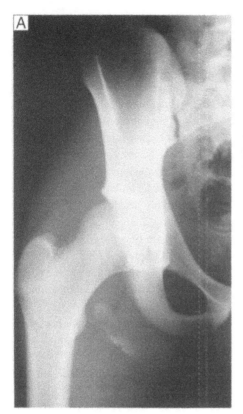
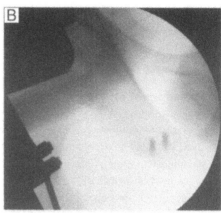

Fig. 9.5. (A) Radiograph of 15-year-old male sprinter who sustained an avulsion of his ischial tuberosity. (B) Due to persistent pain and displacement, this injury was treated with open reduction and internal fixation.

breakdown by anatomic location (Linni *et al.* 2000). The authors reported that 18 patients sustained traumatic avulsions, while four had direct blunt trauma. Plain radiographs confirmed the diagnosis in all cases. Twenty-one patients were treated conservatively, and only one patient underwent operative treatment. Of the 20 patients available for follow-up, none suffered loss of motion or muscular insufficiency. Although all patients were able to return to sports, five had persistent pain at the fracture site during vigorous exercise at a mean of 33 months. Since most patients do well with conservative treatment, referral to a subspecialist is rarely necessary. Treatment usually consists of a short period of rest with the hip positioned comfortably, followed by protected weight-bearing on crutches for approximately two weeks, followed by a progressive rehabilitation program emphasizing gradual strengthening and integration of the involved muscles prior to return to sports (Peck 1995). Ice, compression and anti-inflammatory agents may also be helpful. Surgery is usually reserved for patients with significantly displaced fractures or fractures that heal with excessive, painful callus (Canale and Beaty 1996).

Labral tears and intraarticular injuries can also occur after only minimal trauma, such as twisting or hyperextension of the hip, and patients may not always recall a specific event (Hickman and Peters 2001). Patients frequently complain of hip pain as well as mechanical symptoms, such as clicking, snapping, locking and giving way. These symptoms may be difficult to differentiate from those caused by a snapping iliopsoas tendon riding over an inflamed bursa. If a labral tear is suspected, provocative maneuvers can be employed to produce a palpable click or sharp, catching pain. For instance, acute flexion of the hip with external rotation and abduction, followed by extension, adduction and internal rotation may pinch an anterior labral tear and produce symptoms (Fitzgerald 1995). As with most cases of hip pain, plain radiographs of the pelvis should be obtained, but these may be normal unless the patient has underlying acetabular dysplasia. Plain arthrography, CT arthrography and MRI have been used to try to identify labral tears with limited success; however, MRA, which combines MRI with arthrography, has improved specificity and sensitivity (Hickman and Peters 2001). Patients with labral tears may benefit from two to four weeks of protected weight-bearing and nonsteroidal anti-inflammatory drugs; however, most nonoperative interventions fail (Hase and Ueo 1999, Hickman and Peters 2001). Surgical debridement via open arthrotomy or arthroscopic techniques has been successful; however, the role of labral repair remains unclear (Klaue *et al.* 1991, Fitzgerald 1995, Hickman and Peters 2001). Because hip arthroscopy is technically demanding, candidates for arthroscopic debridement should be referred to specialists with expertise in this field (Berend and Vail 2001).

Hip dislocations
Traumatic hip dislocations may occur in children after significant or minimal trauma. Children under the age of 5 years have soft acetabular cartilage and generalized laxity that may allow the hip to dislocate after only an insignificant fall, whereas adolescents usually require more forceful mechanisms such as athletic injuries or motor vehicle accidents (Canale and Beaty 1996). In a review of 42 patients sustaining traumatic hip dislocations before the age of 16 years, Mehlman *et al.* (2000) found that 64% were attributable to low-energy trauma. Posterior dislocations comprise 87% of all pediatric hip dislocations, and males are affected four times more than females (Petrie *et al.* 1996).

Clinically, patients with posterior hip dislocations typically hold their hip flexed, adducted and internally rotated, whereas anterior dislocations present with the leg extended, abducted and externally rotated. The neurovascular status of the limb should be documented, and radiographs should be obtained before and after any reduction maneuvers (Fig. 9.6). In the study by Melman *et al.*, 17% of patients sustained an ipsilateral hip fracture.

Once the injury has been identified, a closed reduction should be urgently attempted under anesthesia or intravenous sedation. Long-term complications include avascular necrosis, degenerative joint disease and recurrent instability. The incidence of avascular necrosis is about 8–17% (Canale and Beaty 1996, Petrie *et al.* 1996, Melman *et al.* 2000). Poorer prognoses have been associated with dislocations reduced after six to eight hours, high-energy injuries, advanced skeletal maturity, incomplete reductions, and recurrent instability (Canale and Beaty 1996, Hughes and D'Agostino 1996, Petrie *et al.* 1996, Mehlman *et al.* 2000, Kutty *et al.* 2001). For posteriorly dislocated hips, reductions can be performed with the patient in the supine position by applying traction to the affected limb held with the hip and knee flexed or in the prone position with traction applied to the limb hanging over the table's edge with the hip and knee flexed (Petrie *et al.* 1996). Post-reduction radiographs

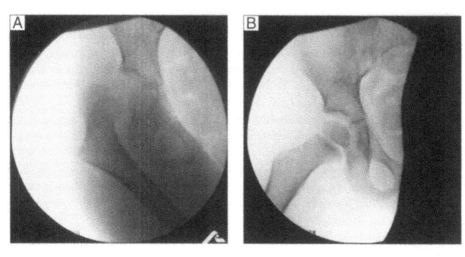

Fig. 9.6. Radiographs of a 4-year-old boy (A) before and (B) after closed reduction of a dislocated hip.

should be obtained, and CT can be useful for identifying interposed fragments or residual displacement. Incomplete reductions or incarcerated fragments usually require an open reduction. Patients should be followed for a minimum of two years looking for evidence of late complications, such as avascular necrosis.

Conclusion

This chapter presents an overview of many of the injuries that can occur to the young hip. The spectrum of hip trauma includes high- and low-energy mechanisms and acute and repetitive insults. Due to the multiple growth centers as well as the precarious blood supply about the immature hip, pediatric patients are particularly susceptible to long-term sequelae following injuries. Careful assessment, including radiographic evaluation, is necessary to identify potential problems, plan appropriate treatment, and achieve the best prognosis. For further study, the reader is directed to the Swiontkowski (1994) and Canale and Beaty (1996).

REFERENCES

Adkins, S.B., Figler, R.A. (2000) 'Hip pain in athletes.' *American Family Physician*, **61**, 2109–2118.
Berend, K.R., Vail, T.P. (2001) 'Hip arthroscopy in the adolescent and pediatric athlete.' *Clinical Sports Medicine*, **20**, 763–778.
Bowyer, S.L., Hollister, J.R. (1984) 'Limb pain in childhood.' *Pediatric Clinics of North America*, **31**, 1053–1081.
Bucholz, R.W., Ezaki, M., Ogden, J.A. (1982) 'Injury to the acetabular triradiate physeal cartilage.' *Journal of Bone and Joint Surgery, American Volume*, **64**, 600–609.
Canale, S.T., Beaty, J.H. (1996) 'Pelvic and hip fractures.' *In:* Rockwood, C.A., Wilkins, K.A., Beaty, J.H. (Eds.) *Fractures in Children*. Philadelphia: Lippincott-Raven, pp. 1109–1193.
Canale, S.T., Bourland, W.L. (1977) 'Fracture of the neck and intertrochanteric region of the femur in children.' *Journal of Bone and Joint Surgery, American Volume*, **59**, 431–443.
Chung, S.M. (1976) 'The arterial supply of the developing proximal end of the femur.' *Journal of Bone and Joint Surgery, American Volume*, **58**, 961–970.

Fitzgerald, R.H. (1995) 'Acetabular labral tears.' *Clinical Orthopaedics and Related Research*, **311**, 60–68.

Hase, T., Ueo, T. (1999) 'Acetabular labral tear: arthroscopic diagnosis and treatment.' *Arthroscopy*, **15**, 138–141.

Hickman, J.M., Peters, C.L. (2001) 'Hip pain in the young adult: Diagnosis and treatment of disorders of the acetabular labrum and acetabular dysplasia.' *American Journal of Orthopedics*, **30**, 459–467.

Hughes, M.J., D'Agostino, J. (1996) 'Posterior hip dislocation in a five-year-old boy: a case report, review of the literature, and current recommendations.' *Journal of Emergency Medicine*, **14**, 585–590.

Ingram, A.J., Bachynski, B. (1953) 'Fractures of the hip in children. Treatment and results.' *Journal of Bone and Joint Surgery, American Volume*, **35**, 867–887.

Key, J.A., Conwell, H.E. (1951) *Management of Fractures, Dislocations, and Sprains*. St. Louis: C.V. Mosby.

Klaue, K., Durnin, C.W., Ganz, R. (1991) 'The acetabular rim syndrome.' *Journal of Bone and Joint Surgery, British Volume*, **73**, 423–429.

Kutty, S., Thornes, B., Curtin, W.A., Gilmore, M.F. (2001) 'Traumatic posterior dislocation of hip in children.' *Pediatric Emergency Care*, **17**, 32–35.

Lambert, M.J., Fligner, D.J. (1993) 'Avulsion of the iliac crest apophysis: a rare fracture in adolescent athletes.' *Annals of Emergency Medicine*, **22**, 1218–1220.

Lazovic, D., Wegner, U., Peters, G., Gosse, F. (1996) 'Ultrasound for diagnosis of apophyseal injuries.' *Knee Surgery, Sports Traumatology, Arthroscopy*, **3**, 234–237.

Linni, K., Mayr, J., Hollwarth, M.E. (2000) 'Apophyseal fractures of the pelvis and trochanter minor in 20 adolescent and 2 young children.' *Unfallchirurg*, **103**, 961–964.

Lombardo, S.J., Retting, A.C., Kerlan, R.K. (1983) 'Radiographic abnormalities of the iliac apophysis in adolescent athletes.' *Journal of Bone and Joint Surgery, American Volume*, **65**, 444–446.

Mehlman, C.T., Hubbard, G.W., Crawford, A.H., Roy, D.R., Wall, E.J. (2000) 'Traumatic hip dislocation in children. Long-term followup of 42 patients.' *Clinical Orthopeadics and Related Research*, **376**, 68–79.

Oveson, O., Arreskov, J., Bellstrom, T. (1989) 'Hip fractures in children: a long-term follow-up of 17 cases.' *Orthopaedics*, **12**, 361–367.

Peck, D.M. (1995) 'Apophyseal injuries in the young athlete.' *American Family Physician*, **51**, 1891–1898.

Petrie, S.G., Harris, M.B., Willis, R.B. (1996) 'Traumatic hip dislocation during childhood. A case report and review of the literature.' *American Journal of Orthopedics*, **25**, 645–649.

Ponseti, I.V. (1978) 'Growth and development of the acetabulum in the normal child.' *Journal of Bone and Joint Surgery, American Volume*, **60**, 575–585.

Price, C.T., Phillips, J.H., DeVito, D.P. (2001) 'Management of fractures.' *In:* Morrissy, R.T., Weinstein, S.L. (Eds.) *Lovell and Winter's Pediatric Orthopaedics. 5th Edn.* Philadelphia: Lippincott, Williams & Wilkins, pp. 1320–1422.

Quinby, W.C. (1966) 'Fractures of the pelvis and associated injuries in children.' *Journal of Pediatric Surgery*, **1**, 353–364.

Raney, E.M., Ogden, J.A., Grogan, D.P. (1993) 'Premature greater trochanteric epiphysiodesis secondary to intramedullary femoral rodding.' *Journal of Pediatric Orthopedics*, **13**, 516–520.

Swiontkowski, M.F. (1994) 'Fractures and dislocations about the hip and pelvis.' *In:* Green, N.E., Swiontkowski, M.F. (Eds.) *Skeletal Trauma in Children*. Philadelphia: W.B. Saunders, pp. 307–343.

Swiontkowski, M.F., Winquist, R.A. (1986) 'Displaced hip fractures in children and adolescents.' *Journal of Trauma*, **26**, 384–388.

Taylor, D.C., Meyers, W.C., Moylan, J.A., Lohnes, J., Bassett, F.H., Garrett, W.E. (1991) 'Abdominal musculature abnormalities as a cause of groin pain in athletes. Inguinal hernias and pupalgia.' *American Journal of Sports Medicine*, **19**, 239–242.

Waters, P.M., Millis, M.B. (1988) 'Hip and pelvic injuries in the young athlete.' *Clinical Sports Medicine*, **7**, 513–526.

Watts, H.G. (1976) 'Fractures of the pelvis in children.' *Orthopedic Clinics of North America*, **7**, 615–624.

10
JUVENILE IDIOPATHIC ARTHRITIS

Janet E. McDonagh

Juvenile idiopathic arthritis (JIA) is the new term unifying the existing classifications for inflammatory arthritis in children (Petty *et al.* 1998). JIA comprises a heterogeneous group of diseases with inclusion criteria of a minimum duration of arthritis of six weeks in a child under 16 years of age. There are seven subtypes of JIA in the World Health Organization/International League Against Rheumatism (ILAR) classification listed in Table 10.1.

The incidence of JIA is 5–18 per 100,000 and the prevalence is 30–150 per 100,000 children (Andersson Gare 1999). The aetiology of JIA is unknown. A genetic predisposition has been suggested through human leukocyte antigen associations (Thomas *et al.* 2000).

Hip involvement

Hip involvement in JIA is common and frequently bilateral. In the literature the incidence of hip-joint involvement in JIA ranges from 38% to 63% (Sairanen 1958, Jacqueline *et al.* 1961, Isdale 1970). The clinical manifestations of hip joint involvement in JIA are pain and a limited range of motion. However, the clinical presentation does not always reveal the true extent of involvement of the hip joint, such that it is possible to have significant abnormalities without patient complaints (Rydholm *et al.* 1986, Koski 1989, Fedrizzi *et al.* 1997). Spencer and Bernstein (2002) recently reviewed hip disease in JIA.

Hip involvement in JIA potentially produces significant functional impairment in a child with polyarticular disease because of the importance of the hip joint itself, as well as the consequences of hip involvement on the pelvis and the entire lower extremity during walking. It must be remembered that impaired mobility during childhood is not just a physical limitation but has serious impact on psychosocial development in terms of schooling, peer interaction and evolving independence as the child reaches adolescence and early adulthood.

Certain variables appear to influence hip involvement in JIA, including age of onset, disease subtype and duration, and functional status.

AGE AT ONSET

Hip involvement has been reported to be especially common in very young children in the early stages of JIA with a polyarticular course (Ansell and Unlu 1970, Fedrizzi *et al.* 1997).

DISEASE SUBTYPE

Hip involvement can occur in any subtype of JIA. Fedrizzi *et al.* (1997) reported that 21% of hips in patients with oligoarticular JIA presented abnormalities on ultrasound despite normal plain X-rays. Hip involvement is most common in the systemic and polyarticular

TABLE 10.1
Subtypes of juvenile idiopathic arthritis
according to the ILAR/WHO classification*

- Systemic
- Oligoarthritis—persistent
- Oligoarthritis—extended
- Polyarthritis—rheumatoid factor negative
- Polyarthritis—rheumatoid factor positive
- Enthesitis-related arthritis
- Psoriatic arthritis

*Petty *et al.* (1998).

types. Systemic-onset JIA (SOJIA) accounts for only 10% of all patients with JIA, but 50% of patients with SOJIA will have a progressive destructive arthritis with significant disability into adulthood (Wallace and Levinson 1991, Flato *et al.* 1998). Predictive factors have been sought in SOJIA in an attempt to identify those children with a worse prognosis, with the aim of offering earlier aggressive therapy. One such factor identified in the literature is 'early hip involvement', *i.e.* at six months of disease (Modesto *et al.* 2001). Modesto and coworkers studied 124 patients with SOJIA and found that early hip involvement (by 6 months) plus the presence of a polyarticular pattern was linked to a poor outcome.

Hip involvement is particularly characteristic of enthesitis-related JIA (this subtype encompasses the previous classification groups. juvenile spondyloarthropathy and juvenile ankylosing spondylitis). Enthesitic points around the hip joint include the greater trochanter, ischial tuberosity and adductor longus insertion. As compared to adult spondyloarthropathies, peripheral joint involvement as a mono- or oligoarticular arthritis is significantly more frequent in juvenile-onset patients, not only as a mode of onset but also during the course of the disease (Garcia-Morteo *et al.* 1983). Those authors reported higher frequencies of hip involvement in juvenile as compared to adult-onset ankylosing spondylitis (87.5% *vs* 49%, $p<0.01$). However, a study of Mexican Mestizo patients failed to confirm this (51.1% *vs* 56.5%, *ns*) (Burgos-Vargas *et al.* 1989). In this subtype of JIA, as in SOJIA, hip-joint involvement has been identified as a predictor of a poor prognosis (Burgos-Vargas *et al.* 1989).

DISEASE DURATION AND FUNCTIONAL STATUS
Hip involvement is most common in those with longer duration of disease and in those who have poor functional status (Fedrizzi *et al.* 1997).

Hip involvement at initial presentation
It is very uncommon for JIA to begin with isolated hip arthritis, and the other differential diagnoses must be considered (Table 10.2).

Rarely, enthesitis-related arthritis in an older child might present with monoarticular hip involvement. Some authors have proposed that idiopathic chondrolysis actually represents a form of oligoarticular JIA (van der Hoeven *et al.* 1989), but Bleck (1983) found no histological evidence of significant synovial inflammation.

131

TABLE 10.2 Differential diagnosis of hip pain in children	TABLE 10.3 Consequences of hip synovitis in JIA
Early childhood Sepsis Congenital dislocation	Pain Muscle spasm Contractures
Middle childhood Perthes' disease Transient synovitis/irritable hip	Increased intra-articular pressure Damage of articular cartilage Regional osteopaenia Muscle weakness
Late childhood/adolescence Slipped capital femoral epiphyses Tumour—osteoid osteoma Idiopathic chondrolysis Juvenile idiopathic arthritis	Relative immobility Localized growth abnormalities Bone erosions Subluxation Avascular necrosis

Consequences of hip synovitis in JIA

In a study of 35 children with JIA followed over periods of three to 22 years, four categories of hip involvement were identified (Harris and Baum 1988): (i) mild disability with slight radiographic changes (n=13); (ii) episodic disability that correlated with disease activity (n=2); (iii) progressive disability and radiographic changes (n=14); (iv) dramatic clinical and radiographic findings but little functional disability (n=6).

In any joint, inflammatory synovitis leads to pain and muscle spasm (Table 10.3). The patient with synovitis of the hip will tend to hold the joint in about 45° of flexion and neutral or slight external rotation to maximize intracapsular capacity, thereby reducing the intra-articular pressure (Rydholm *et al.* 1986). If the inflammation is uncontrolled, the articular cartilage then becomes damaged. This is exacerbated by the stiff contracted nature of the joint, which leads to increased loading over a small area of articular cartilage and impairs the normal mechanisms of cartilage nutrition. In addition, periarticular inflammation induces regional osteopaenia, which is compounded by the muscle weakness and relative immobility of these patients. Localized growth abnormalities also occur due to under- or overdevelopment of the bones (see below). These result from changes in epiphyseal growth secondary to synovitis, hyperaemia and abnormal mechanical forces.

With cartilage loss, narrowing and irregularity of the joint space occurs with bone erosions, destruction and sometimes subluxation of the femoral head, and/or avascular necrosis (see below).

The typical established deformity of the affected hip is one of fixed flexion, adduction and internal rotation. If both hips become involved and one hip is severely adducted, the other may develop an abduction deformity, the so-called 'windswept' appearance. Consequences of hip deformity include excessive lumbar lordosis. Svantesson *et al.* (1981) also highlighted the association between hip involvement and the development of scoliosis in JIA patients. Fixed flexion deformity of the hips is also associated with a tendency towards fixed flexion deformities of the knees. The fixed adduction of the hip leads to the development of a genu valgum deformity. The internal rotation may lead to external tibial torsion.

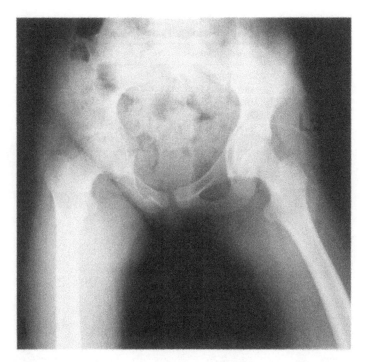

Fig. 10.1. X-ray of patient with JIA showing periarticular osteopaenia, narrowing of the joint space and subchondral erosions of the right hip.

Leg length discrepancy may be seen as a result of either premature epiphyseal fusion or stimulation at either hip or knee.

Imaging
X-Ray
The earliest radiographic change with hip synovitis in JIA is periarticular osteoporosis. As the disease progresses, the inflammatory process results in erosion of the cartilage and subchondral bone of the femoral heads and acetabuli, narrowing the joint spaces (Fig. 10.1). Such changes generally occur late in the disease and are uncommon in children below the age of 4 years. Fedrizzi *et al.* (1997) reported a time lapse for the development of such changes of six years (range 2–11 years). Jacobsen *et al.* (1992) reported that such destruction was rare in the oligoarticular subtype but occurred in 10% of patients with polyarticular or systemic arthritis after five years of disease. Weight-bearing anteroposterior X-rays may show subluxation of the hip with upward and lateral displacement of the femoral head.

A combination of regional hyperaemia and abnormal mechanical forces on the hip induces growth abnormalities and a failure of the normal remodelling process of the proximal femur (Table 10.4). The exact pattern of the deformity is related to the age of onset and the duration of the disease (Rombouts and Rombouts-Lindemans 1971. In the child

TABLE 10.4
Localized growth abnormalities of the hip joint in JIA

Age of child	Growth abnormality
<9 years	Coxa magna
	Long valgus femoral neck with marked anteversion
	Dysplastic acetabulum
>9 years	Coxa magna
	Short and varus femoral neck
	Protrusio acetabuli in the older child

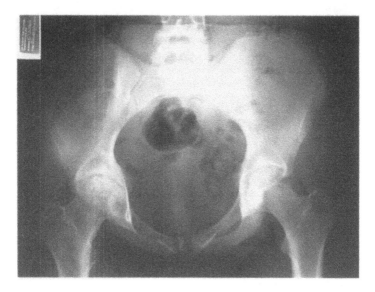

Fig. 10.2. X-ray showing coxa magna and protrusio acetabuli of right hip in JIA.

below the age of 9 years, coxa magna develops due to stimulation of the femoral capital epiphysis, leading to valgus, elongation and anteversion of the femoral neck. In children of this age with very severe disease, however, a generally underdeveloped hip may also be seen. In older children (>9 years), coxa magna is also seen (Fig. 10.2), but as the growth plate will close by the age of 13 years in 50% of patients, the femoral neck will be short. Due to continued growth at the trochanteric epiphysis, the short femoral neck is often in varus. In older children who develop hip disease towards the end of growth, overdevelopment of both the femoral head and acetabulum is common. Hastings *et al.* (1994) also reported a more unusual deformity in this age group of a small femoral head in a capacious acetabulum.

Protrusio acetabuli may also develop and, in some patients, rapidly progress (Hughes *et al.* 1988) (Fig. 10.2). Acetabular development is determined in large part by the development of the femoral head and neck. A valgus, anteverted femoral neck as seen in younger patients will lead to a shallow dysplastic acetabulum and subluxation of the hip. Coxa

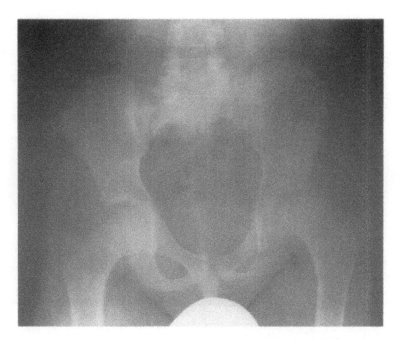

Fig. 10.3. X-ray showing avascular necrosis of left femoral head.

magna will lead to a large acetabulum, although the femoral head may remain uncovered. Gusis *et al.* (1993) reported acetabular protrusion in 12% of JIA patients, predominantly in those with older age at onset (8 *vs* 4.2 years; p<0.001). Jacqueline *et al.* (1961) reported overdevelopment of the femoral head and acetabulum in mild cases of hip involvement commencing in children between 8 and 14 years.

Avascular necrosis of the femoral head can occur (Fig. 10.3) but less frequently than in systemic lupus erythematosus. Kobayakawa *et al.* (1989) reported radiographic signs of ischaemic necrosis of the femoral head in terms of abnormal epiphysis and caput indices in 30/72 hips in 36 children with hip pain or limitation of motion among 206 children, consecutively admitted during 15 months because of JIA. Nine out of 10 hips with obvious signs of femoral head necrosis showed a sclerotic rim at the base of the femoral neck, confirming an earlier episode of ischaemic damage to the epiphysis and growth plate. A more recent study reported a lower frequency of avascular necrosis in SOJIA (Lang *et al.* 1995).

Possible causes of avascular necrosis include circulatory disturbance secondary to increased intraarticular pressure due to synovitis and/or effusion (N.B. the nutrient vessels to the capital epiphyses are largely intracapsular), treatment with passive extension of the hip, and concurrent steroid therapy.

ULTRASOUND
Ultrasound is more sensitive than conventional radiographs in diagnosing early changes in the hip joint in JIA in terms of effusion and synovitis (Fedrizzi *et al.* 1997) (Fig. 10.4), although

135

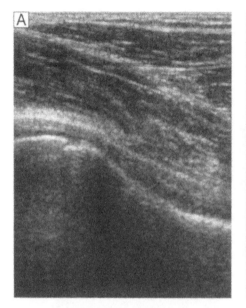
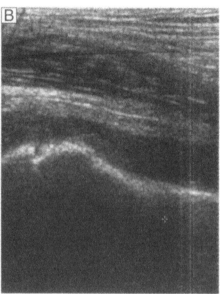

Fig. 10.4. Ultrasound of the hip joint in patient with JIA: (A) normal left hip, (B) right hip with effusion and (C) synovitis.

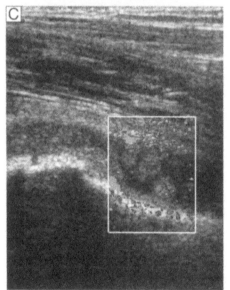

baseline X-rays remain important in view of differential diagnosis as well as long-term monitoring. Ultrasound may demonstrate increased intra-articular fluid or synovial hypertrophy, particularly between the femoral head and the medial margin of the acetabulum.

MAGNETIC RESONANCE IMAGING
MRI is extremely useful in determining the extent of synovitis, articular cartilage damage

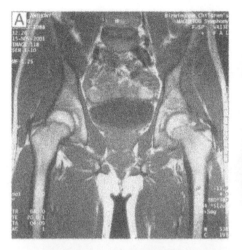

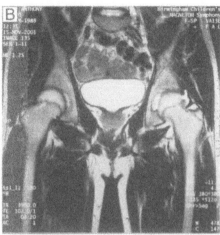

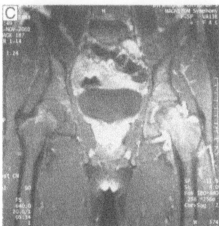

Fig. 10.5. MRI of synovitis of the left hip joint in patient with JIA: (A) T₁ spin–echo without gadolinium enhancement; (B) T₂ spin–echo high signal without gadolinium enhancement; (C) T₁ fat saturated with gadolinium with synovial enhancement.

(Fig. 10.5) and avascular necrosis (Fig. 10.6), particularly in the early stages. Murray *et al.* (1996) evaluated 14 hips in seven children with mean disease duration of seven years. The importance of contrast enhancement in the evaluation of synovium was shown because inflamed synovium was underestimated in 75% of the unenhanced MR images (Fig. 10.5).

DEXA

Several studies have reported reduced bone mineral density (BMD) in children and adolescents with JIA (Pepmueller *et al.* 1996; Henderson *et al.* 1997, 2000; Kotaniemi 1997; Brik *et al.* 1998; Kotaniemi *et al.* 1999; Zak *et al.* 1999; Haugen *et al.* 2000; Murray *et al.* 2000). BMD in the hip (and lumbar spine) has also been reported to be significantly lower in young adults with JIA compared to healthy controls matched for age, sex, height and weight (Zak *et al.* 1999). Low bone mass is not restricted to the severe end of the disease spectrum nor is it restricted to those treated with corticosteroids. Henderson *et al.* (2000)

137

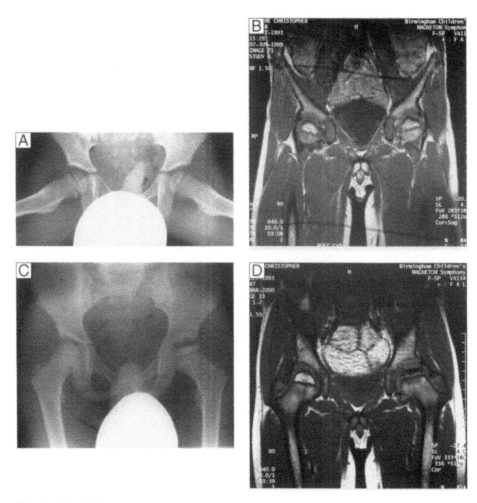

Fig. 10.6. Serial X-rays and MRI of avascular necrosis of left femoral head. (A) X-ray of hips at presentation. (B) MRI at presentation showing subtle irregularity and loss of signal in left femoral head. (C) X-ray showing established avascular necrosis of left femoral head. (D) Coronal T_1-weighted MRI showing established avascular necrosis with flattening and sclerosis of left femoral head and small effusion.

reported that 30% of postpubertal female patients with mild-to-moderate non-corticosteroid treated juvenile rheumatoid arthritis (JRA) had low bone mass. Since a third of young adults with JIA continue to have active inflammation into adulthood, the relationship with disease activity is not restricted to childhood. Haugen *et al.* (2000) reported significantly lower BMD in young adults (male and female) with persistent, active disease compared with healthy subjects. However, in cases where the disease went into remission, there was an interesting difference in BMD at the spine compared to the hip in female patients. In the presence of quiescent disease, female patients attained the same BMD as healthy subjects in the lumbar spine (and radius) but significantly lower BMD in the femoral neck. This has obvious implications to arthroplasty surgery in such patients in terms of bone stock and risk of fracture.

Management
THE ROLE OF THE MULTIDISCIPLINARY TEAM
Ideally, successful management of childhood arthritis is achieved by a multidisciplinary team of medical experts working in close partnership with the young person and their family. Such a team is composed of a paediatric rheumatologist, rheumatology nurse specialists, occupational therapists, physiotherapists, orthotists, social workers, dietitian, psychologists, ophthalmologist and othopaedic surgeon. Liaison with schoolteachers and community resources is also important, acknowledging the reciprocal influences of a chronic illness like JIA on cognitive and psychosocial development.

DRUG THERAPY AND INTRA-ARTICULAR INJECTION THERAPY
Initial management of hip involvement in JIA includes analgesics and anti-inflammatory medication combined with a physical therapy programme (including prone lying to help prevent fixed flexion deformity). For hip joints with no fixed deformity and persisting synovitis, an injection of intra-articular steroid under X-ray screening will improve mobility, and rapidly reduce pain and effusions (Boehnke *et al.* 1994). Triamcinolone hexacetonide (1 mg/kg) is the drug of choice, with a period of 24 hours non-weight-bearing post-procedure. Sparling *et al.* (1990) expressed concern regarding radiographic deterioration in hip joints post-injection in a retrospective study, although avascular necrosis was seen in only one hip of 12 injected in this study. However, these authors also stated that X-rays prior to joint injection had showed rapid changes. Prospective studies in this area are needed. In polyarticular disease, whatever the subtype, systemic drug therapy is imperative to control the joint inflammation, control pain, and maintain normal growth and development: *e.g.* methotrexate, oral or subcutaneous (0.5–1.0 mg/kg/week to a maximum total dose of 30 mg (Wallace 1998); etanercept (0.4 mg/kg twice weekly to a maximum dose of 25 mg) (Lovell *et al.* 2000); steroids (intra-articular triamcinolone hexacetonide, 1 mg/kg for large joints, 0.5 mg/kg for small joints); or intermittent intravenous pulse therapy (methylprednisolone, 10–30 mg/kg to maximum of 1 g per dose). With the advent of methotrexate and etanercept, daily oral steroids are less frequently used and usually only as an interim measure (prednisolone 0.5–2 mg/kg/day).

ANTERIOR SOFT-TISSUE RELEASE PROCEDURES
For those hips with a fixed deformity, limited range of movement and functional impairment but normal joint space, a soft-tissue release of the tight adductors and the psoas through a small incision in the groin can correct deformity, relieve pain and improve function (Swann and Ansell 1986, Morenzo Alvarez *et al.* 1993). For more severe fixed flexion deformities (>25°), a more extensive procedure has been described in which the muscles are stripped from the ilium and combined with a partial synovectomy. Witt and McCullough (1994) reported the results of this procedure in a study of 31 hips in 17 patients with JIA. A reduction

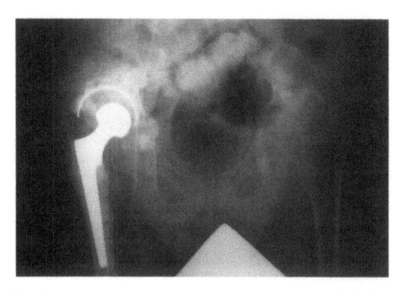

Fig. 10.7. Severe destruction of the hips in SOJIA with unilateral total hip replacement.

of fixed flexion was noted one year postoperatively, with improvement maintained at five years. At follow-up of five to 12 years, 14 hips had maintained an acceptable range of motion with no further requirement for surgery. Radiographic improvement was reported in some hips postoperatively, with a reduction in osteopaenia, a clearer definition and widening of the joint line.

A postoperative physiotherapy programme is vital for these patients in order to maintain the range of motion and may include traction in abduction and hydrotherapy.

TOTAL HIP ARTHROPLASTY
The main indications for total hip arthroplasty (THR) in patients with JIA are primarily the relief of pain and the restoration of function (Fig. 10.7). THR in the younger child, especially the pre-adolescent, must be carefully considered and usually only for severe disease and disability. Other indications include ankylosis of the hip in a suboptimal position leading to functional impairment and secondary deformity of other joints and/or progressive protrusio acetabulae as seen on serial X-rays. If there is hip and knee disease, the hips should be replaced before the knees. The results in several studies have demonstrated a marked reduction in pain and improvement in functional ability and improved quality of life following hip arthroplasty (Roach and Paradies 1984, Ruddlesdin *et al.* 1986, Gudmundsson *et al.* 1989, Witt *et al.* 1991, Cage *et al.* 1992, Maric and Haynes 1993, Chmell *et al.* 1997, Haber and Goodman 1998, Rahimtoola *et al.* 2000). However, the rate of loosening and subsequent revision in the long term are of concern. In a study of 186 patients with JIA followed for 22 years (Lehtimaki *et al.* 1997), survivorship of the Charnley THR was 91.9% at 10 years and 83% at 15 years. Survivorship of the femoral component was 95.6% at 10 years and 91.9% at 15 years, and that of the acetabulum was 95% and 87.8% respectively.

In a study of 92 primary THRs in patients with JIA, a revision procedure was required in 25% of hips after an average follow-up of 11.5 years (Witt *et al.* 1991). An increased rate of aseptic loosening in THR performed with cement in young patients with JIA, especially during the second decade after the procedure, has been reported by several authors (Lachiewicz *et al.* 1986, Ruddlesdin *et al.* 1986, Witt *et al.* 1991, Cage *et al.* 1992, Maric and Haynes 1993, Chmell *et al.* 1997, Lehtimaki *et al.* 1997). Furthermore, the relative reduced durability of the acetabular component as compared to the femoral component has been reported in various long-term studies of THR performed with cement in patients with JIA as well as other conditions; *e.g.* Cage *et al.* (1992) recorded rates of 61% and 85% respectively at 15 years. In view of these rates of medium term loosening in cemented arthroplasties, consideration has being given to the use of customized uncemented femoral components in this group of patients (Lachiewicz *et al.* 1986, Maric and Haynes 1993, Kumar and Swann 1998). These implants have a porous coating applied to them to allow bone ingrowth to occur or have a hydroxyapatite coating that bonds directly to bone. Initial results are excellent in the short term but failure rates were considerably higher on later follow-up (Kumar and Swann 1998). Other more conservative alternatives to THR in JIA patients include a hybrid total hip arthroplasty (one component fixed with cement, the other without). Bipolar hemiarthroplasty is another potential conservative alternative, which may allow for the preservation of often limited acetabular bone stock. However, migration of the socket is a complication two to five years postoperatively (Wilson and Scott 1989), and the results of this procedure need to be compared with those of total hip arthroplasty in a long-term follow-up study of a large group of patients.

As in patients with adult-onset ankylosing spondylitis, ectopic ossification after THR was found to occur with increased frequency in patients with enthesitis-related JIA than in those with other subtypes of JIA (Garcia-Morteo *et al.* 1983). Functional capacity was not impaired, regardless of the severity of the ectopic ossification.

The reduced durability of total hip prosthesis in the long term in JIA populations (Chmell *et al.* 1997) as compared to patients with adult rheumatoid arthritis may be due to various factors:
• In many patients with JIA, implants may need to be custom-made for individuals to allow for variation in skeletal size and such growth disturbances as detailed above. In some small patients even this may not always be possible.
• Unlike adult rheumatoid arthritis, JIA affects a growing skeleton and therefore may cause localized growth disturbances in the lower limb and pelvis, which may then alter the usual magnitude and direction of forces borne by the implant postoperatively. There may also be a mismatch between the sizes of the metaphysis and diaphysis that precludes an adequate fit of the femoral component. Contractures of the lower extremity may also have similar effects.
• The dynamic state of skeletal remodelling may interfere with the maintenance of fixation due to femoral cortical hypertrophy, seen in 37% of THRs in one study (Chmell *et al.* 1997).
• Osteopaenia of varying severity can pose a particular problem with insertion of the femoral component without cement. Osteopaenia in JIA is multifactorial including factors such

as steroid therapy, disuse, nutritional status and disease activity (Pepmueller *et al*. 1996; Henderson *et al*. 1997, 2000; Kotaniemi 1997; Brik *et al*. 1998; Kotaniemi *et al*. 1999; Zak *et al*. 1999; Haugen *et al*. 2000; Murray *et al*. 2000).

• Adolescent patients with JIA may make more demands on the implant as compared to adults with rheumatoid arthritis in terms of their education, career, sporting activities, etc. Moreover, they have a longer life expectancy at the time of surgery.

Age and developmentally appropriate information about hip surgery should be provided for these young people to enable informed consent and shared decision-making as well as to enhance their self-efficacy. Consideration must be made for the impact of THR on various aspects of their young lives, *e.g.* education and future careers, driving a car or indeed learning to drive (important for their sense of independence), sporting activities, and current or future sexual activity. Giving a 16-year-old patient a booklet designed for older patients with osteoarthritis or rheumatoid arthritis is not appropriate. Involvement of the multidisciplinary team, especially the physiotherapist and occupational therapist, is imperative in preoperative counselling and preparation. If possible, timing of surgical intervention should take into account school examinations and where possible be scheduled for early summer to enable rehabilitation over the summer months.

Outcome

Current literature reports that at least one-third of children with JIA will continue to have active inflammatory disease into their adult years and that up to 60% of all patients continue to have some limitation of their activities of daily living into adulthood (David *et al*. 1994, Gare and Fasth 1995, Peterson *et al*. 1997, Ruperto *et al*. 1997). Information on long-term impact of the new drug therapies and earlier use of established drugs like methotrexate in the course of the disease is eagerly awaited from prospective studies.

The prognosis of hip involvement in oligoarticular JIA is less good in the patients in the enthesitis-related subgroup (Garcia-Morteo *et al*. 1983, Jacobsen *et al*. 1992). In SOJIA, patients with a younger age of onset have a worse prognosis and more frequent radiographic changes than those with later onset (Jacobsen *et al*. 1992). An interesting phenomenon of hip-joint remodelling in SOJIA has been reported (Banks and Ostrov 2000).

Early diagnosis and management by an appropriate multidisciplinary team, expert in the management of such children will hopefully go a long way to limiting if not preventing much of the damage and deformity that is observed when inflammation remains uncontrolled over time.

Summary

Although JIA rarely presents as monoarticular hip disease, hip involvement is common especially in those with longer duration of disease. Hip involvement is a predictor for poor outcome. Advances in imaging techniques, *e.g.* MRI and ultrasound, have made early diagnosis of hip synovitis easier. With the advent of new biological therapies including anti-TNFa therapy (*e.g.* etanercept, a soluble TNFa receptor fusion protein—Lovell *et al*. 2000), the need for hip arthroplasty in the second and third decades will hopefully become a rare occurrence in this population of young people.

REFERENCES

Andersson Gare, B. (1999) 'Juvenile arthritis – who gets it, where and when? A review of current data on incidence and prevalence.' *Clinical and Experimental Rheumatology*, **17**, 367–374.

Ansell, B.M., Unlu, M. (1970) 'Hip involvement in juvenile chronic polyarthritis.' *Annals of the Rheumatic Diseases*, **29**, 687–688.

Banks, S., Ostrov, B.E. (2000) 'Clinical Images: Hip joint remodeling in systemic-onset juvenile rheumatoid arthritis.' *Arthritis and Rheumatism*, **43**, 2856.

Bleck, E.E. (1983) 'Idiopathic chondrolysis of the hip.' *Journal of Bone and Joint Surgery, American Volume*, **65**, 1266–1275.

Boehnke, M., Behrend, R., Dietz, G., Kuster, R.M. (1994) 'Intraarticular hip treatment with triamcinolone hexacetonide in juvenile chronic arthritis.' *Acta Universitatis Carolinae. Medica*, **40**, 123–126.

Brik, R., Keidar, Z., Schapira, D., Israel, O. (1998) 'Bone mineral density and turnover in children with systemic juvenile chronic arthritis.' *Journal of Rheumatology*, **25**, 990–992.

Burgos-Vargas, R., Naranjo, A., Castillo, J., Katona, G. (1989) 'Ankylosing spondylitis in the Mexican Mestizo: patterns of disease according to age of onset.' *Journal of Rheumatology*, **16**, 186–191.

Cage, D.J., Granberry, W.M., Tullos, H.S. (1992) 'Long-term results of total arthroplasty in adolescents with debilitating polyarthropathy.' *Clinical Orthopaedics*, **283**, 156–162.

Chmell, M.J., Scott, R.D., Thomas, W.H., Sledge, C.B. (1997) 'Total hip arthroplasty with cement for juvenile rheumatoid arthritis. Results at a minimum of ten years in patients less than thirty years old.' *Journal of Bone and Joint Surgery, American Volume*, **79**, 44–52.

David, J., Cooper, C., Hickey, L., Lloyd, J., Dore, C., McCullough, C., Woo, P. (1994) 'The functional and psychological outcomes of juvenile chronic arthritis in young adulthood.' *British Journal of Rheumatology*, **33**, 876–881.

Fedrizzi, M.S., Ronchezel, M.V., Hilario, M.O., Lederman, H.M., Sawaya, S., Goldenberg, J., Sole, D. (1997) 'Ultrasonography in the early diagnosis of hip joint involvement in juvenile rheumatoid arthritis.' *Journal of Rheumatology*, **24**, 1820–1825.

Flato, B., Aasland, A., Vinje, O., Forre, O. (1998) 'Outcome and predictive factors in juvenile spondyloarthropathy.' *Journal of Rheumatology*, **25**, 366–375.

Garcia-Morteo, O., Maldonado-Cocco, J.A., Babini, J.C. (1983a) 'Ectopic ossification following total hip replacement in juvenile chronic arthritis.' *Journal of Bone and Joint Surgery, American Volume*, **65**, 812–814.

Garcia-Morteo, O., Maldonado-Cocco, J.A., Suarez-Almazor, M.E., Garay, E. (1983b) 'Ankylosing spondylitis of juvenile onset: comparison with adult onset disease.' *Scandinavian Journal of Rheumatology*, **12**, 246–248.

Gare, B.A., Fasth, A. (1995) 'The natural history of juvenile chronic arthritis. A population based cohort study. II. Outcome.' *Journal of Rheumatology*, **22**, 308–319.

Gudmundsson, G.H., Harving, S., Pilgaard, S. (1989) 'The Charnley total hip arthroplasty in juvenile rheumatoid arthritis patients.' *Orthopaedics*, **12**, 385–388.

Gusis, S.E., Maldonado Cocco, J.A., Rivero, E.M., Babini, J.C., Gagliardi, S.A. (1993) 'Protrusio acetabuli in juvenile rheumatoid arthritis.' *Clinical Rheumatology*, **12**, 36–40.

Haber, D., Goodman, S.B. (1998) 'Total hip arthroplasty in juvenile chronic arthritis: a consecutive series.' *Journal of Arthroplasty*, **13**, 259–265.

Harris, C.M., Baum, J. (1988) 'Involvement of the hip in juvenile rheumatoid arthritis. A longitudinal study.' *Journal of Bone and Joint Surgery, American Volume*, **70**, 821–833.

Hastings, D.E., Orsini, E., Myers, P., Sullivan, J. (1994) 'An unusual pattern of growth disturbance of the hip in juvenile rheumatoid arthritis.' *Journal of Rheumatology*, **21**, 744–747.

Haugen, M., Lien, G., Flato, B., Kvammen, J., Vinje, O., Sorskaar, D., Forre, O. (2000) 'Young adults with juvenile arthritis in remission attain normal peak bone mass at the lumbar spine and forearm.' *Arthritis and Rheumatism*, **43**, 1504–1510.

Henderson, C.J., Cawkwell, G.D., Specker, B.L., Sierra, R.I., Wilmott, R.W., Campaigne, B.N., Lovell, D.J. (1997) 'Predictors of total body bone mineral density in non-corticosteroid-treated prepubertal children with juvenile rheumatoid arthritis.' *Arthritis and Rheumatism*, **40**, 1967–1975.

Henderson, C.J., Specker, B.L., Sierra R.I., Campaigne, B.N., Lovell, D.J. (2000) 'Total-body bone mineral content in non-corticosteroid-treated postpubertal females with juvenile rheumatoid arthritis: frequency of osteopenia and contributing factors.' *Arthritis and Rheumatism*, **43**, 531–540.

143

Hughes, R.A., Tempos, J., Ansell, B.M. (1988) 'A review of the diagnoses of hip pain presentation in the adolescent.' *British Journal of Rheumatology*, **27**, 450–453.

Isdale, I.C. (1970) 'Hip disease in juvenile rheumatoid arthritis.' *Annals of the Rheumatic Diseases*, **29**, 603–608

Jacobsen, F.S., Crawford, A.H., Broste, S. (1992) 'Hip involvement in juvenile rheumatoid arthritis.' *Journal of Pediatric Orthopedics*, **12**, 45–53.

Jacqueline, F., Boujot, A., Canet, L. (1961) 'Involvement of the hips in juvenile rheumatoid arthritis.' *Arthritis and Rheumatism*, **4**, 500–513.

Kobayakawa, M., Rydholm, U., Wingstrand, H., Pettersson, H., Lidgren, L. (1989) 'Femoral head necrosis in juvenile chronic arthritis.' *Acta Orthopaedica Scandinavica*, **60**, 164–169.

Koski, J.M. (1989) 'Ultrasonographic evidence of hip synovitis in patients with rheumatoid arthritis.' *Scandinavian Journal of Rheumatology*, **18**, 127–131.

Kotaniemi, A. (1997) 'Growth retardation and bone loss as determinants of axial osteopenia in juvenile chronic arthritis.' *Scandinavian Journal of Rheumatology*, **26**, 14–18.

Kotaniemi, A., Savolainen, A., Kroger, H., Kautiainen, H., Isomaki, H. (1999) 'Weight-bearing physical activity, calcium intake, systemic glucocorticoids, chronic inflammation, and body constitution as determinants of lumbar and femoral bone mineral in juvenile chronic arthritis.' *Scandinavian Journal of Rheumatology*, **28**, 19–26.

Kumar, M.N., Swann, M. (1998) 'Uncemented total hip arthroplasty in young patients with juvenile chronic arthritis.' *Annals of the Royal College of Surgeons of England*, **80**, 203–209.

Lachiewicz, P.F., McCaskill, B., Inglis, A., Ranawat, C.S., Rosenstein, B.D. (1986) 'Total hip arthroplasty in juvenile rheumatoid arthritis. Two to eleven-year results.' *Journal of Bone and Joint Surgery, American Volume*, **68**, 502–508.

Lang, B.A., Schneider, R., Reilly, B.J., Silverman, E.D., Laxer, R.M. (1995) 'Radiologic features of systemic onset juvenile rheumatoid arthritis.' *Journal of Rheumatology*, **22**, 168–173.

Lehtimaki, M.Y., Lehto, M.U., Kautiainen, H., Savolainen, H.A., Hamalainen, M.M. (1997) 'Survivorship of the Charnley total hip arthroplasty in juvenile chronic arthritis. A follow-up of 186 cases for 22 years.' *Journal of Bone and Joint Surgery, British Volume*, **79**, 792–795.

Lovell, D.J., Giannini, E.H., Reiff, A., Cawkwell, G.D., Silverman, E.D., Nocton, J.J., Stein, L.D., Gedalia, A., Ilowite, N.T., Wallace, C.A., Whitmore, J., Finck, B.K. (2000) 'Etanercept in children with polyarticular juvenile rheumatoid arthritis. Pediatric Rheumatology Collaborative Study Group.' *New England Journal of Medicine*, **342**, 763–769.

Maric, Z., Haynes, R.J. (1993) 'Total hip arthroplasty in juvenile rheumatoid arthritis.' *Clinical Orthopaedics*, **290**, 197–199.

Murray, J.G., Ridley, N.T.F., Mitchell, N., Rooney, M. (1996) 'Juvenile chronic arthritis of the hip: value of contrast-enhanced MR imaging.' *Clinical Radiology*, **51**, 99–102.

Modesto, C., Woo, P., Garcia-Consuegra, J., Merino, R. (2001) 'Systemic onset juvenile chronic arthritis, polyarticular pattern and hip involvement as markers for a bad prognosis.' *Clinical and Experimental Rheumatology*, **19**, 211–217.

Moreno Alvarez, M.J., Espada, G., Maldonado-Cocco, J.A., Gagliardi, S.A. (1993) 'Longterm followup of hip and knee soft tissue release in juvenile chronic arthritis.' *Clinical Rheumatology*, **12**, 36–40.

Murray, K.J., Boyle, R.J., Woo, P. (2000) 'Pathological fractures and osteoporosis in a cohort of 103 systemic onset juvenile idiopathic arthritis patients.' *Arthritis and Rheumatism*, **43**, S119.

Pepmueller, P., Cassidy, J., Allen, S., Hillman, L. (1996) 'Bone mineralization and bone mineral metabolism in children with juvenile rheumatoid arthritis.' *Arthritis and Rheumatism*, **39**, 746–757.

Peterson, L.S., Mason, T., Nelson, A.M., O'Fallon, W.M., Gabriel, S.E. (1997) 'Psychosocial outcomes and health studies of adults who have had juvenile rheumatoid arthritis: a controlled, population-based study.' *Arthritis and Rheumatism*, **40**, 2235–2240.

Petty, R.E., Southwood, TR., Baum, J., Bhettay, E., Glass, D.N., Manners, P., Maldonado-Cocco, J., Suarez-Almazor, M., Orozco-Alcala, J., Prieur, A.M. (1998) 'Revision of the proposed classification criteria for juvenile idiopathic arthritis: Durban, 1997.' *Journal of Rheumatology*, **25**, 1991–1994.

Rahimtoola, Z.O., Finger, S., Imrie, S., Goodman, S.B. (2000) 'Outcome of total hip arthroplasty in small-proportioned patients.' *Journal of Arthroplasty*, **15**, 27–34.

Roach, J.W., Paradies, L.H. (1984) 'Total hip arthroplasty performed during adolescence.' *Journal of Pediatric Orthopedics*, **4**, 418–421.

Rombouts, J.J., Rombouts-Lindemans, C. (1971) 'Involvement of the hip in juvenile rheumatoid arthritis.' *Acta Rheumatologica Scandinavica*, **17**, 248–267.

Ruddlesdin, C., Ansell, B.M., Arden, G.P., Swann, M. (1986) 'Total hip replacement in children with juvenile chronic arthritis.' *Journal of Bone and Joint Surgery, British Volume*, **68**, 218–222.

Ruperto, N., Levinson, J.E., Ravelli, A., Shear, E.S., Link Tague B., Murray, K., Martini, A., Giannini, E.H. (1997) 'Long-term health outcomes and quality of life in American and Italian inception cohorts of patients with juvenile rheumatoid arthritis. I. Outcome status.' *Journal of Rheumatology*, **24**, 945–951.

Rydholm, U., Wingstrand, H., Egund, N., Elborg, R., Forsberg, L., Lidgren, L. (1986) 'Sonography, arthroscopy, and intracapsular pressure in juvenile chronic arthritis of the hip.' *Acta Orthopaedica Scandinavica*, **57**, 295–298.

Sairanen, E. (1958) 'On rheumatoid arthritis in children. A clinicoroentgenological study.' *Acta Rheumatologica Scandinavica Supplementum*, **2**, 1–79.

Sparling, M., Malleson, P., Wood, B., Petty, R. (1990) 'Radiographic followup of joints injected with triamcinolone hexacetonide for the management of childhood arthritis.' *Arthritis and Rheumatism*, **33**, 821–826.

Spencer, C.H., Bernstein, B.H. (2002) 'Hip disease in juvenile rheumatoid arthritis' *Current Opinion in Rheumatology*, **14**, 536–541.

Svantesson, H., Marhaug, G., Haeffner, F. (1981) 'Scoliosis in children with juvenile rheumatoid arthritis.' *Scandinavian Journal of Rheumatology*, **10**, 65–68.

Swann, M., Ansell, B.M. (1986) 'Soft-tissue release of the hips in children with juvenile chronic arthritis.' *Journal of Bone and Joint Surgery, British Volume*, **68**, 404–408.

Thomas, E., Barrett, J.H., Donn, R.P., Thomson, W., Southwood, T.R. (2000) 'Subtyping of juvenile idiopathic arthritis using latent class analysis. British Paediatric Rheumatology Group.' *Arthritis and Rheumatism*, **43**, 1496–1503.

van der Hoeven, H., Keessen, W., Kuis, W. (1989) 'Idiopathic chondrolysis of the hip. A distinct clinical entity?' *Acta Orthopaedica Scandinavica*, **60**, 661–663.

Wallace, C.A. (1998) 'The use of methotrexate in childhood rheumatic diseases.' *Arthritis and Rheumatism*, **41**, 381–389.

Wallace, C.A., Levinson, J.E. (1991) 'Juvenile rheumatoid arthritis: Outcome and treatment for the 1990s.' *Rheumatic Disease Clinics of North America*, **17**, 891–905.

Williams, W.W., McCullough, C.J. (1993) 'Results of cemented total hip replacement in juvenile chronic arthritis. A radiological review.' *Journal of Bone and Joint Surgery, British Volume*, **75**, 872–874.

Wilson, G.M., Scott, R.D. (1989) 'The bipolar socket in juvenile rheumatoid arthritis: a two- to five-year follow-up study.' *Journal of Orthopaedic Rheumatology*, **2**, 133–143.

Witt, J.D., McCullough, C.J. (1994) 'Anterior soft-tissue release of the hip in juvenile chronic arthritis.' *Journal of Bone and Joint Surgery, British Volume*, **76**, 267–270.

Witt, J.D., Swann, M., Ansell, B.M. (1991) 'Total hip replacement for juvenile chronic arthritis.' *Journal of Bone and Joint Surgery, British Volume*, **73**, 770–773.

Zak, M., Hassager, C., Lovell, D.J., Nielsen, S., Henderson, C.J., Pedersen, F.K. (1999) 'Assessment of bone mineral density in adults with a history of juvenile chronic arthritis: a cross-sectional long-term followup study.' *Arthritis and Rheumatism*, **42**, 790–798.

11
GAIT ANALYSIS IN DOCUMENTING AND UNDERSTANDING HIP FUNCTION

Sylvia Õunpuu

The hip joint and hip musculature are involved in many pathologies of children that ultimately affect hip motion. For example, abnormal hip motion is a common sequela in patients with neuromuscular disorders such as cerebral palsy (Tylkowski 1982, Gage 1991), myelomeningocele (Duffy *et al.* 1996, Õunpuu *et al.* 1996), femoral head avascular necrosis, and the so-called miserable malalignment of the lower extremities (see below). Abnormal hip motion may also be a compensation for abnormalities in the motion at other joints, for example circumduction to prevent clearance problems due to reduced sagittal plane knee motion. The documentation of hip motion using three-dimensional gait analysis techniques not only provides objective information about hip motion in three planes, which is very hard to visualize, but it can also assist the clinician in understanding the mechanical basis of abnormal hip motion. This will ultimately provide more information with which to make informed treatments, and in the long-term allow objective documentation of treatment and eventually improve treatment outcome.

The function and status of the hip joint in many cases need to be monitored in several ways: for example, using imaging techniques and clinical examination estimates to document bony anomalies and abnormal torsions (Ruwe *et al.* 1992); physical examination to document muscle abnormalities such as weakness and spasticity; and motion analysis techniques to document dynamic function. The purpose of this chapter is to describe the role of three-dimensional gait analysis techniques in the objective documentation of hip function during gait and to highlight how the addition of gait analysis data to the more traditional tools leads to a better documentation and ultimately understanding of hip motion. Gait analysis output will be used in each case example. Readers are encouraged to take the time to understand the gait "plot" so that they may see the benefit of this added information. However, for each case the written explanations alone provide background information in a variety of hip pathologies that will assist in the visual observation of gait when that is the only tool available.

Understanding the complexity of hip motion
There are two ways of documenting hip motion during dynamic activity, by observation and by use of three-dimensional gait analysis techniques. The latter do not preclude the important role of observational gait analysis. The initial pathology is usually noted through observation, but three-dimensional gait analysis techniques provide information not possible

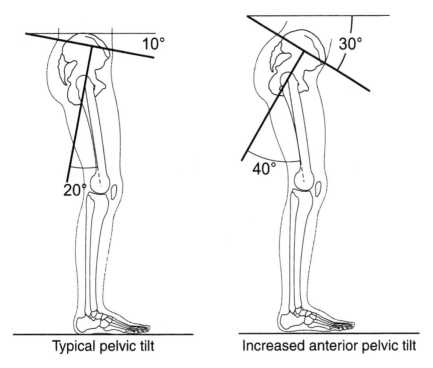

Fig. 11.1. Example of the effect of pelvic position on hip motion with thigh segment remaining stationary. Hip angle cannot be estimated without appreciation for the position of the pelvis.

with visual analysis alone. Understanding the importance of the additional information provided by three-dimensional gait analysis includes understanding the limitations of visual observation of gait. When analyzing hip motion visually, it is typical to focus only on the orientation of the thigh segment in space. That is, the clinician judges the position and motion of the hip on the position and motion of the thigh segment alone. For example, if the distal portion of the thigh segment is anterior to the proximal portion (typical in knee flexion), we assume that the hip is in flexion. Similarly, if the thigh segment is vertical, we assume that the hip is neutral (Fig. 11.1). In both these examples, we are not considering the orientation of the pelvis segment. This would be a reasonable assumption if the pelvis were positioned normally or did not move during gait. This is not the case in many pathologies where the pelvis moves significantly to assist or permit thigh motion or may be asymmetrical, that is, retracted and/or depressed.

The definition of a joint angle is the relative orientation of the two segments that form the joint. The hip joint is the relative angle between the pelvis and thigh segments. Therefore, we must have an appreciation for the position and motion of both the pelvis and thigh segments to evaluate hip function. This is difficult in most clinic settings where the position of the pelvis is "hidden" by clothing or very difficult to observe because of large motions in three planes. In Figure 11.1, for example, there is an increase in hip flexion when the

147

pelvis is more anterior. In clinical settings where three-dimensional gait analysis is not available, keeping these concepts and the examples presented in this chapter in mind when observing patients will assist the clinician in making more appropriate observations. As well, observations of hip motion can be improved by having the patient clothed in such a way that the majority of the thigh and pelvic segments are visible.

Keeping in mind the definition of the hip angle, one can begin to appreciate the impact of pelvic position on hip angle. Pelvic position and motion during gait, however, are not only affected by the function of the hip joint but also show positioning and motion related to balance issues, spinal deformity, contralateral hip function and muscle weakness. In cases where there is an excessive anterior pelvic tilt due to abdominal weakness, hip flexion is increased; similarly, when the pelvis is tilted posteriorly due to severe hamstring contracture, the hip flexion is decreased. Hip angle may also be affected by knee position. That is, increasing knee flexion will result in increasing hip flexion, and conversely, increasing knee extension will result in hip extension. Therefore, understanding hip motion involves appreciating abnormalities both proximal and distal to the hip joint.

The clinician needs also to appreciate that abnormal hip motion goes beyond the sagittal plane in many pathologies and includes abnormalities in the coronal and transverse planes of motion. Adding to this already complex picture in many cases is the pelvis that could be moving through a large range of motion in all three planes. These issues are best understood with the use of gait analysis data, that is, hip kinematic plots that describe the angular motion of the hip in three planes as in the examples given below.

Gait analysis and the documentation of hip motion
The best way to document and ultimately appreciate and understand hip motion is through the use of three-dimensional gait analysis techniques, which allow documentation of hip motion in three planes. The angular changes of the hip (kinematics) during gait are typically represented using a plot of hip angle versus time (initial contact to the following initial contact of one foot). Understanding a hip kinematic plot requires some insight into how this information is obtained and the angle definitions used to define each plot. The routine methods used in clinical gait analysis are well described in the literature (Davis and DeLuca 1996). In brief, reflective segment markers are aligned to bony landmarks. The three-dimensional location of these markers is then determined by a motion capture system. The relationships between these balls and the segments they represent are calculated using the Euler's equations of motion (Greenwood 1965). An example of a subject with the reflective marker system in place for a full body motion analysis is given in Figure 11.2.

As mentioned previously, the hip joint angle is the relative angle between the pelvis and thigh segments. The angle definition for the hip in the three planes of motion is illustrated in Figure 11.3. In the sagittal plane (Fig. 11.3A), the hip angle is the relative angle between the long axis of the thigh and a perpendicular to the pelvic plane as viewed by an observer looking along a line connecting the anterior superior iliac spines (ASISs). In the coronal plane (Fig. 11.3B), the hip angle is the relative angle between the long axis of the thigh and a perpendicular to the pelvic plane as viewed from the front of and in the pelvic plane. In the transverse plane (Fig. 11.3C), the hip angle is the motion of the thigh (as

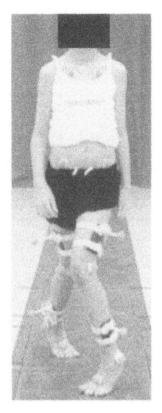

Fig. 11.2. Example of a typical patient equipped for a motion analysis study. Reflective markers are aligned to specific bony landmarks on the trunk, pelvis and both lower extremities.

defined by the knee flexion extension axis) relative to the ASIS–ASIS line as viewed by an observer above the pelvic plane. Typical hip motion using the above definitions can then be defined and used as a reference for pathological gait (Fig. 11.4). Typical hip motion in the coronal plane (Fig. 11.4A) shows adduction during loading response (weight acceptance), followed by abduction in mid-stance to toe-off, followed by adduction in swing. The overall range of motion in the coronal plane is about 13°. In the sagittal plane (Fig. 11.4B), the hip is flexed at about 35° at initial contact and continues to extend through terminal stance when it starts to flex again just before toe-off. The hip then flexes in initial through mid-swing and extends slightly in terminal swing. The overall range of motion in the sagittal plane is about 43°. In the transverse plane (Fig. 11.4C), hip rotation is minimal with a few degrees of internal rotation in loading response followed by external rotation throughout the remainder of stance. The overall range of motion in the transverse plane is about 8°.

The relationship between gait analysis and clinical examination measures
Another aspect of understanding hip motion is the appreciation of how hip angles measured during gait relate to the assessment of the hip angle on the examination table, enabling us to determine the potential impact of muscle contractures and torsional deformities of the femur. In the sagittal plane, the interpretation of hip motion during gait requires an appre-

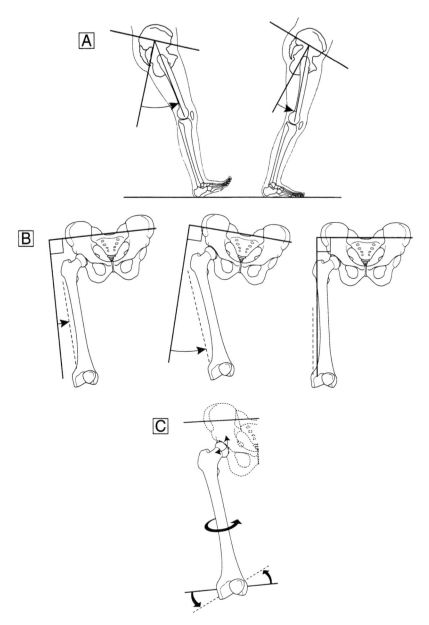

Fig. 11.3. Illustration of joint angles for the hip in (A) sagittal, (B) coronal, and (C) transverse planes.

ciation of the presence or absence of a hip flexion contracture. Positive hip extension is typically measured in one of two ways, the Thomas test and the Staheli method (Bleck 1987). Irrespective of the method, the hip angle definition in both the gait analysis and the clinical examination must be the same in order to correlate results. That is, the segments that make

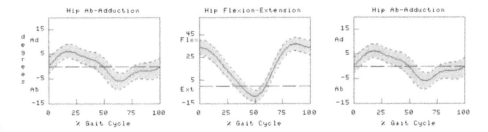

Fig. 11.4. Typical hip motion in coronal (left), sagittal (centre), and transverse (right) planes. The gray band represents the mean ±1 SD.

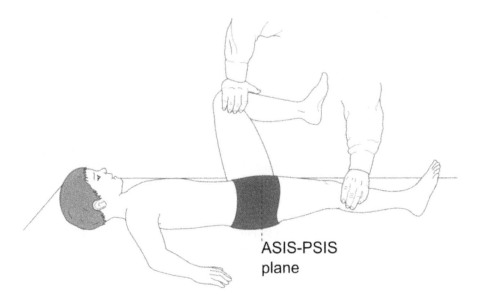

ASIS-PSIS
plane

Fig. 11.5. The modified Thomas test where the pelvic position is oriented so that it is consistent with the angle definition commonly used in gait analysis. That is, a line connecting the anterior (ASIS) and posterior (PSIS) superior iliac spines is vertical or perpendicular to the table. The hip flexion angle measured becomes the angle between the long axis of the thigh and the surface of the table.

up the angle (in this case the pelvis and thigh) must be represented in the same way. Therefore, the Thomas test will only directly correlate with the motion data if the orientation of the pelvis is such that the ASIS and posterior superior iliac spine (PSIS) are aligned vertically so that the line connecting the two is perpendicular to the table (Fig. 11.5). This has been referred to as the modified Thomas test. If during the Thomas test the opposite limb is moved toward the trunk so that the pelvis tilts posteriorly, the angle definitions are no longer the same and the measured "flexion contracture" may be more than the minimum hip flexion during gait, suggesting an inconsistency. Understanding the implications of angle definitions is critical in the interpretation of gait analysis data in all three planes.

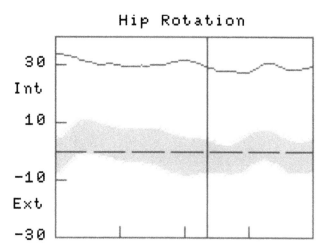

Fig. 11.6. Example of excessive internal hip rotation (solid line) at approximately 30° over the gait cycle in comparison to typical rotation (gray band).

Pathological hip function

In this section, a variety of hip pathologies will be described in terms of gait function. Gait analysis data, specifically kinematic plots, will be used to describe abnormal hip motion in all planes of motion. The role of gait analysis in understanding abnormal hip function will be emphasized.

ABNORMAL ROTATIONAL PROFILES IN PERSONS WITH NORMAL MUSCLE TONE
Three-dimensional gait analysis data and estimates of bony torsions will provide the clinician with a complete picture of hip pathology and allow us to better determine whether abnormal hip motion is a primary deviation or secondary compensation. The examples below represent abnormal hip motion that is primarily due to excessive femoral anteversion and secondarily as compensation for a tibial deformity.

In-toeing gait
In-toeing gait is typically described as excessively internally pointing feet during ambulation. This not only causes an abnormal visual presentation but may also result in functional issues. In-toeing may result from rotational abnormalities at many levels including bony deformity (internal femoral and tibial torsion and fixed forefoot adductus) and dynamic deformity (internal hip rotation, internal knee rotation, forefoot adduction). Determining the contribution of these various causes is critical to deciding upon the appropriate treatment and predicting outcome. In many cases, an in-toeing gait can be a result of bilateral excessive internal hip rotation (Fig. 11.6), which is correlated with increased femoral anteversion. Typically, a patient with bilateral increased internal hip rotation has in-pointing knees as well, if the pelvic position is symmetrical. The visual impression is typically consistent with the gait data, as would be expected. In this case, the gait data may confirm the impression

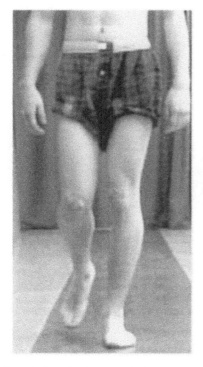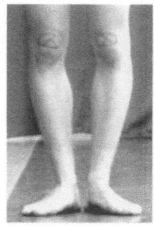

Fig. 11.7. Frontal view of male patient during gait (A) and standing with the knees aligned forward (B). During gait, foot progression is typical and knees are in-pointing consistent with excessive internal hip rotation however, this does not have a major visual impact due to full knee extension in stance. The standing view with knees aligned forward reveals significant bilateral external tibial torsion. (Reproduced by permission from Õunpuu 2002.)

of bilateral internal hips, but also confirm the presence or absence of rotational issues distal to the knees that may also contribute to in-pointing feet.

In-pointing knees during gait
In many circumstances, a combination of deformity and compensatory rotation in the transverse plane can lead to a visually "typical" gait pattern in spite of abnormal bone alignment, as illustrated in Figure 11.7. Although this patient has in-pointing knees, they are not so obvious without excessive knee flexion in stance, and the less experienced observer may not note this abnormality. A comprehensive clinical examination including tibial and femoral torsion estimates and three dimensional gait analysis, allows us to better understand the rotational profile of this patient. An estimate of excessive external tibial torsion and normal femoral anteversion on clinical examination indicates that the primary pathology is in the tibia, bilaterally. Gait analysis data including transverse plane rotational information (Fig. 11.8) allows us to determine the degree of associated compensatory internal hip rotation that results in the in-pointing knees. This combination of deformity has been termed

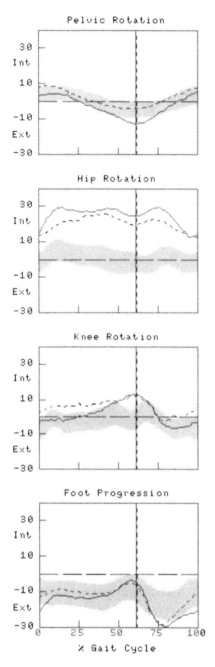

Fig. 11.8. Bilateral transverse plane kinematics for the pelvis, hip, knee and foot progression. The data show increased internal hip rotation on the right (solid lines) and left sides (broken lines), and normal foot progression bilaterally in comparison to typical patterns (gray bands). Related clinical examination indicated external tibial torsion, consistent with the rotational profile. (Reproduced by permission from Õunpuu 2002.)

"miserable malalignment" and can lead to a variety of problems including knee pain (Meister and James 1995, Delgado *et al.* 1996).

GAIT ANALYSIS IN UNDERSTANDING HIP MOTION IN CEREBRAL PALSY
There are many possible abnormalities in hip function in the patient with cerebral palsy. These may occur in one or a combination of all planes of motion and are a result of any one or a combination of issues such as postural demand, muscle contracture, abnormal muscle tone, abnormal control, muscle weakness and bone deformity. The first step in understanding abnormal hip function is a clinical examination to assess any of the above-mentioned potential abnormalities. These issues, however, will only allow one to determine the primary cause of abnormal hip motion, yet this may also result from problems distal or proximal to the hip joint or from problems on the opposite limb. A systematic evaluation of the entire patient including documentation of the trunk, pelvic and bilateral lower extremity motion using gait analysis techniques will help the clinician better understand what are the primary problems and the secondary compensations. With this knowledge, more informed treatment decisions are possible. A complete analysis of function in this manner, over time, allows the clinician to begin to understand that reduced hip extension in stance may be a result of a hip flexion contracture, but may also be a result of hip extensor weakness, knee flexion contracture, severe hamstring tightness/spasticity and/or ankle plantar flexor weakness that results in crouch (excessive knee flexion). Therefore, correction of the hip flexion contracture alone may not lead to an increase in hip extension in stance if abnormal. Without addressing the entire problem, the contracture may reoccur if walking continues in the same manner over the long term. The following examples are just a few cases where gait analysis has provided information not available through observation and clinical examination alone.

Transverse plane asymmetry in patients with cerebral palsy
In many cases, the observational profile represents symmetry, that is, bilateral in-pointing knees and in-pointing feet (Fig. 11.9). However, the transverse plane profile may be much more asymmetrical than supposed without appreciation of pelvic asymmetry. For example, pelvic asymmetry is a typical finding in patients with hemiplegia or asymmetric diplegia. The transverse plane kinematic data for the patient in Figure 11.9 reveal significant asymmetries (Fig. 11.10). The left hemipelvis is retracted (externally rotated) with associated protraction (internal rotation) of the right side throughout the gait cycle. Hip rotation is also asymmetrical, with excessive internal rotation of the left hip and normal rotation of the right. Understanding of the hip angle definition will help explain the inconsistency between visual impression and kinematic data. Visually, this child appears to have bilateral internal hip rotation (Fig. 11.9). However, she has normal rotation of the right hip. This is consistent with the fact that the right hemipelvis in protracted throughout the gait cycle. As a result, the neutral right hip to the pelvis shows an in-pointing knee. This example illustrates the complexity of transverse plane hip motion and the limitations of a visual assessment alone. Again, appreciation of pelvic position in the transverse plane is critical to understanding hip position in this case.

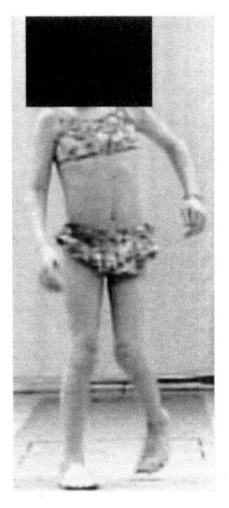

Fig. 11.9. Front view of a typical child with spastic diplegic cerebral palsy. She presents with bilateral in-pointing knees and internal foot progression (in-pointing feet). (Reproduced by permission from Õunpuu 2002.)

Reduced hip extension in terminal stance in cerebral palsy
Reduced hip extension in terminal stance may be a result of primary problems such as hip flexor spasticity and hip flexion contracture (Perry 1992), which can be determined on a clinical examination. Reduced hip extension in terminal stance may also be a result of problems more proximal or distal to the hip joint. As a result, there is a poor correlation between maximum hip extension in gait and the degree of hip flexion contracture. For example, it is not uncommon to find limited hip extension in terminal stance with no hip flexion contracture present. Keeping in mind the angle definition of the hip joint, any abnormality that results in increased knee flexion such as hip extensor weakness, hamstring contracture and/or ankle plantar flexor weakness will increase hip flexion (Fig. 11.11). Therefore, correction of the primary problem with subsequent increase in knee extension during stance will result in improved hip extension during stance.

156

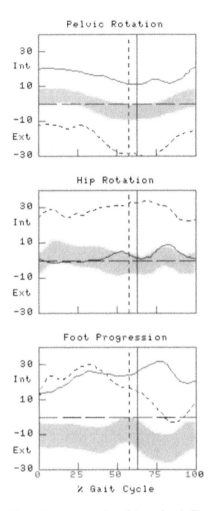

Fig. 11.10. Transverse plane kinematic representation of the patient in Figure 11.9. Asymmetry is noted in the pelvis and hips with symmetrical foot progression (right side—solid lines, left side—broken lines). (Reproduced by permission from Õunpuu 2002.)

UNDERSTANDING THE IMPACT OF HIP FUSION

Hip fusion in some cases is the procedure of choice in painful hip disease such as avascular necrosis (Fulkerson 1977, Roberts and Fetto 1990). It is important to understand the implications of hip fusion on the contralateral hip. Although hip fusion is only possible as a unilateral procedure, the contralateral hip may also have pathology. The increased sagittal plane range of motion of the contralateral hip, which is a secondary effect of the hip fusion was not appreciated prior to examination of sagittal plane hip kinematics. To compensate for the hip fusion, during ambulation, the pelvis moves through an increased arc of motion to allow the thigh segment to rotate from a distal portion of the segment anterior at initial

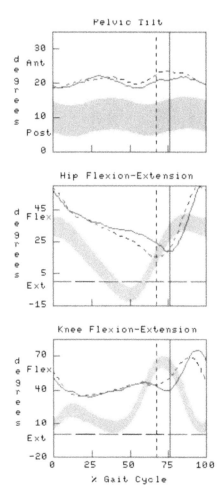

Fig. 11.11. The sagittal plane motion of the pelvis, hip, knee and ankle in comparison to normal patterns. Excessive knee flexion due to excessive ankle dorsiflexion results in associated skewing of hip motion towards flexion.

contact to posterior at toe-off during stance, with the reverse in swing. The pelvis thus shows its point of maximum anterior tilt at toe-off and posterior tilt at initial contact (Fig. 11.12). The opposite hip is in maximum flexion during the time of maximum anterior pelvic tilt and in maximum extension during the time of maximum posterior pelvic tilt. As a result, the opposite hip shows greater than normal motion consistent with the increase in pelvic motion. There is a mean increase in sagittal plane pelvic motion of 15° (SD 3°) in persons with hip fusion (Õunpuu *et al.* 1998). The associated increase in contralateral hip motion may explain some of the contralateral hip-joint pain reported in these patients. In this case, gait analysis data allowed the clinician to appreciate the secondary affect of surgery and understand one of the common postoperative sequalae of hip fusion.

158

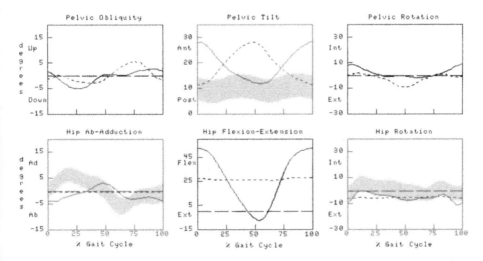

Fig. 11.12. A comparison of coronal, sagittal and transverse plane motion of the pelvis and hip for the involved (broken lines) and non-involved (solid lines) sides of a patient with unilateral hip fusion. Due to the fusion, there is no motion of the hip joint in the three planes. On the contralateral side (solid line), there is increased motion in the sagittal plane as a secondary effect of the fusion and associated required pelvic motion.

HIP MOTION IN PERSONS WITH MYELOMENINGOCELE (L4 FUNCTIONAL LEVEL)

Significant muscular weakness is associated with L4 functional level myelomeningocele, and motion at the hip is a direct result of this weakness and the associated trunk/pelvic motion needed to attain forward progression (Õunpuu *et al.* 1996). The abnormal hip motion occurs in primarily the coronal and transverse planes (Fig. 11.13). In the coronal plane, the hip shows progressive abduction in stance and adduction in swing. This is counterintuitive initially as these patients have minimal to no hip abductor strength and visually we see adduction as the knee rotates medially during loading response. Understanding hip motion in this case comes through examination of the pelvis and trunk segment motion in the same plane. During loading response, there is a lateral trunk lean to minimize or eliminate the requirement for hip abductor force (strength). A joint kinetic analysis substantiates this need. To allow for the lateral trunk lean, the pelvis is elevated on the swing side with a relative depression (drop) on the stance side. During this pelvic elevation on the swing side, the stance hip moves into abduction, not under the force of hip abductors but due to the lateral momentum of the trunk.

In the transverse plane, hip motion shows a significant increase in range with progressive internal rotation in stance and external rotation in swing. This motion is not produced by the hip rotators, but is secondary to the increased transverse plane rotations of the pelvis and trunk. In swing, there is a large internal rotation of the trunk and pelvis to assist as a "motor" in forward progression with an associated external rotation in stance. During the internal rotation of the trunk and pelvis, there is an associated external rotation of the hip that allows the knee to continue to point forward. Similarly, in stance, along with the

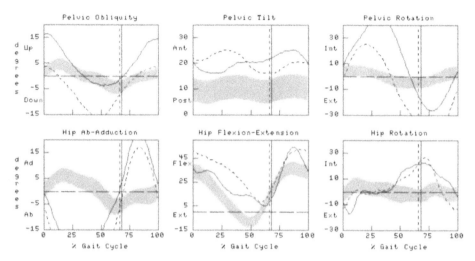

Fig. 11.13. The coronal, sagittal and transverse plane rotations of the pelvis and hip for a person with L4 level myelomeningocele. Increased hip range of motion in comparison to typical values (gray band) is seen primarily in the coronal and transverse planes.

external rotation of the trunk and pelvis, there is an associated internal rotation of the hip that again allows the knee to continue to point in the forward direction. Having an appreciation of these large ranges of motion may have an impact on our treatment decision-making because of the improved understanding of hip motion and ultimately may make us question the longevity of the hip joint functioning in this manner over time.

THE LIMPING GAIT PATTERN

The "limping" gait pattern is a common gait abnormality with a wide variety of etiologies. The clinician's focus, at least initially, tends to be on the most visual abnormality, which in many cases may be the compensation for the primary problem. This can often lead to a missed or delayed diagnosis and delay in needed treatment. One classic example is in the child with the unilateral toe initial contact gait with early heel rise in stance, which is the secondary compensation in children with unilateral dislocated hip prior to onset of hip pain. The toe contact and early heel rise is the first abnormality that is noted, as clothing typically "hides" the primary deviation: abnormal pelvic motion during gait. In patients with unilateral hip dislocation, there is functional weakening of the ipsilateral hip abductors with an associated drop of the contralateral pelvis during single limb stance (Fig. 11.14). To compensate for this functional shortening of the stance limb and lengthening of the swing limb, the child will develop an early heel rise to allow clearance of the swing limb and minimize vertical excursion of the center of gravity. Over time, this walking pattern can lead to heel-cord tightness on the involved side. Full-body three-dimensional gait analysis or at minimum good simultaneous video recording in the sagittal and frontal planes with the pelvis (ASISs) exposed and marked allows the clinician to differentiate between the primary problems and the secondary compensations.

160

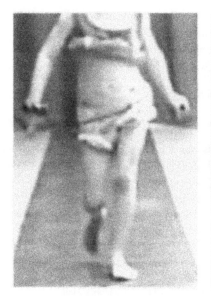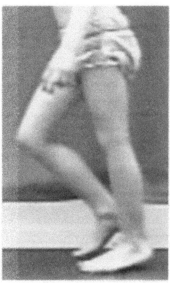

Fig. 11.14. Frontal and side views of a patient walking with unilateral left hip dislocation. The lateral view shows an early heel rise as compensation for the functional lengthening of the swing limb. This is required as the swing side of the pelvis drops as seen in the frontal view. The early heel rise allows for better clearance of the swing limb and is the secondary compensation for the primary problem, left hip dislocation. (Reproduced by permission from Õunpuu 2002.)

Conclusion

Hip pathology can lead to a variety of abnormalities in hip motion during gait. An understanding of hip motion is important in the assessment of the severity of pathology and in many cases the initial diagnosis. Careful observation of hip motion with the patient in appropriate clothing to allow appreciation of the pelvis and thigh segment motion is critical. Drawing relationships between hip motion and related clinical examination measures can further complete the clinical picture. In many cases, however, visual observation may be difficult and misleading, and a three-dimensional gait analysis will be necessary.

One of the roles of gait analysis is to provide objective documentation of hip function in three dimensions during motion. With hip-joint rotation profiles (kinematics) and in many cases joint kinetic data (not discussed in this chapter), the clinician can better understand the biomechanical basis of gait abnormalities and thus better differentiate between the primary problems and secondary compensations. With this information, the clinician can make more informed treatment decisions, which are ultimately based on their philosophy of treatment, as gait analysis data do not dictate a particular treatment protocol. Finally, gait analysis provides the clinician with an objective measurement of outcome related to dynamic function. Objective measurement of outcome leads not only to improved understanding of the biomechanical basis of movement abnormalities, but ultimately to new treatment protocols when we observe that a particular treatment approach leads to unexpected outcomes. Clinicians have benefited significantly from the knowledge gained through gait analysis and can apply that knowledge to new patients, some of whom may not need a full three-dimensional approach. However, systematic use of three-dimensional gait analysis in treatment decision-making and evaluation in all of our patients will lead to new insights. The only possible long-term consequence with this approach is improved outcomes.

REFERENCES

Bleck, E.E. (1987) *Orthopaedic Management in Cerebral Palsy. Clinics in Developmental Medicine No. 99/100.* London: Mac Keith Press.

Davis, R., DeLuca, P. (1996) 'Clinical gait analysis: current methods and future directions.' *In:* Harris, G., Smith, P. (Eds) *Human Motion Analysis: Current Applications and Future Directions.* Piscataway, NJ: IEEE Press, pp. 17–42.

Delgado, E., Schoenecker, P.L., Rich, M.M., Capelli, A.M. (1996) 'Treatment of severe torsional malalignment syndrome.' *Journal of Pediatric Orthopedics*, **16**, 484–488.

Duffy, C.M., Hill, A.E., Cosgrove, A.P., Corry, I.S., Mollan, R.A., Graham, H.K. (1996) 'Three-dimensional gait analysis in spina bifida.' *Journal of Pediatric Orthopedics*, **16**, 786–791.

Fulkerson, J.P. (1977) 'Arthrodesis for disabling hip pain in children and adolescents.' *Clinical Orthopaedics and Related Research*, **128**, 296–302.

Gage, J.R. (1991) *Gait Analysis in Cerebral Palsy. Clinics in Developmental Medicine No. 121.* London: Mac Keith Press.

Greenwood, D.T. (1965) *Principles of Dynamics.* Englewood Cliffs, NJ: Prentice-Hall.

Meister, K., James, S. (1995) 'Proximal tibial derotational osteotomy for anterior knee pain in the miserably malaligned extremity.' *American Journal of Orthopedics*, **24**, 149–155.

Õunpuu, S. (2002) 'Gait analysis in orthopaedics.' *In:* Fitzgerald, R.H., Kaufer, H., Malkani, A.L. (Eds.) *Orthopaedics.* St Louis: C.V. Mosby, pp. 86–107.

Õunpuu, S., Davis, R., DeLuca, P.A. (1996) 'Joint kinetics: methods, interpretation and treatment decision-making in children with cerebral palsy and myelomeningocele.' *Gait and Posture*, **4**, 62–78.

Õunpuu, S., R. B. Davis, DeLuca, P.A., Kimball. H., Mencio, G., Gorton, G., Masso, P. (1998) 'Surgical hip fusion: gait kinematics and kinetics.' *Gait and Posture*, **7**, 159.

Perry, J. (1992) *Gait Analysis: Normal and Pathological Function.* Thorofare, NJ: Slack.

Roberts, C., Fetto, J. (1990) 'Functional outcome of hip fusion in the young patient: Follow-up study of 10 patients.' *Journal of Arthroplasty*, **5**, 89–96.

Ruwe, P.A., Gage, J.R., Ozonoff, M.B., DeLuca, P.A. (1992) 'Clinical determination of femoral anteversion. A comparison with established techniques.' *Journal of Bone and Joint Surgery, American Volume*, **74**, 820–830.

Tylkowski, C.M. (1982) 'Internal rotation gait in spastic cerebral palsy.' *In:* Nelson, J.P. (Ed.). *The Hip: Proceedings of the 10th Open Scientific Meeting of the Hip Society.* St. Louis: C.V. Mosby, pp. 89–125.

12
CEREBRAL PALSY

J. Mark H. Paterson

Cerebral palsy (CP) is the name given to a group of disorders occurring in young children in which disease of the brain causes impairment of motor function (Ingram 1995). Although the central lesion is non-progressive, the resulting disorders of movement and posture and their peripheral effects on the musculoskeletal system of the child typically change with growth and development of the child.

The characteristic motor disorder is spasticity, defined as a hyperexcitable stretch reflex, which gives rise to increased tone in muscles and ultimately reduced muscle growth and contractures. To this pyramidal lesion are frequently added elements of extrapyramidal dysfunction giving rise to movement disorders such as athetosis and dystonia (Rymer 1992). This results in a wide spectrum of physical disability ranging from mild hemiplegia to severe spastic quadriplegia. The latter is now frequently referred to as total body involvement (TBI) cerebral palsy as it helps to remind us that these children have other problems in addition to the motor dysfunction in their limbs. For instance, muscle imbalance may cause scoliosis or spinal curvature in the coronal plane. In addition, some of these children have major difficulties with swallowing or a seizure disorder, with implications for surgical management (Stanley *et al.* 2000).

Spasticity leads to reduced excursion of muscles and hence reduced range of joint movement. Furthermore, some muscle groups are inevitably affected more than others, leading to the possibility of joints being drawn into increasingly deformed and fixed positions. This will clearly have an adverse effect on function of that segment. If the deformity exceeds the stable range of that joint's function, there is a risk of progressive dislocation. This risk is greatest in children with TBI cerebral palsy and least in those children with unilateral or bilateral CP who develop good functional walking ability.

Why should we be concerned about hips dislocating in children who do not have standing or walking potential? As will be seen in the following sections, such displacement is often associated with pain. Increasing restriction of abduction makes cleaning and toileting difficult. Seating and lying posture is increasingly affected, and ultimately there are adverse effects on the pelvis and spine.

In this chapter we will firstly explore the mechanisms by which the hip is affected in CP, then move on to consider what can be done to prevent these problems developing. As will be seen, this is not always successful, and further sections will cover the management of both early hip displacement and established hip dislocation. Finally, and on a somewhat different note, hip problems in the walking child with CP will be discussed.

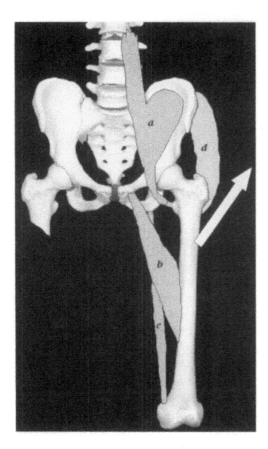

Fig. 12.1. Key muscles stabilizing the hip. In cerebral palsy, the iliopsoas (a), adductors (b) and hamstrings (c) often overcome the power of the abductors (d), causing displacement of the hip.

Pathology of the hip in CP

The hip joint is a ball-and-socket joint. It has some inherent stability on account of its bony structure, with additional protection against displacement provided by a fibrous rim or acetabular labrum. Further stability is provided by the tough fibrous capsule that surrounds the joint. Finally, there is the stability provided by the muscles acting around the joint. It is these latter structures which are responsible for the hip problems in CP.

Figure 12.1 shows the key muscles involved in retaining the hip in its normal or reduced position. In children with normal neuromuscular development the actions and power of these muscles is balanced. Unfortunately, in children with CP this is not necessarily the case.

Normally the hip joint is reasonably stable at birth. The acetabulum develops further within the first four years of life to provide greater depth and hence greater stability. This acetabular development only occurs if the femoral head is in normal apposition with the acetabulum. Any tendency for the femoral head to drift away from a fully reduced position in the first few years of life will reduce the stimulus for acetabular growth. This may give rise to a secondary acetabular dysplasia in which the socket is shallower and less constraining than would normally be the case.

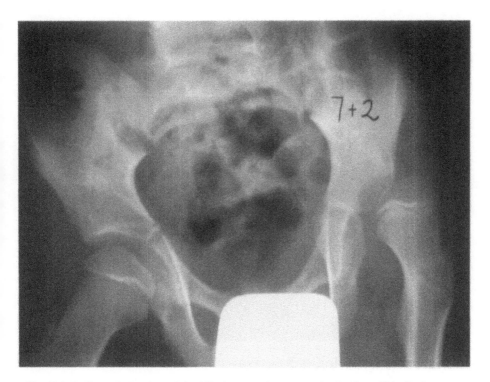

Fig. 12.2. Radiograph showing pelvic obliquity occurring as a result of unilateral hip displacement.

Prenatal development of the hip is generally normal in children with CP. As spasticity develops, it generally affects certain muscle groups more than others. At the hip, the muscles most often affected are the adductors and iliopsoas. These muscles resist stretch, and although they may not be particularly powerful, they become functionally short and easily overcome the less-affected abductor and extensor muscles. Thus, there is a tendency for the hip to be displaced laterally and proximally. The precise direction of displacement depends to a certain extent on the individual child and his or her postural preferences. The hip increasingly lies in an adducted and flexed posture with reduction in range of abduction and extension. This leads to increased uncovering of the femoral head. Further muscle imbalance and contracture of the deforming adductors and flexor causes the hip joint to lose its congruency, and the femoral head will start to move out of the acetabulum. This is known as subluxation of the hip.

The situation is complicated greatly by the fact that we have two hips, and that symmetrical involvement is the exception rather than the rule in CP. The pelvis may be pulled into an oblique position by the adduction contractures on the more heavily involved side, while the less involved side may be quite abducted. With further adduction and flexion contractures, tilt and rotational deformities also occur in the pelvis (Fig. 12.2).

The consequences of these pelvic events are seen in the spine, which will tend to become distorted by the torsional and angulatory forces emanating from the pelvis. This may

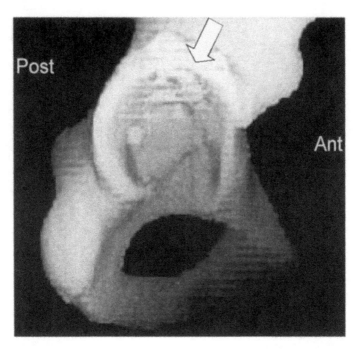

Fig. 12.3. CT scan of 9-year-old girl with femur subtracted: the acetabulum is usually deficient superiorly.

exacerbate pre-existing scoliosis. However, this is not always the case, and some children dislocate both hips in a symmetrical fashion, maintaining a level pelvis and a straight spine.

Subluxation occurs at a variable rate, depending on many factors. These include the degree of asymmetry as mentioned above, skeletal growth, and importantly, the posture of the child.

As the hip joint loses congruency, there will be increasing deformity of both the femoral head and the acetabulum. The area of articular surface of the femoral head no longer in contact with its acetabular counterpart will become worn and damaged by continuous pressure against a stretched hip capsule and surrounding gluteal muscles, and this damage may in some long-standing cases preclude consideration of surgical reconstruction. The direction of the displacement varies from child to child, and may reflect individual postural characteristics. Commonly, however, the head moves superiorly or postero-superiorly out of the socket, wearing away the rim of the acetabulum as it does so (Fig. 12.3).

Eventually, the displaced femoral head or heads leave the acetabulum behind and ride up the side of the pelvic wall. In the established case of dislocation the femoral head may actually be palpable in the soft tissues of the buttock.

Hip displacement is detected radiologically on anteroposterior radiographs of the pelvis (Fig. 12.4). Serial films should demonstrate if the subluxation is progressive, but if these films are to be meaningful these radiographs must be made in a standardized manner. This involves making sure that the lower limbs are in neutral rotation and that the effects on pelvic

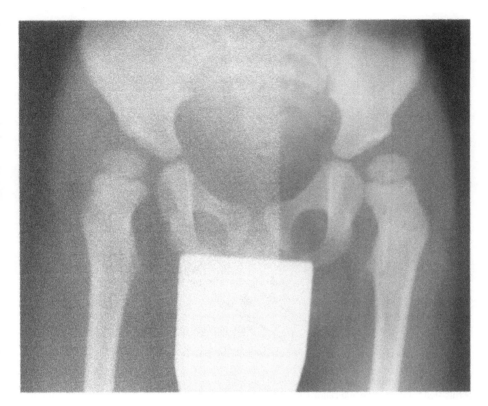

Fig. 12.4. Radiograph showing bilateral symmetrical hip subluxation in a non-walking child with total body involvement.

tilt of flexion contracture at the hips are neutralized by supporting the limbs in flexion (Fig. 12.5). Hip displacement is quantified by using Reimer's migration percentage (MP) (Reimers 1980). In addition, acetabular development is monitored by serial measurements of the acetabular index (AI) (Fig. 12.6).

Preventing hip dislocation in cerebral palsy

Scrutton *et al.* (2001) showed that hip migration occurs early in children with CP. By the age of 18 months, the MP and AI in this population were found to be significantly different from those found in normally developing children. It is thought that this may be due to poor movement ranges in infancy.

However, not every child with abnormal radiological parameters at this early age need go on to develop frank dislocation. There is evidence that if the femoral head can be centralized within the acetabulum by the age of 4 years, long-term stability is likely.

It is important to identify those hips at risk of progressive subluxation. This can only be achieved by instituting a formal surveillance protocol. Scrutton *et al.* (2001) have recommended that all children with bilateral CP have an anteroposterior radiograph of the

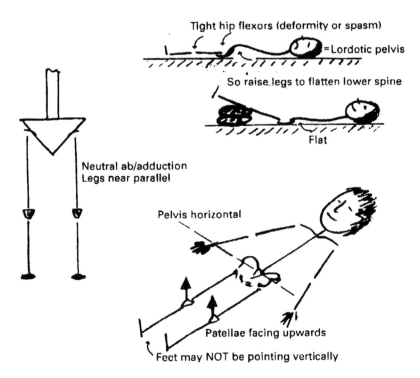

Fig. 12.5. Standardized radiographs enable meaningful comparisons of serial films. (Reproduced by permission from Scrutton and Baird 1997.)

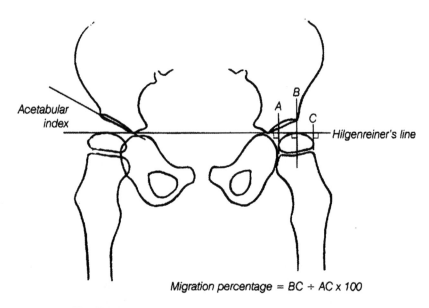

Migration percentage = BC ÷ AC x 100

Fig. 12.6. Reimer's migration percentage and the acetabular index.

pelvis made in a standardized position at the age of 30 months. Radiographs at an earlier age result in a high false-positive rate as they will show up cases that will continue to stabilize spontaneously.

Children with hip migration of less than 15% at 30 months of age and who are able to walk at least a few steps unassisted are at little risk of subsequent significant hip displacement. On the other hand, a migration percentage of greater than 33% at this age is indicative of certain progressive subluxation.

Having identified those children whose hips are showing signs of displacement, it is essential that close attention is paid to achieving and maintaining full ranges of hip movement, and to achieving and maintaining appropriate posture in sitting, lying and assisted standing where appropriate. Pountney *et al.* (2000) have written on postural management of children in this situation. The programmes involve positioning in equipment, active exercise, hands-on therapy, and education of parents and carers. A recurring theme is the need to maintain symmetry in lying, sitting or standing without restricting movement. A retrospective study has demonstrated that the timely introduction of 24-hour postural management may reduce the incidence of progressive hip subluxation (Pountney *et al.* 2002).

Orthopaedic management of early or mild displacement

Despite the best efforts of therapists and carers, some children's hips will continue relentlessly on their course towards dislocation. In addition, there will inevitably be cases that for some reason have escaped earlier surveillance. The orthopaedic surgeon is thus confronted with a child who has one or both hips in a displaced position and in whom joint ranging and postural management have failed to stabilize the joint(s). For the purposes of this discussion, early or mild displacement is taken as meaning an MP of up to 50%.

In some children, it is possible to show that on abduction the hip becomes centralized. In these cases it is tempting simply to prescribe an abduction brace (Fig. 12.7). Although one might take some comfort from the knowledge that the hips are enlocated when the brace is being worn, such orthoses are frequently poorly tolerated, and there is the problem of not knowing how long such treatment should continue.

There may be greater enthusiasm for a combined use of bracing plus myoneural blockade in the form of botulinum toxin A injections or ethanol injections. Injection treatment of the adductors can help to increase abduction range and improve tolerance of an abduction orthosis (Fig. 12.8).

Recently there has been increased enthusiasm for selective dorsal root rhizotomy to reduce the tone in muscles innervated by the lower lumbar and upper sacral nerve roots. The resultant decrease in muscle tone has improved functional ambulation in children whose gait pattern is severely restricted by spasticity (Steinbok 2001).

The standard surgical treatment for hips that are showing mild but progressive subluxation is a soft tissue surgery involving lengthening of the tendons of the contracted deforming muscles. The adductor longus can safely be divided in the groin near its origin on the pubis (Fig. 12.9), together with the gracilis muscle. In the non-walking child, tenotomy of the iliopsoas can safely be performed through the same groin incision (complete defunctioning of the iliopsoas muscle is contraindicated in children with walking potential—see below).

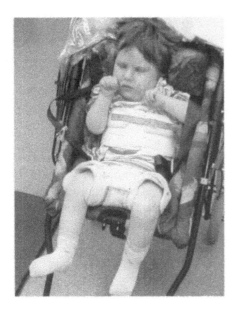

Fig. 12.7. One type of abduction brace, here combined with a spinal orthosis.

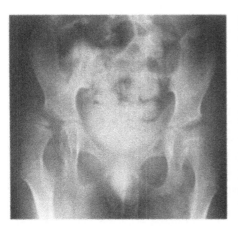 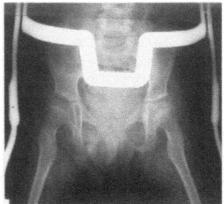

Fig. 12.8. Radiographs before and after botulinum toxin injection of the adductors and institution of an abduction brace, showing satisfactory reduction of the subluxated right hip.

Traditionally the above procedure was combined with a division of the anterior branch of the obturator nerve in order to defunction permanently both the adductor longus and adductor brevis. However, this is associated with a definite incidence of subsequent abduction contracture in which the hips are fixed in wide abduction. This makes seating, transport and care difficult, and many surgeons do not now add the neurectomy.

Many surgeons advise bilateral soft-tissue surgery even if only one hip is subluxed. The reason for this is shown in Figure 12.10. It is not uncommon to see a rebound flexion

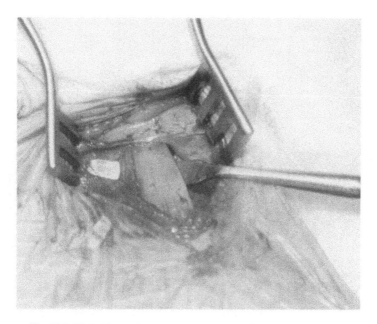

Fig. 12.9. The adductor longus tendon in the groin just prior to division.

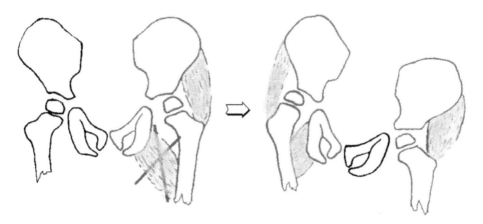

Fig. 12.10. The perils of unilateral soft-tissue surgery. The diagram shows how a secondary abduction contracture can swing the pelvis back the other way, promoting adduction contracture on the contralateral hip, the so-called 'seesaw' or 'teeter-totter' pelvis.

and adduction contracture of the contralateral hip following unilateral adductor and psoas release.

Postoperative management varies from unit to unit. The author's personal preference is for a short period (about three weeks) of immobilization in an abduction 'broomstick' cast followed by a vigorous return to daily stretches and joint ranging. Close attention must

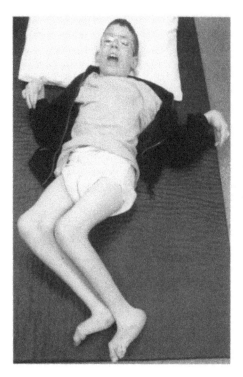

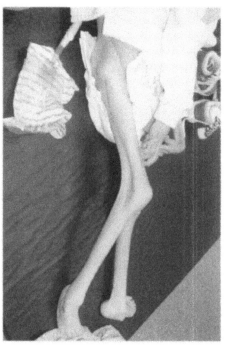

Fig. 12.11. 'Windswept' posture characteristic of unilateral hip displacement in severe CP.

Fig. 12.12. This cachectic child with poor gag reflex and seizure disorder represents a serious operative risk for hip reconstruction surgery.

be paid at this time to arrangements for seating and lying; simple measures such as seat pommels to maintain abduction and symmetry can be beneficial, and consideration should be given to provision of lying support systems.

Therapists often express concern about the amount and extent of physical activity that should be allowed for children with threatened or actual hip dislocation. Orthopaedic surgeons are commonly asked whether a particular patient with a subluxed hip should go on using a standing frame. There are no good data on whether or not this kind of activity provokes further subluxation. One should remember that the hip joint is subject to substantial forces even when lying down, and the author's personal attitude is that children with subluxed hips should be permitted to continue with their standing activity as long as it is comfortable and as long as placement in the frame is easy to achieve.

Orthopaedic management of severe displacement
As subluxation of the hip or hips continues, there is an increasing likelihood of pain. There will be increasing restriction of hip abduction, making cleaning and dressing difficult. If the dislocation is unilateral, the child will assume an increasingly 'windswept' posture (Fig. 12.11) that creates major problems with both lying and sitting positions. Contact pressures on chair and bed are concentrated on abnormal sites causing pain and tissue damage.

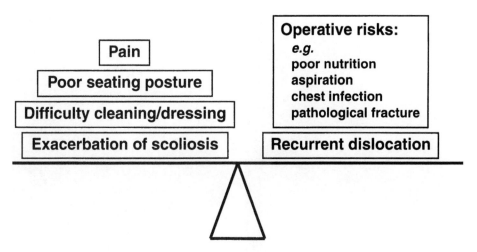

Fig. 12.13. A difficult balance: the 'pros and cons' of hip reconstruction.

As explained above, the pelvic asymmetry will ultimately translate into spinal deformity. If the child was previously able to use a standing frame, this ability will be jeopardized.

The whole issue of pain in the dislocating hip is a complex one. The intensity of pain experienced is very variable; some children appear to be able to dislocate, their hips without any significant discomfort whereas others have almost intractable pain. In severely disabled children it may be very difficult to know if they are actually in pain, or if the pain they are in is in fact coming from the hip. In some children, pain is a relatively transient phenomenon experienced as the hip teeters on the brink of dislocation; once completely free of the confines of the acetabulum it may become painless. However, this cannot be relied upon to happen.

Surgery to reduce and reconstruct the severely subluxated and the frankly dislocated hip should not be undertaken lightly. The surgery involves a combination of extensive soft-tissue releases (often on both hips) as well as bony realignment in the proximal femur and the pelvis (Root *et al.* 1995). It is tempting to reduce the surgical burden by missing out one or more of these elements of the procedure, but this will lead to poor results and recurrence of the dislocation. On the other hand, surgery of this nature is very extensive and would constitute a significant risk even in able-bodied children. In the case of a child with TBI cerebral palsy, the risks are greatly increased. These children are frequently in a poor general condition (Fig. 12.12). They may be malnourished and this will have an adverse effect on wound healing and overall recovery from this major surgery. Impaired swallowing and cough reflexes increase the risk of aspiration and postoperative chest infection. There may be exacerbation of seizure disorder. Cast immobilization is accompanied by a risk of pathological fractures in osteopaenic bones.

When one considers all these points, it becomes clear that the decision to proceed to reconstructive surgery is a difficult one. The various issues are summarized in diagrammatic form in Figure 12.13.

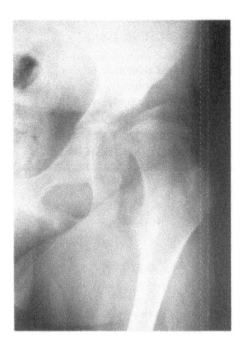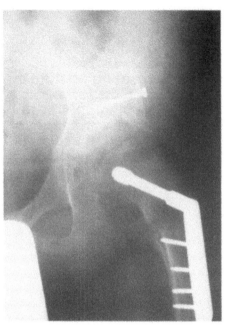

Fig. 12.14. Eleven-year-old boy with severely subluxed hip treated by soft-tissue releases, varus and rotational femoral osteotomy and acetabular shelf augmentation.

The aims of reconstructive surgery of the dislocated hip in CP are firstly to obtain a concentric reduction of the femoral head in the acetabulum, and then to achieve as much stability as possible so as to minimise the risk of recurrent dislocation (Fig. 12.14).

Preoperative preparation is extremely important. The child needs to be assessed fully by a paediatrician. There is no urgency for this surgery, and if necessary it should be deferred until steps have been taken to ensure that the child's nutritional status and respiratory function have been optimized.

The operation starts with extensive soft-tissue releases. This includes lengthening of the adductors and hamstrings proximally, together with iliopsoas tenotomy if this is still intact. The next stage of the procedure is the proximal femoral osteotomy. Fluoroscopy will help to determine whether varus angulation or external rotation of the femur is indicated to achieve reduction of the hip, and how much of each is required. Although it may initially appear that decreasing the neck–shaft angle by performing a varus femoral osteotomy is going to be the prime procedure, the hip is commonly reduced more convincingly by internally rotating the limb, thereby neutralizing the marked femoral anteversion seen in these hips (Fig. 12.15). If this is the case, an appropriate amount of rotation is built into the osteotomy.

Having reduced the hip by the proximal femoral osteotomy, a decision has to be made with respect to the acetabulum. In a few cases, it may be that the femoral procedure alone has produced a concentric reduction with adequate cover by the acetabulum (Fig. 12.16).

174

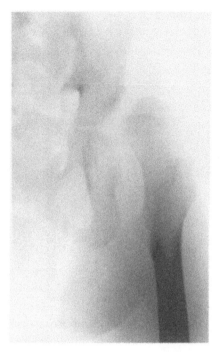

Fig. 12.15. The apparently high neck–shaft angle (valgus neck) is an illusion; this appearance is due to marked femoral anteversion. This hip reduced on full internal rotation and was therefore managed by an external rotation femoral osteotomy. Note the deficient acetabulum which also required attention.

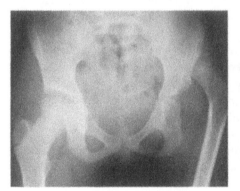 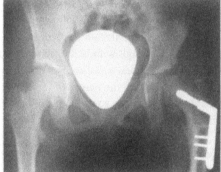

Fig. 12.16. Complete unilateral dislocation treated by soft-tissue releases and femoral osteotomy (combined varus and rotational). In this case no acetabular procedure was required for maintenance of stable reduction.

More commonly, there will still be a deficiency of cover that needs to be filled in order to prevent re-dislocation. Many bony procedures have been used for this purpose. Some, such as the shelf procedure seen in Figure 12.14, aim to augment a deficient acetabulum by fashioning an extension to the roof of the acetabulum with bone from the adjacent wing of the ilium. Others achieve the objective of hip stabilization by altering the shape of the

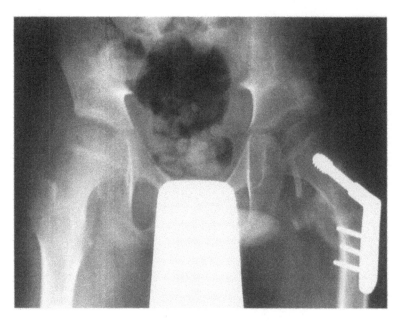

Fig. 12.17. Results of combined femoral osteotomy and Dega-type pelvic osteotomy.

socket through osteotomies around the acetabulum (*e.g.* the Pemberton and Dega procedures—Fig. 12.17). It may well not be necessary to open the hip joint itself, although some surgeons like to tighten the stretched joint capsule.

In unilateral dislocations there may be an abduction contracture on the opposite hip. Unless this is dealt with at the same time as the hip reconstruction, pelvic obliquity will remain uncorrected and there is a real threat of recurrent dislocation.

Depending on the nature of the pelvic procedure a full hip spica may or may not be employed. However, some degree of immobilization to maintain hip abduction is generally indicated for the first six weeks after surgery.

Postoperative recovery has been revolutionized by the use of epidural analgesia. This removes the need for respiratory-depressant opiate analgesia and reduces postoperative spasm and associated distress.

The risk of recurrent subluxation and dislocation is a real one, even when all components of the surgery are performed. Most surgeons would accept a recurrence rate of about 20%.

Heroic reconstructive surgery may well be inappropriate in certain cases. In a long-standing dislocation, the femoral head may be too deformed to consider reduction. In the event of recurrent dislocation after major reconstructive surgery there may be an understandable lack of enthusiasm on the part of all concerned for revision reconstruction. Under these circumstances, painful dislocation in a non-walker can be treated by proximal femoral excision. In this surgery, the proximal femur is removed up to and including the lesser trochanter (Fig. 12.18). This leaves a 'flail hip' which is generally comfortable and mobile and which can be positioned appropriately for sitting and lying. This procedure has devel-

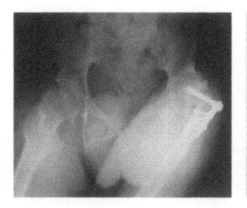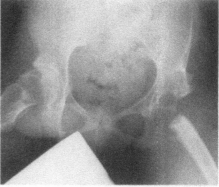

Fig. 12.18. Proximal femoral excision performed for intractable pain and poor position following failed hip containment surgery in a 16-year-old boy with severe total body involvement CP. Note the extensive resection required for a good result.

oped a bad reputation in some quarters for failing to relieve pain. However, in many cases this appears to be because insufficient femur was removed; this is not the Girdlestone femoral head and neck resection of the pre-hip arthroplasty era. Provided an adequate resection is made and steps are taken to reduce the incidence of heterotopic bone formation (nonsteroidal anti-inflammatory medication, postoperative traction), satisfactory pain relief can be expected in 80% of cases.

The hip in children who walk

The same pathological principles apply to the walking child with CP as to the TBI nonwalker. However, weight bearing appears to confer a stability to the joint which is absent in the child who is unable to stand and walk. Thus, it is unusual for a child with walking ability to dislocate a hip.

In the walking child, the muscle imbalance and consequent contractures manifest themselves not so much as a deforming force on the hip joint but rather as a derangement of the normal complex sequence of muscle activity that comprises normal gait.

In CP it is a mistake to consider any joint in isolation, and this is particularly so in the child with walking ability. Abnormalities of ankle and knee motion have a direct effect on hip function, and vice-versa.

In the sagittal plane, the principal problems are those of excessive hip flexion (often with a fixed flexion contracture) and inadequate hip extension. These are frequently seen in association with a stiff flexed knee and foot, and ankle deformities arising from contractures of the triceps surae. Fixed flexion deformity of the hip leads to a forward tilt of the pelvis, which in turn will cause an increase in the lumbar lordosis.

In the coronal plane, the spastic adductor muscles make it difficult to separate the lower limbs in gait and may give rise to 'scissoring' of the lower limbs. This is a major impediment to forward progression and makes for an extremely inefficient gait pattern.

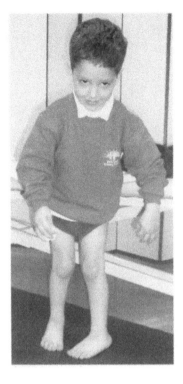

Fig. 12.19. Marked femoral anteversion in a walking child with diplegia.

In the transverse plane, the main problem is usually excessive internal rotation of the lower limb (Fig. 12.19). This is due to increased anteversion of the femoral neck and is thought to develop as a result of abnormal and unbalanced muscle action.

These abnormalities cannot properly be assessed by conventional static 'on couch' examination. CP is a disorder of movement and posture, and accurate evaluation of its problems demands a dynamic assessment. Some form of gait analysis is mandatory if surgical intervention is to be considered (Õunpuu *et al.* 2002).

Such analysis may be used to determine the appropriate surgical approach. At the hip this might include lengthening of the adductors and iliopsoas tendons. Adductor release will allow separation of the limbs, improves balance, and reduces the frequency of knee collisions in gait. Iliopsoas should be lengthened rather than divided completely in walking CP patients; some preservation of hip flexion is required to initiate gait. The lengthening is best performed as an intramuscular lengthening within the pelvis (Novachek *et al.* 2002).

It is not uncommon for any child to have increased femoral anteversion, leading to an in-toed gait pattern. In the absence of neuromuscular disorder, this is not a major problem and the majority of such children do not require any treatment. However, in the child with CP, the fact that the knee and ankle are angled inwards from the line of gait progression throws additional strains on an already compromised sequence of movements in gait.

Consideration should therefore be given to restoring a more normal rotational profile to the lower limbs by performing derotation osteotomies in the femur. This may be done at either the proximal or distal ends of the femur. This bony surgery may be combined with any of the above soft-tissue surgery, but care must be exercised in a proximal osteotomy as the change in rotational profile can alter the mechanics of the muscles acting around the hip. Modern internal fixation techniques make prolonged immobilization unnecessary, and the child may be allowed to bear weight almost immediately.

These hip operations may be performed together with other procedures designed to address problems at knees and ankles as well. The success of so-called multilevel CP surgery depends on high quality preoperative dynamic assessment, careful patient selection, and the commitment and comprehension on the part of the patient to undergo prolonged and intensive postoperative rehabilitation (Cooperman *et al.* 1987, Bagg *et al.* 1993).

REFERENCES

Bagg, M.R., Farber, J., Miller, F. (1993) 'Long-term follow-up of hip subluxation in cerebral palsy patients.' *Journal of Pediatric Orthopedics*, **13**, 32–36.
Cooperman, D.R., Bartucci, E., Dietrick, E., Millar, E.A. (1987) 'Hip dislocation in spastic cerebral palsy: Long term consequences.' *Journal of Pediatric Orthopedics*, **7**, 268–276.
Ingram, T.T.S. (1955) 'A study of cerebral palsy in the childhood population of Edinburgh.' *Archives of Disease in Childhood*, **30**, 85–98.
Novachek, T.F., Trost, J.P., Schwartz, M.H. (2002) 'Intramuscular psoas lengthening improves dynamic hip function in children with cerebral palsy.' *Journal of Pediatric Orthopedics*, **22**, 158–164.
Õunpuu, S., DeLuca, P., Davis, R., Romness, M. (2002) 'Long-term effects of femoral derotation osteotomies: An evaluation using three-dimensional gait analysis.' *Journal of Pediatric Orthopedics*, **22**, 139–145.
Pountney, T.E., Mulcahy, C.M., Clarke, S.M., Green, E.M. (2000) *The Chailey Approach to Postural Management.* Birmingham, England: Active Design.
Pountney, T., Mandy, A., Green, E., Gard, P. (2002) 'Management of hip dislocation with postural management.' *Child: Care, Health and Development*, **28**, 179–185.
Reimers, J. (1980) 'The stability of the hip in children. A radiological study of the results of muscle surgery in cerebral palsy.' *Acta Orthopaedica Scandinavica Supplementum*, **184**, 1–100.
Root, L., LaPlaza, F.J., Brourman, S.N., Angel, D.H. (1995) 'The severely unstable hip in cerebral palsy. Treatment with open reduction, pelvic osteotomy, and femoral osteotomy with shortening.' *Journal of Bone and Joint Surgery, American Volume*, **77**, 703–712.
Rymer, W.Z. (1992) 'The neurophysiological basis of spastic muscle hypertonia.' *In:* Sussman, M. (Ed.) *The Diplegic Child: Evaluation and Management. Shriners Hospital for Crippled Children Symposium.* Rosemont, IL: American Academy of Orthopaedic Surgeons, pp. 21–29.
Scrutton, D, Baird, G. (1997) 'Surveillance measures of the hips of children with bilateral cerebral palsy.' *Archives of Disease in Childhood*, **76**, 381–384.
Scrutton, D., Baird, G., Smeeton, N. (2001) 'Hip dysplasia in bilateral cerebral palsy: incidence and natural history in children aged 18 months to 5 years.' *Developmental Medicine and Child Neurology*, **43**, 586–600.
Stanley, F., Blair, E., Alberman, E. (2000) *The Cerebral Palsies: Epidemiology and Causal Pathways. Clinics in Developmental Medicine No. 151.* London: Mac Keith Press.
Steinbok, D. (2001) 'Outcomes after selective dorsal rhizotomy for spastic cerebral palsy.' *Child's Nervous System*, **17**, 1–18.

13
MYELOMENINGOCELE

John V. Banta

Spina bifida is the most commonly encountered form of neural-tube defect (NTD), with an incidence of approximately 0.5–1 per 1000 pregnancies in the USA (American Academy of Pediatrics 1999). Worldwide, NTDs are estimated to occur in around 300,000 fetuses per year, with the highest recorded incidence being in northern China where the estimated incidence is 4.8 per thousand pregnancies of at least 20 weeks gestation (Berry *et al.* 1999). Technically, the term myelomeningocele refers to an NTD in which the lesion consists of a failure of closure of the neural tube resulting in an open lesion in the midline that represents a herniation of the meninges through a defect in the posterior neural arch (a bifid spine), and which contains neural elements (Fig. 13.1). NTDs constitute a wide spectrum of conditions ranging from anencephaly that is uniformly fatal, to the commonly encountered myelomeningocele and less common disorders including lipomeningocele, meningocele (an open defect with herniation of only the meninges without any neural elements in the sac), myelocystocele (a cystic expansion of the spinal cord into a meningocele defect), and occult lesions such as spinal cord lipomas and diastematomyelia (split cord malformation) (Shurtleff and Lemire 1995). The last mentioned conditions are of increasing importance today since the discovery of the preventative benefit of folate supplementation, and prenatal detection and termination of pregnancy have reduced the incidence of myelomeningocele in many countries throughout the developed world. In this chapter I will first describe the classic findings in the child with myelomeningocele and the impact of varying degrees of paralysis on the hip joint before describing in detail the more occult disorders, followed by a discussion of the surgical rationale for treatment of the hip in these conditions (Lindseth 1976).

Embryonic development of the neural tube
In the developing embryo a neural groove appears at stage 8 (post- ovulatory day 18), and neural folds begin fusion at the junction of the brain and the spinal cord as neural crest cells arise from the neural ectoderm. Final closure of the neural tube occurs at the somite level 31, which corresponds to the second sacral level at four weeks of embryonic development. A second stage of secondary neurulation occurs with differentiation of the tail bud (O'Rahilly and Muller 1994). Closure of the neural folds is still incompletely understood but is thought to include three cellular mechanisms; interactions of cell surface glycoproteins, interdigitation of cell surface filopodia, and formation of intercellular junctions (Dias and Pang 1995). For a detailed description of the neural development of the spinal cord and the various congenital malformations the reader is directed to Pang (1995).

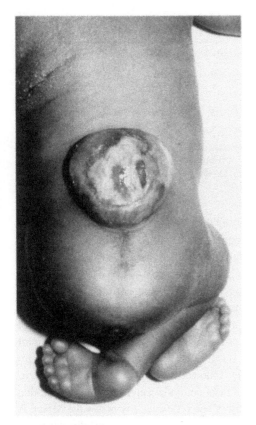

Fig. 13.1. Newborn infant with a mid-lumbar level myelomeningocele prior to surgical repair. Note the exposed dura surrounded at the periphery by early granulation and epithelialization. The hips are contracted and there is bilateral talipes equinovarus foot deformity.

Hydrocephalus occurs in approximately 90% of patients with myelomeningocele. The cause of hydrocephalus is related to numerous mechanisms including obliteration of the subarachnoid space and aqueductal blockage that is associated with the Chiari II malformation. Type II includes three components: the cerebellum, the hindbrain and the fourth ventricle, with herniation of the caudal brainstem in the foramen magnum (Dias and Pang 1995). The survival rate of children born with open lesions accompanied by hydrocephalus was less than 10% prior to the development of modern shunt techniques to control the hydrocephalus (van Gool and van Gool 1986, Shurtleff and Lemire 1995, Banta 1996).

Clinical assessment
The location of the level of the NTD, in general, determines the level of the neurologic involvement, which can range from complete paralysis of the lower trunk and lower extremities in high thoracic lesions to varying degrees of paralysis of the lower extremities in lesions located in the lumbar and sacral levels. The neurosegmental level of muscle activity in the lower extremity is most commonly classified as noted in Table 13.1.

By convention the muscle strength is graded by the definitions laid down in the Medical Research Council report on investigation of peripheral nerve injuries (University of Edinburgh 1943) (Table 13.2).

181

TABLE 13.1

Neurosegmental level of muscle activity in the lower extremity*

Level	Function
Thoracic	Flail lower extremities
Lumbar 1–2	Hip flexion/adduction
Lumbar 3	Knee extension
Lumbar 4	Knee flexion
Lumbar 5	Ankle dorsiflexion
Sacral	Ankle plantar flexion or more

*Asher and Olson (1983).

TABLE 13.2

MRC muscle strength grading system*

Grade	Function
0	Flail
1	Trace
2	Full range with gravity eliminated
3	Full range against gravity
4	Full range against some resistance
5	Normal strength

*University of Edinburgh Department of Surgery (1943).

The Chiari II malformation poses a significant threat to the newborn infant since hindbrain herniation can cause respiratory stridor, apnea, vocal changes, aspiration pneumonia, feeding disorders and shunt malfunction. Chiari II complications are the most common cause of death during the first four years of life (Guthkelch 1986).

In evaluating the neurologic status of the child with myelomeningocele it is generally accepted that the most precise assessment of motor function cannot be ascertained until the child is at least 3–4 years of age (Beaty and Canale 1990). The initial assessment is further complicated by the fact that as many as 30% of affected individuals have an upper motor neuron component to the paralysis. Stark and Baker (1967) evaluated the neurological involvement of the lower limbs of newborn infants followed for two years and described four distinct types of spinal cord involvement. The most common pattern was that of a lesion causing complete or partial loss of motor, sensory and reflex activity below the defect. A second type of lesion may spare terminal portions of the spinal cord such that distal isolated portions of the cord may function causing hypertonic muscle tone, exaggerated reflex activity or absence of spontaneous movement but lower-limb movement in response to stimulation above the level of the lesion. Prior to the advent of newer imaging techniques, they also correctly proposed that the lower-extremity functional loss might result from a cerebral rather than a spinal cord abnormality (Fig. 13.2). Furthermore, the ability to precisely determine the level of the neurologic lesion is further compounded by the fact that movement of one lower extremity may cause reflex or synergistic movement of the contralateral extremity on the basis of a reflex arc in the lower cord. With the emergence of magnetic resonance imaging techniques the pathological findings of the spinal cord in patients with myelomeningocele have been noted to include hydromyelia, diastematomyelia, lipomas and spinal cord atrophy, all of which can contribute to upper motor neuron lesions superimosed upon the paralytic segment of the spinal cord (Szalay et al. 1987). Recent long-term studies of older children confirm that spasticity can adversely affect the function of not only the lower but also the upper extremities. Mazur et al. (1986) evaluated 101 patients of whom 31% were identified as having thoracic level involvement, 56% lumbar level, and 13% sacral. A total of 54% of these cases presented with flaccid lower and normal upper extremities, 9% with flaccid lower and spastic upper extremities, 24% spastic lower, and 13% with spastic lower and upper extremities. In certain instances of high-level involvement this spasticity

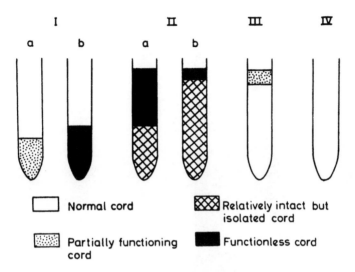

Fig. 13.2. Stark and Baker's hypothetical lesions of the myelodysplastic spinal cord, illustrating the various possibilities for a superimposed upper motor neuron lesion superimposed upon the paralytic component. (Reproduced by permission from Stark and Baker 1967.)

TABLE 13.3
Classification of functional ambulatory skills in the individual with myelomeningocele*

Community	Walks indoors and outdoors for *most* activities, and may need crutches or braces, or wheelchair for long distances
Household	Walks only indoors with appliances. Self-transfers from chair to bed with little or no assistance
Non-functional	Ambulates in home therapy sessions only
Non-ambulatory	Wheelchair dependent. *Usually* can transfer from chair to bed

*Hoffer *et al.* (1973).

interferes with the patient's ability to function to such a degree that intraspinal rhizotomy and distal cordectomy is sometimes indicated (McLaughlin *et al.* 1986).

The most common concern of parents of a newborn child with a paralytic defect is whether or not their child will be able to ambulate as s/he matures. Hoffer *et al.* (1973) established the classic definition of functional ambulatory skills in the patient with myelomeningocele, based upon long-term evaluation of 55 patients followed over a period of five years at the Rancho Los Amigos Hospital (Table 13.3).

Several authors have noted the relative prognostic significance of the strength of the quadriceps muscle function as it relates to future walking ability. Schopler and Menelaus (1987) evaluated 109 children and concluded that those with motor grade 4 or 5 at age 3 years have a high probability of retaining community ambulatory skill at a later age. However, it has been noted that those children with preservation of at least medial hamstring function have a much better prognosis for retained walking ability (Banta 2002). This is due

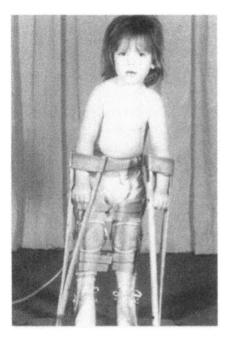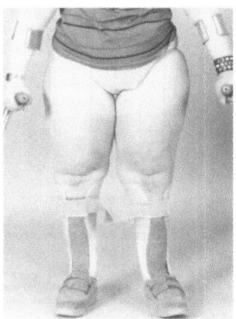

Fig. 13.3. Clinical photographs of the same patient at ages 3 and 15 years demonstrating the "law of mass" in which the body increases in strength by the square (the cross-sectional measurements of the intact muscles) while the mass increases as the cube measured as width, depth and height.

primarily to the fact that the additional one or two motor levels provide not only some knee flexor control but more importantly also offer some weak extensor motor power at the hip joint, since the hamstring origins from the ischial tuberosity are located posterior to the axis of flexion and extension of the hip joint. Further recent multivariate statistical analysis of factors affecting ambulation by Samuelsson and Skoog (1988) showed that the neurologic level, age, and the presence of scoliosis but not hip reduction were major predictive factors.

Asher and Olson (1983) evaluated the factors affecting ambulatory potential in 98 patients at an average age of 14 years and concluded that the functional motor level, age, obesity, musculoskeletal deformity and motivation were the most important factors. However, the most significant determinant was the cost of energy expenditure.

The underlying principle of a person's strength relative to their size was first elucidated by Galileo in 1631 as the "law of mass", which simply stated: "volume expands as the cube of bodies' dimensions, while strength increases only as much as their square" (Sobel 2000). Thus it is evident that with further growth, a child who is capable of walking with assistive devices with permanent paralysis of some lower extremity muscles will eventually exceed their functional strength as their weight increases. Clinically this is reflected in the fact that most children by the second decade of life recognize the relative cost of their energy expenditure with reciprocal walking with crutches and/or orthoses compared to the relative efficiency of a wheelchair for mobility (Fig. 13.3).

Finally, all clinicians treating children with NTDs must be aware of the risk of latex allergy in this unique patient population. It is recognized that up to 30% of children with NTDs will have a heightened sensitivity to latex, which in the worst case can be fatal with an acute anaphylactic reaction. It is now recommended that these patients be treated in both the clinical and surgical setting in a totally latex-free environment (Birmingham *et al.* 1996, Michael *et al.* 1996, Drennan 1999).

There have been few long-term studies of the outcome of patients with spina bifida. Barden *et al.* (1975) reviewed 143 patients, of whom 63 were followed long-term. Twenty-nine were still alive at ages 20 to 43 years. Only two of nine with thoracic-level paralysis ambulated, whereas 19 of 20 with a third lumbar motor level did so. Of interest, the status of the hip did not correlate with their ability to walk. One-third were self-supporting, yet one-half of the patients had scoliosis. Kinsman and Doehring (1996) reviewed 98 adult patients and noted that 47% of the hospitalizations these patients incurred were preventable. The most common admitting diagnoses were urologic, renal calculi, pressure ulcers and osteomyelitis. Brinker *et al.* (1994) reviewed 36 adults aged 19 to 51 years who functioned in their youth at the sacral level and noted that 11 lost ambulatory skill, 14 lost plantar flexion, 15 lost sensation, and 27 developed skin breakdown. Given the fact that these patients have significant problems that affect their neurologic, urologic, social and orthopaedic function, it has been recommended that they be followed in an interdisciplinary setting in which all of the appropriate health-care specialists can coordinate their care (Kaufman *et al.* 1994).

Prenatal detection and prevention

Beginning in the mid-1970s maternal serum alphafetoprotein determination was developed to detect open NTDs. Unfortunately only approximately 75% of affected fetuses were detected, due in part to the fact that (a) the maternal serum levels were dependent upon the fetal age (as determined by ultrasound measurement techniques with less resolution), and (b) other congenital anomalies also caused elevated levels, hence it lacked both sensitivity and specificity. Detection improved to approximately 99% by the additional test of amniotic fluid for the presence of acetylcholinesterase (Brock *et al.* 1985). However, amniocentesis carries approximately a 1% risk of abortion following the intrauterine test aspiration procedure. (Milunsky *et al.* 1980, Seller 1994). Figure 13.4 demonstrates the comparison of the fetal ultrasound image with the clinical findings of a terminated fetus as well as the radiographic appearance of an extremely large dysraphic defect extending from the mid-thoracic spine to the sacrum. More recently, high-resolution maternal prenatal ultrasound techniques have been perfected such that currently the diagnosis of NTDs can be most accurately determined by examination of the fetal brain. Characteristic dilatation of the fetal brain with the recognition of the "lemon" and "banana" signs has proved more specific than the evaluation of the thoracic and lumbar spine for NTDs (Van den Hof *et al.* 1990, Seller 1994, Babcock 1995). Prenatal detection thus introduces ethical and moral issues, so that no single approach will be uniformly adopted by all societies. Boyd *et al.* (2000) evaluated the status of prenatal diagnosis of NTDs by ultrasonographic means in major European centers and noted a high prenatal detection of anencephaly but a large variation in prenatal detection

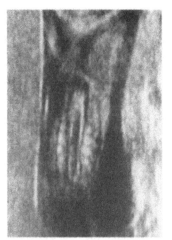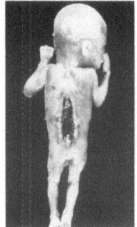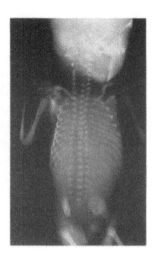

Fig. 13.4. The high-resolution ultrasound on the left illustrates the spinal defect prior to elective termination. The center photograph demonstrates the extent of the lesion in the fetus, with the radiograph on the right showing the magnitude of the spinal dysraphism extending from the upper thoracic region of the spine to the sacrum.

and termination rates between centers that reflected the current cultural and ethical differences in various populations.

In the latter half of the 20th century there were many studies suggesting that NTDs were caused by a vitamin deficiency. A major breakthrough occurred in 1991 with the reporting of the results of a randomized, double-blind trial in the UK by the Medical Research Council of women who had a previous history of an affected pregnancy (Lancet 1991). Those women receiving a daily dose of 4µg folic acid had up to 75% fewer affected offspring than women receiving minerals, vitamins, or vitamins plus a lower dose of folic acid. A further study in 1992 demonstrated the same protective effect of periconceptional folate in a group of 2500 women without a history of a previous affected pregnancy (Czeizel and Dudas 1992). A collaborative study was conducted in China with the United States Centers for Disease Control (Berry *et al.* 1999). Women in northern China who did not take folic acid had a 4.8 per 1000 pregnancy incidence of NTDs compared to 1.0 per 1000 pregnancies in women taking supplemental folate. The mean reduction in risk was measured at 41%, with a 95% confidence interval of 3–64%.

Honein *et al.* (2001) reported a 19% reduction in NTD birth prevalence following fortification of the US food supply in which the average fortifying dose was 100µg of folate. The fortifying dose was deliberately set low as reasoned by the Federal Drug Administration in fear that elderly women might develop a delay in the diagnosis of pernicious anemia. A major public health debate continues at this time regarding fortification of the food supply versus folate supplementation (American Academy of Pediatrics 1999, Oakley 2001).

Many clinical studies have noted a relationship between elevated plasma homocysteine levels and the development of arteriosclerosis comparable to the risks of hypercholesterolemia and smoking. (McCully 1998, Bostom *et al*. 1999). Rimm *et al*. (1998) reported a 14-year study suggesting that intake of folate and vitamin B$_6$ appears to reduce the incidence of coronary heart disease in females. In summary the evidence for folate supplementation reducing the incidence of NTDs is clear and there is highly suggestive evidence that it may also have a role in the reduction in arteriosclerosis in the adult population.

In the past three years there has been renewed interest in intrauterine surgery for the repair of the myelomeningocele in selected fetuses. The concept has evolved from an animal model in which it was shown that intrauterine repair of the open spinal defect resulted in prevention of hydrocephalus (see Bannister 2000). As Bannister stated:

> "If the brain defects arise in the embryonic period and undergo no further change and if the spinal cord is so deformed that it is functionless from the start, then operative intervention before birth will have no significant effect on the ultimate neurological defect. If, on the other hand, the brain lesions evolve during gestation and the deformed spinal cord has some useful function that can be lost by contact with the amniotic fluid or is susceptible to mechanical damage, then intrauterine surgery may have a beneficial role."

Clinical trials are now under way at several medical centers in the USA, although it will be several years before a sufficient number of cases can be followed in a randomized treatment setting.

Orthopaedic management of the hip

Based upon review of the pathophysiology of the myelomeningocele defect it is understandable that there has been great controversy concerning the best management for hip subluxation and dislocation in these children. Based upon the enormous clinical experience at the Sheffield Children's Hospital following the development of successful shunt implants, Sharrard (1967, 1983) analyzed the problem of hip dislocation seen there in many of the newborn infants and attributed this to the motor imbalance resulting from active hip flexor and adductor power in the presence of weak or absent hip extension and abduction power. He described a muscle transfer of the iliopsoas muscle (a primary hip flexor) through a window prepared in the ilium to insert into the tip of the greater trochanter to convert a primary hip flexor to provide hip abductor–extensor function. Subsequent analyses by other surgeons cast doubt on the validity of the proposal that motor imbalance alone was the cause of hip dislocation. Broughton *et al*. (1993) examined 802 patients of whom 28% had thoracic-level paralysis, 30% L1–L2 level, 36% L3, 22% L4, 7% L5, and 1% sacral-levels paralysis. They concluded that hip dislocation was not inevitable even with documented muscle imbalance. Furthermore, hip flexion contractures were commonly seen by the age of 9–11 years in patients with high thoracic-level paralysis, reflecting the fact that patients with high levels of paralysis spend much of their time seated in wheelchairs which over time without upright standing is known to lead to flexion contractures. Fraser *et al*. (1992) in a review of 55 children stated that all hips that developed instability due to motor imbalance did so within the first year of life, and they concluded that the neurologocal level of paralysis was the most valid predictor of walking potential. Carroll and Sharrard (1972) along with Menelaus (1976) reviewed 57 patients following an iliopsoas transfer and determined that the psoas muscle transfer alone would not produce hip extension in the absence of any gluteal (abductor and extensor) muscle power. Their conclusion was that "A child with poorly controlled hydrocephalus, poor balance, a high paraplegia, a lumbar kyphosis, and poor renal function, will never walk, no matter how many operations are done to stabilize his hips" (Carroll and Sharrard 1972).

The first evaluation of ambulatory function in children with bilateral hip dislocation was reported by Feiwell et al. (1978) with a review of 76 children over the age of 5 years comparing 41 cases with no hip reconstruction and 35 who underwent one or more surgical procedures. They concluded that surgery did not result in any increase in hip range of motion or walking ability or reduction in level of bracing. The best function was found in those patients with a good hip range of motion and a level pelvis. Sherk et al. (1991) compared 30 patients with untreated hip dislocation and 11 who had undergone surgical stabilization procedures. The untreated patients were pain free, with good motion and sitting ability. The operative group incurred numerous postoperative complications and three of them developed poor sitting balance. Heeg (1998) reviewed 19 patients with bilateral hip dislocation at an average age of 21 years at the time of review and concluded that dislocated hips should not be reduced.

Today there is consensus that teratologic dislocations noted at birth should not be subjected to attempted relocation, and bilateral dislocated hips should also be left out to avoid the serious problems of postoperative stiffness, and imbalance with a unilateral location and contralateral dislocation resulting in pelvic obliquity and loss of function. It should also be mentioned that treating a neonatal unstable hip with paralytic imbalance as if it were a developmental dysplasia of the hip with abduction orthoses is ill advised. Placing the child's hip in a flexed abducted splinted position will only lead to abduction and flexion contracture in the absence of hip abductor and extensor motor function.

The treatment objectives for all children with myelomeningocele should be to enhance mobility including self-transfer skills. In many instances this will require conversion from orthotic devices in the first decade of life to the use of a wheelchair in the second decade. In addition to mobility, interdisciplinary treatment should be directed to optimum upper-extremity function, education and, most importantly, social continence of bowel and bladder function, so that these individuals will be able to contribute to society to the greatest extent possible (Kaufman et al. 1994, Banta 2002).

Children presenting with mid- and low-lumbar motor function with active quadriceps and medial hamstring function are potential candidates for reconstructive surgery, which may include release of contractures, selected tendon transfers and osteotomies about the femoral neck and acetabulum (Phillips and Linseth 1992, Greene 1999, Schoenecker 2001, Banta 2002) (Fig. 13.5) Menelaus (1976) and (Stillwell and Menelaus 1984) recognized the problem of postoperative contractures, disuse osteopenia, cast-induced pressure sores, and loss of developmental skills with prolonged hospitalizations, and recommended careful preoperative planning and management directed toward a minimum number of operations and minimum periods of immobilization.

Current management of the child with paralysis about the hip is directed toward providing an upright experience for the young child with appropriate orthotic support to promote growth and development and self-transfer skills (Phillips et al. 1995) (Fig. 13.6). When

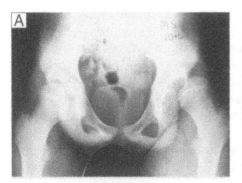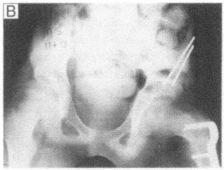

Fig. 13.5. (A) Anteroposterior view of the pelvis of a child aged 10 years 6 months with L5 level with progressive paralytic dysplasia of the left hip. (B) Postoperative radiograph demonsrating six months later the result of a varus intertrochanteric femoral osteotomy to redirect the femoral head into the acetabulum and an innominate osteotomy of the ilium to increase the acetabular coverage of the hip joint.

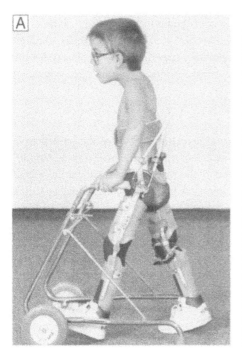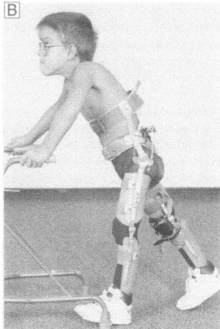

Fig. 13.6. (A) Child with L1 motor level (intact hip flexors) in a reciprocating type of hip–knee–ankle orthosis with a thoracic extension. This design is intended to let the patient initiate hip flexion with the swing leg while the posterior cable provides an extension moment to the weight-bearing stance leg.

(B) Upon initiation of the gait cycle the patient relies on the walker to provide upright support and the extensor effect of the reciprocating device is compromised as the trunk shifts forward with the ground reaction force anterior to the left foot. The energy cost of such an orthotic device for a high-level paraplegia is high.

necessary, selected release of soft-tissue contractures is approriate so long as both the treating physicians and the patient's family are appraised of the realistic long-term goals for their child's mobility (Greene 1999, Schoenecker 2001). With lower levels of paralysis, in children with predictable future community ambulatory skills, varus producing osteotomies to redirect the hip into the acetabulum (Dias and Hill 1980), adductor transfer to the ischium (London and Nichols 1975, Phillips and Lindseth 1992) and pelvic osteotomies to increase the acetabular coverage of the femoral head (Mannor *et al.* 1996) are sometimes indicated in selected cases (Fig. 13.5).

With increasing survival rates, surgeons have become aware of the serious problem of paralytic scoliosis. According to Raycroft and Curtis (1972), developmental scoliosis (paralytic) can be attributed to infra pelvic, intrapelvic and suprapelvic factors. Contractures about the hip joint can directly affect pelvic obliquity and contribute to progressive spinal deformity. The presence of a hip abduction contracture directly relates to the development of pelvic obliquity and subsequent scoliosis (Locke *et al.* 2001). Unilateral hip dislocation in the absence of contracture, however, does not contribute to pelvic obliquity and subsequent scoliosis (Keggi *et al.* 1992). A progressive hip-flexion contracture of the down-side pelvis frequently contributes to the progression of increased lordosis and scoliosis (Banta 1990). Even minor pelvic obliquity in a patient with insensate skin over the buttocks and lower extremities often leads to pressure sore formation (Drummond *et al.* 1985) For these reasons, children with upper levels of paralysis who are non ambulatory must be followed closely for the development of pelvic obliquity and progressive spinal deformity, which increases in direct proportion to the degree of motor paralysis.

Occult dysraphic lesions

It is evident from the recent advances in prenatal detection as well as the preventative potential of folate supplementation that the incidence of open NTDs will continue to fall. There is no evidence to date that the incidence of the more unusual congenital spinal anomalies is declining. Therefore it is important to review the less obvious anomalies which potentially can cause paralysis and if left untreated, adversely affect hip function and ambulation. Wilkinson and Sedgwick (1988) first described occult spinal dysraphism in a consecutive series of 117 children with established "congenital dislocation of the hip" (or developmental dysplasia of the hip as is now the preferred terminology—see Chapter 4) Three cases presented with abnormal cutaneous findings: a lumbosacral pigmented nevus; abnormal hair distribution; and a subcutaneous lipoma. All showed spina bifida occulta on radiographs of the lumbosacral spine. An additional five cases subsequently failed conventional treatment for a dislocated hip, and at the age of 2 years showed atrophy of the foot in the affected extremity and most suffered nocturnal enuresis. Although magnetic resonance imaging was not yet available at that time, abnormal somatosensory evoked potentials were noted in 57% of the 42 cases with occult or overt spinal dysraphism.

The most common so-called occult lesion is the *spinal cord lipoma*. The exact embryology of this lesion is incompletely understood but is thought to be associated with the formation of the caudal end of the spinal cord, which develops from the recanalization of the tail bud that is responsible for the caudal spinal cord formation, estimated to be between the second

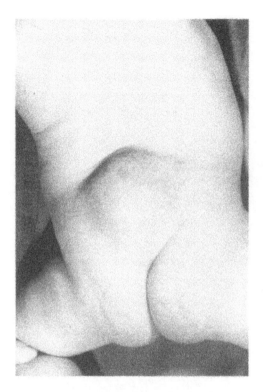

Fig. 13.7. Newborn infant with an obvious lipoma with eccentric swelling in the lumbo-sacral region. Note the hemangioma at the apex of the lesion. At surgery, a tract leading directly through the bifid posterior element to a large intradural lipoma was resected with the aid of an operating microscope and a laser. The child retained urologic and lower-extremity function.

lumbar segment and the conus (Pang 1995). Affected children show symptoms by the age of 2 years, since in all cases there is tethering of the filum terminale at the end of the spinal cord. Most cases show some cutaneous signs: subcutaneous lipoma, capillary hemangioma, skin dimple or skin tag, or rarely a hairy patch (Fig. 13.7). In some instances multiple signs are noted. The patient often shows neurologic deficits with lower-extremity weakness, and then bladder and bowel symptoms become evident as toilet training is attempted. Pain is an uncommon symptom; however, atrophy of the foot and calf musculature is clinically discernable in some cases (Fig. 13.8). Failure to diagnose the lesion leads to progressive neurologic loss that cannot be recovered after surgical release of the cord and removal of the lipoma (Pang 1995). Experimental studies in the cat have shown that traction on the distal spinal cord adversely affects the oxidative metabolism of the nerve cells, which with progressive tension result in further reduction of spinal cord perfusion leading to histologic damage and permanent neorologic loss (Yamada *et al.* 1981).

Lhowe (1987) reported clinical findings in 29 patients with congenital intraspinal lipomas who presented at an average age of 12.8 years. Only five cases were neurologically normal at presentation and these were all less than 6 months of age. The most common orthopedic problem was foot deformity, for which reconstructive surgery was only successful in those children who had resection of the lipoma prior to the foot surgery.

Diastematomyelia refers to the rare congenital abnormality of a double spinal cord that is divided by a cartilaginous or bony spur most often found in the thoracolumbar to the

191

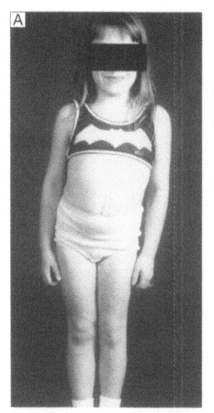

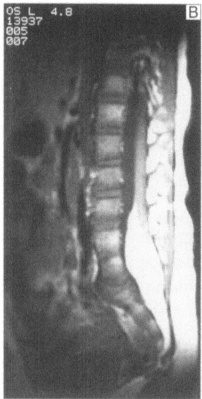

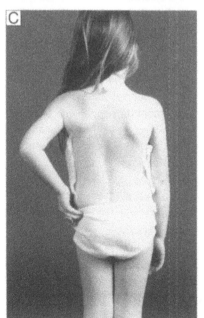

Fig. 13.8. (A) This child presented at age 3 years 6 months with limb-length inequality, left leg weakness, a club foot, congenital scoliosis and early bladder dysfunction. (B) MR image illustrating the massive intradural lipoma as well as the low-lying conus medullaris. (C) Posterior view of the patient following lipoma excision and hemivertebrectomy and spinal fusion at the lumbosacral level. Mild paralytic acetabular dysplasia is now developing and may require surgery. She had been treated for three years for the club-foot deformity without recognition of the underlying congenital spinal anomaly.

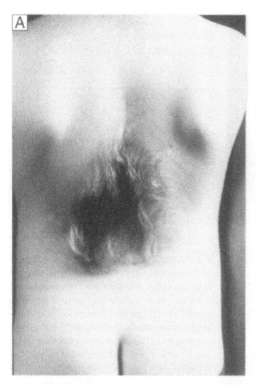

Fig. 13.9. (A) Hypertrichosis overlying a lower thoracic diastematomyelia.

(B) Radiograph *(left)* shows the midline bone spur together with widening of the inter-pedicular space. MR image *(right)* illustrates the midline diastematomyelia with duplication of the spinal cord.

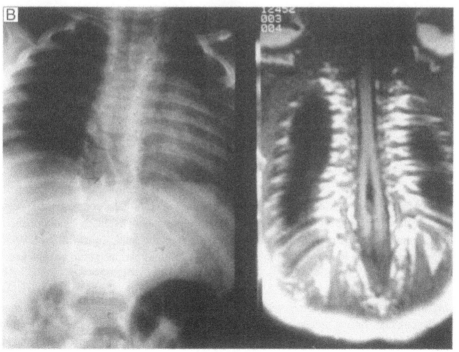

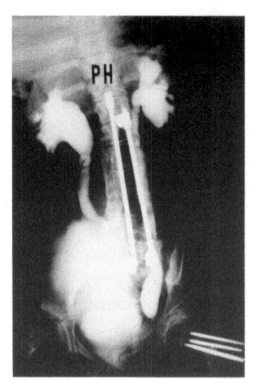

Fig. 13.10. Radiograph of an 11-year-old male with upper lumbar paralysis who previously had undergone operative pin fixation of a left hip fracture, as well as a successful posterior spinal fusion for paralytic scoliosis with Harrington instrumentation. Unfortunately this patient never received adequate urological evaluation and treatment, and he died of renal failure four months following this radiograph.

lumbosacral level of the spine. It is not uncommon in cases of myelomeningocele and is readily identified by conventional MRI. Pang (1995) has referred to diastematomyelia as representing one component of what he has described as a unified theory "split cord malformation", which he postulates is due to "the formation of an abnormal fistula through the midline embryonic disc that maintains communication between yolk sac and amnion, and enables continued contact between ectoderm and endoderm with the fistula." The fistula thus causes the split spinal cord, and variable motor loss may occur with lower-extremity weakness and sphincter disturbance.

Diastematomyelia is found in up to 30% of cases of myelomeningocele and is easily identified now by MRI. Other children present at birth with no neurologic findings but with a hairy patch over the midline of their spinal column (Fig. 13.9) Less common is the presence of an hemangioma or, rarely, a skin dimple. In the presence of a split-cord malformation, with spinal growth there is often increasing tension upon the spinal cord with subsequent neurologic loss that may affect sphincter function, as well as peripheral motor weakness.

Conclusion

In summary, the newborn infant with myelomeningocele presents a formidable challenge to the clinician since a precise classification of the neurologic deficit is often difficult to delineate within the first three to four years of life and may consist of both a lower and an upper motor neuron component. Ambulatory potential remains a major concern for the parents, and the most effective medical and surgical care can be provided by a coordinated team that includes not only the pediatrician, neurosurgeon and orthopaedist, but also, and of equal importance, a urologist and physical and occupational therapists as well as nursing and social service support (Fig. 13.10). The hip pathology demands a thorough understanding of currently accepted goals and objectives. Finally, pediatricians and general practitioners must be aware of the subtle more occult dysraphic lesions that may arise in what is thought to be an otherwise normal neonate.

REFERENCES

American Academy of Pediatrics: Committee on Genetics (1999) 'Folic acid for the prevention of neural tube defects.' *Pediatrics*, **104**, 325–327.
Asher, M., Olson, J. (1983) 'Factors affecting the ambulatory status of patients with spina bifida cystica.' *Journal of Bone and Joint Surgery, American Volume*, **65**, 325–356.
Babcock, C.J. (1995) 'Ultrasound evaluation of the prenatal and neonatal spina bifida.' *Neurosurgery Clinics of North America*, **6**, 203–218.
Bannister, C.M. (2000) 'The case for and against intrauterine surgery for myelomeningocele.' *European Journal of Obstetrics, Gynecology, and Reproductive Biology*, **92**, 109–113.
Banta, J.V. (1990) 'Combined anterior and posterior fusion for spinal deformity in myelomeningocele.' *Spine*, **15**, 946–952.
Banta, J.V. (1996) 'The orthopaedic history of spinal dysraphism. II. The modern surgical treatment.' *Developmental Medicine and Child Neurology*, **38**, 954–960.
Banta, J.V. (2002) 'Myeolmeningocele.' *In:* Fitzgerald, R.H., Kaufer, H., Malkani, A.L. (Eds.) *Orthopaedics.* St Louis: C.V. Mosby, pp. 1555–1566.
Barden, G.A., Meyer, L.C., Stelling, F.H. (1975) 'Myelodysplastics—Fate of those followed for twenty years or more.' Journal of Bone and Joint Surgery, American Volume, **57**, 643–647.
Beaty, J.H., Canale, S.T. (1990) 'Orthopaedic aspects of myelomeningocele.' *Journal of Bone and Joint Surgery, American Volume*, **72**, 626–630.
Berry, R.J., Li, Z., Erickson, J.D., Li, S., Moore, C.A., Wang, H., Mulinare, J., Zhao, P., Wong, L.Y., Gindler, J., Hong, S.X., Correa, A. (1999) 'Prevention of neural tube defects with folic acid in China. China–U.S. Collaborative Project for Neural Tube Defect Prevention.' *New England Journal of Medicine*, **341**, 1485–1490.
Birmingham, P.K., Dsida, R.M., Grayhack, J.J., Han, J., Wheeler, M., Pongracic, J.A., Cote, C.J., Hall, S.C. (1996) 'Do latex precautions in children with myelodysplasia reduce intraoperative allergic reactions?' *Journal of Pediatric Orthopedics*, **16**, 799–802.
Bostom, A.G., Silbershatz, J., Rosenberg, I.H., Jacques, P.F., Selhub, J., D'Agostino, R.B., Wilson, P.W., Wolf, P.A. (1999) 'Nonfasting plasma total homocysteine levels and all-case and stroke incidence in elderly persons. The Framingham Study.' *Annals of Internal Medicine*, **131**, 352–355.
Boyd, P.A., Weilesley, D.G., De Walle, H.F., Tenconi, R., Garcia-Minaur, S., Anwijken, G.R., Stoll, C., Czementi, M. (2000) 'Evaluation of the prenatal diagnosis of neural tube defects by fetal ultrasonographic examination in different centers across Europe.' *Journal of Medical Screening*, 7, 169–174.
Brinker, M.R., Rosenfeld, S.R., Feiwell, E., Granger, S.P., Mitchell, D.C., Rice, J.C. (1994) 'Myelomeningocele at the sacral level: Long-term outcomes in adults.' *Journal of Bone and Joint Surgery, American Volume*, **76**, 1293–1300.
Brock, D.J., Barron, L., van Heyningen, V. (1985) 'Prenatal diagnosis of neural-tube defects with a monoclonal antibody specific for acetylcholinesterase.' *Lancet*, **1**, 5–8.
Broughton, N.S., Menelaus, M.B., Cole, W.G., Shurtleff, D.B. (1993) 'The natural history of hip deformity in myelomeningocele.' *Journal of Bone and Joint Surgery, British Volume*, **75**, 760–763.
Carroll, N.C., Sharrard, W.J.W. (1972) 'Long term followup of posterior iliopsoas transplantation for paralytic dislocation of the hip.' *Journal of Bone and Joint Surgery, American Volume*, **54**, 551–560.
Czeizel, A.E., Dudas, I. (1992) 'Prevention of the first occurrence of neural-tube defects by periconceptional vitamin supplementation.' *New England Journal of Medicine*, **327**, 1832–1835.

195

Dias, L.S., Hill, J.A. (1980) 'Evaluation of treatment of hip subluxation in myelomeningocele by intertrochanteric varus derotation femoral osteotomy.' *Orthopedic Clinics of North America*, **11**, 31–37.

Dias, M.S., Pang, D. (1995) 'Human neural embryogenesis: A description of neural morphogenesis and a review of embryonic mechanisms.' *In:* Pang, D. (Ed.) *Disorders of the Pediatric Spine*. New York: Raven Press, pp. 1–23.

Drennan, J.C. (1999) 'Current concepts in myelomeningocele.' *Instructional Course Lectures*, **48**, 548–550.

Drummond, D., Breed, A.L., Narechania, R. (1985). 'Relationship of spine deformity and pelvic obliquity on sitting pressure distribution and decubitus ulceration.' *Journal of Pediatric Orthopedics*, **5**, 396–402.

Feiwell, E., Sakai, D., Blatt, T. (1978) 'The effect of hip reduction on function in patients with myelomeningocele.' *Journal of Bone and Joint Surgery, American Volume*, **60**, 169–173.

Fraser, R.K., Hoffman, E.B., Sparks, L.T., Buccimazza, S.S. (1992) 'The unstable hip and mid-lumbar myelo-meningoceles.' *Journal of Bone and Joint Surgery, British Volume*, **74**, 143–146.

Greene, W.B. (1999) 'Treatment of hip and knee problems in myelomeningocele.' *Instructional Course Lectures*, **48**, 563–574.

Guthkelch, N. (1986) 'Aspects of the surgical management of myelomeningoceles.' *Developmental Medicine and Child Neurology*, **28**, 525–532.

Heeg, M., Broughton, N.S., Menelaus, M.B. (1998) 'Bilateral dislocation of the hip in spina bifida: A long-term follow-up study.' *Journal of Pediatric Orthopedics*, **18**, 434–436.

Hoffer, M.M., Feiwell, E., Perry, J., Bonnet, C. (1973) 'Functional ambulaton in patients with myelomeningocele.' *Journal of Bone and Joint Surgery, American Volume*, **55**, 137–148.

Honein, M.A., Paulozzi, L.J., Mathews, T.J., Erickson, J.D., Wong, L.Y. (2001) 'Impact of folic acid fortification of the US food supply on the occurrence of neural tube defects.' *Journal of the American Medical Association*, 285, 2981–2986.

Kaufman, B.A., Terbrock, A., Winters, N., Ito, J., Klosterman, A., Park, T.S. (1994) 'Disbanding a multidisciiplinary clinic: Effects on the health care of myelomeningocele patients.' *Pediatric Neurosurgery*, **21**, 36–44.

Keggi, J.M., Banta, J.V., Walton, C. (1992) 'The myelodysplastic hip and scoliosis.' *Developmental Medicine and Child Neurology*, **34**, 240–246.

Kinsman, S.L., Doehring, M.C. (1996) 'The cost of preventable conditions in adults with spina bifida.' *European Journal of Pediatric Surgery*, **6**, Suppl. 1, 17–20.

Lancet (1991) 'Prevention of neural tube defects. Results of the Medical Research Council Vitamin Study. MRC Vitamin Study Research Group.' *Lancet*, **338**, 131–137.

Lhowe, D., Ehrlich, M.G., Chapman, P.H., Zaleske, D.J. (1987) 'Congenital intraspinal lipomas: Clinical presentation and response to treatment.' *Journal of Pediatric Orthopedics*, **7**, 531–537.

Lindseth, R.E. (1976) 'Myelomeningocele.' *Instructional Course Lectures*, **25**, 77.

Locke, M.D., Dias, L.S., Sarwark, J.E. (2001) 'The relationship between infrapelvic obliquity and scoliosis.' *In:* Sarwark, J.F, Lubicky, J. (Eds.) *Caring for the Child with Spina Bifida*. Rosemont, IL: American Academy of Orthopaedic Surgeons, p. 105.

London, J.T., Nichols, O. (1975) 'Paralytic dislocation of the hip in myelodysplasia. The role of the adductor transfer.' *Journal of Bone and Joint Surgery, American Volume*, **57**, 501–506.

Mannor, D.A., Weinstein, S.L., Dietz, F.R. (1996) 'Long-term follow-up of Chiari pelvic osteotomy in myelo-meningocele.' *Journal of Pediatric Orthopedics*, **16**, 769–773.

Mazur, J.M., Stillwell, A., Menelaus, M.B. (1986) 'The significance of spasticity in the upper and lower limbs in myelomeningocele.' *Journal of Bone and Joint Surgery, British Volume*, **68**, 213–217.

McCully, K.S. (1998) 'Homocysteine, folate, vitamin B6 and cardiovascular disease.' *Journal of the American Medical Association*, **279**, 392–393. *(Editorial.)*

McLaughlin, T.P., Banta, J.J., Gahm, N.H., Raycroft, J.E. (1986) 'Intraspinal rhizotomoy and distal cordectomy in patients with myelomeningocele.' *Journal of Bone and Joint Surgery, American Volume*, **68**, 88–94.

Menelaus, M.B. (1976) 'The hip in myelomeningocele. Management directed towards a minimum number of operations and a minimum period of immobilization.' *Journal of Bone and Joint Surgery, British Volume*, **58**, 448–452.

Michael, T., Niggemann, B., Moers, A., Seidel, U., Wahn, U., Scheffner, D. (1996) 'Risk factors for latex allergy in patients with spina bifida.' *Clinical and Experimental Allergy*, **26**, 934–939.

Milunsky, A., Alpert, E., Neff, R.K., Frigoletto, F.D. (1980) 'Prenatal diagnosis of neural tube defects. IV. Maternal serum alfa-fetoprotein screening.' *Obstetrics and Gynecology*, **55**, 60–66.

Oakley, G.P. (2001) 'Folic acid-preventable spina bifida.' *In:* Sarwark, J.F., Lubicky, J.P. (Eds.) *Caring for the Child with Spina Bifida: Shriners Hospitals for Children Symposium*. Rosemont, IL: American

Academy of Orthoapedic Surgeons, pp. 19–28.

O'Rahilly, R., Muller, F. (1994) 'Neurulation in the normal human embryos.' *In:* Bock, G., Marsh, J. (Eds.) *Ciba Foundation Symposium No. 181. Neural Tube Defects.* New York: John Wiley, pp. 70–89.

Pang, D. (1995) 'Split cord malformation: unified theory.' *In:* Pang, D. (Ed.) *Disorders of the Pediatric Spine.* New York: Raven Press, pp. 206–207.

Phillips, D.L., Field, R.E., Broughton, N.S., Menelaus, M.B. (1995) 'Reciprocating orthoses for children with myelomeningocele. A comparison of two types.' *Journal of Bone and Joint Surgery, British Volume,* **77,** 110–113.

Phillips, D.P., Lindseth, R.E. (1992) 'Ambulation after transfer of adductors, external oblique, and tensor fascia lata in myelomeningocele.' *Journal of Pediatric Orthopedics,* **12,** 712–717.

Raycroft, J.F., Curtis, B.H. (1972) 'Spinal curvature in myelomeningocele: Natural history and etiology.' *In:* *American Academy of Orthopaedic Surgeons Symposium on Myelomeningocele.* St Louis: C.V. Mosby, pp. 186–201.

Rimm, E.B., Willett, W.C., Hu, F.B., Sampson, L., Colditz, G.A., Manson, J.E., Hennekens, C., Stampfer, M.J. (1998) 'Folate and vitamin B6 from diet and supplements in relation to risk of coronary heart disease among women.' *Journal of the American Medical Association,* **279,** 359–364.

Samuelsson, L., Skoog, M. (1988) 'Ambulation in patients with myelomeningocele: A multivariate statistical analysis.' *Journal of Pediatric Orthopedics,* **8,** 569–575.

Schoenecker, P.L. (2001) 'Surgical management of the hip problems in children with myelomeningocele.' *In:* Sarwark, J.F., Lubicky, J.P. (Eds.) *Caring for the Child with Spina Bifida. Shriners Hospitals for Chlldren Symposium.* Rosemont, IL: American Academy of Orthopaedic Surgeons, pp. 130–135.

Schopler, S.A., Menelaus, M.B. (1987) 'Significance of the strength of the quadriceps muscles in children with myelomeningocele.' *Journal of Pediatric Orthopedics,* **7,** 507–512.

Seller, M.J. (1994) 'Risks in spina bifida.' *Developmental Medicine and Child Neurology,* **36,** 1021–1025.

Sharrard, W.J.W. (1967) 'Paralytic deformity in the lower limb.' *Journal of Bone and Joint Surgery, British Volume,* **49,** 731–747.

Sharrard, W.J.W. (1983) 'Management of paralytic subluxaton and dislocation of the hip in myelomeningocele.' *Developmental Medicine and Child Neurology,* **25,** 374–376.

Sherk, H.H., Uppal, G.S., Lane, G, Melchionni, J. (1991) 'Treatment versus non-treatment of hip dislocation in ambulatory patients with myelomeningocele.' *Developmental Medicine and Chlld Neurology,* **33,** 491–494.

Shurtleff, D.B., Lemire, R.J. (1995) 'Epidemiology, etiologic factors, and prenatal diagnosis of open spinal dysraphism.' *Neurosurgery Clinics of North America,* **6,** 183–193.

Sobel, D. (2000) *Galileo's Daughter.* Harmondsworth: Penguin.

Stark, G.D., Baker, G.C. (1967) 'The neurological involvement of the lower limbs in myelomeningocele.' *Developmental Medicine and Child Neurology,* **9,** 732–740.

Stillwell, A., Menelaus, M.B. (1984) 'Walking ability after transplantation of the iliopsoas: A long-term follow-up.' *Journal of Bone and Joint Surgery, British Volume,* **66,** 656–659.

Szalay, E.A., Roach, J.W., Smith, H., Maravilla, K., Partain, C.L. (1987) 'Magnetic resonance imaging of the spinal cord in spinal dysraphisms.' *Journal of Pediatric Orthopedics,* **7,** 541–545.

University of Edinburgh Department of Surgery (1943) *Aids to the Investigation of Peripheral Nerve Injuries: Medical Research Council War Memorandum No. 7, 2nd Edn, Revised.* London: HMSO.

Van den Hof, M.C., Nicolaides, K.H., Campbell, J., Campbell, S. (1990) 'Evaluation of the lemon and banana signs in one hundred thirty fetuses with open spina bifida.' *American Journal of Obstetrics and Gynecology,* **162,** 322–327.

Van Gool, J.D., van Gool, A.B. (1986) *A Short History of Spina Bifida.* Utrecht: Society for Research into Hydrocephalus and Spina Bifida.

Wilkinson, J.A., Sedwick, E.M. (1988) 'Occult spinal dysraphism in established congenital dislocation of the hip.' *Journal of Bone and Joint Surgery, British Volume,* **70,** 741–749.

Yamada, S., Zinke, D.E., Sanders, D. (1981) 'Pathophysiology of "tethered cord syndrome".' *Journal of Neurosurgery,* **54,** 494–503.

14
MUSCLE WEAKNESS DISORDERS

Brian G. Smith

Muscle diseases in children adversely impact gross motor function and can cause significant impairment in ambulation. Muscle weakness disorders frequently involve the proximal musculature, specifically the hip and shoulder girdle areas. Many children with muscle diseases in the USA are managed in clinics sponsored by the Muscular Dystrophy Association (MDA). These MDA programs provide disabled children with multidisciplinary care in the outpatient setting from pediatric subspecialists, including a neurologist, an orthopedist, and both physical and occupational therapists. This chapter will review the common muscle weakness disorders seen in the MDA clinic and their impact on the hip joint and its function. [For further information, the reader is referred to the textbook Muscular Disorders edited by Younger (1999).]

Muscular dystrophy

Duchenne's muscular dystrophy (DMD) is a progressive muscle wasting disorder usually inherited via an X-linked recessive mode. The incidence is about 1 in 3500 male births (Thompson and Berenson 2001). The natural history is one of gradual progression of muscle weakness and functional decline. Typically the boys cease ambulation around age 9–12 years, develop scoliosis often managed with spinal fusion from 11 to 14 years, and succumb to sequelae of respiratory or cardiac dysfunction at 16–24 years.

ETIOLOGY
The genetic defect in DMD is a deletion at the p21 locus on the X chromosome in an area coding for the protein dystrophin. In about 65% of patients a positive family history is present, although because the gene is relatively large, the mutation rate is high.

Dystrophin is a large protein but comprises only 1% of protein in skeletal muscle. Dystrophin has a critical role in regulation of calcium metabolism. A lack of dystrophin results in muscle cell membrane instability, causing excessive calcium accumulation within the muscle fiber and ultimately producing necrosis of the muscle cell. Muscle membrane instability in dystrophinopathies results in leakage of creatine phosphokinase (CPK) into the serum, with affected patients often demonstrating elevated CPK levels of over 10,000.

A dystrophin level below 1% of normal results in the diagnosis of DMD, while a level of 1–10% of normal is characterized as Becker's muscular dystrophy (BMD).

DIAGNOSIS
About 65% of patients can now be diagnosed by DNA analysis of a blood sample with

identification of a deletion in the X chromosome. The remaining patients presenting with motor weakness and an elevated creatine kinase (CK) level with a negative blood test for the deletion require a muscle biopsy in which dystrophin levels can be measured for confirmation of the diagnosis of DMD.

PRESENTATION AND DIFFERENTIAL DIAGNOSIS

Boys who have the subsequent diagnosis of DMD may have normal gross motor development in the first year or two of life. Frequent tripping and falling, toe-walking, difficulty climbing stairs, clumsiness and trouble keeping up with peers in sports are the complaints parents often cite in their boys aged 2–4 years at the time of presentation (Sussman 2002). Occasionally, calf enlargement is present as well, the manifestation of calf pseudohypertrophy that typically occurs in DMD patients.

The differential diagnosis includes BMD, dermatomyositis, spinal muscular atrophy (SMA), and the limb–girdle muscular dystrophies, including Emery–Dreifuss dystrophy. BMD can often be distinguished from DMD by the age at presentation, with DMD manifesting between 2 and 4 years and BMD commonly not presenting until age 8 or older. BMD and DMD are also distinguished based on the amount of dystrophin identified on muscle biopsy (Sussman 2002). Muscular dystrophy should always be included in the differential diagnosis of a boy who presents with toe-walking between the ages of 2 and 4 years.

CLINICAL COURSE

The gait pattern of DMD patients is characterized by a wide-based, stiff-kneed pattern that evolves over time to include excessive lordosis of the lumbar spine and toe-walking. As the weakness progresses over time, individuals with DMD fall more frequently and demonstrate the Gower's maneuver on attempting to arise from the floor (Fig. 14.1). Difficulty picking them up off the floor because of shoulder girdle weakness demonstrates the so-called "slip-through" sign.

With the weakness progressing over the years, contractures of the lower extremities develop in DMD patients. The muscles most commonly affected include the gastroc-soleus complex, hamstrings, hip flexors and tensor fascia lata. As the contractures worsen and the weakness of proximal musculature progresses, ambulation declines and usually ceases around the age of 10–13 years. Subsequently, DMD patients are dependent upon wheelchairs for mobility.

Typically within a year of utilizing a wheelchair, scoliosis will develop. It will progress because of growth and progressive weakness, compromising upright sitting position, exacerbating respiratory dysfunction, and limiting upper-extremity function in these patients. Spinal fusion surgery is the preferred management of the spinal deformity in these patients, and is typically recommended when the scoliosis reaches 20–30° and before the pulmonary function declines below 35%. Stabilization of the spine prevents progression of deformity and greatly enhances the quality of life of DMD patients by preserving sitting balance and avoiding pain.

The use of oral glucocorticoids, such as prednisone at a dose of 0.75 mg/kg/day, has been found to delay the progression of weakness in patients with DMD. Oral steroids are

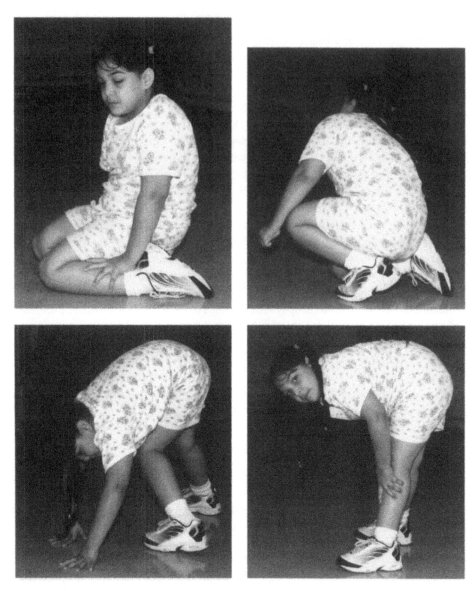

Fig. 14.1. Series of photos of an 8-year-old girl with limb–girdle muscular dystrophy rising from the floor, depicting the Gower's sign of using her body as a scaffolding to assist in attaining upright stance.

very commonly used in Europe and Canada as a means of medical management for this disorder. The side-effects of prednisone, including weight gain, osteopenia, delayed skeletal growth and mood changes, have limited its use in the USA. The US Food and Drug Administration has not yet approved some of the newer steroids (e.g. deflazacort) that have fewer of the above side-effects (Sussman 2002).

Hip Involvement

Boys with DMD will typically develop hip flexion–abduction contractures that make standing difficult but help to preserve and maintain the femoral head in the acetabulum. Consequently, hip subluxation and dislocation are rarely reported in these patients, who spend the last portion of their lives sitting in wheelchairs.

Hip flexion contractures are one of the lower-extremity deformities acquired by these patients, which may make recumbency difficult late in their lives. Minimizing contractures requires significant ongoing efforts by the patient's family and physical therapists to maintain hip extension. Frequent periods out of the wheelchair in a prone position for optimal stretching of hip flexors help to maintain hip range of motion (Drennan 1990).

Hip Physical Examination Findings

Many patients with DMD tend to gain excessive weight because they are wheelchair bound and relatively immobile. This makes transfer out of the wheelchair to an examining table difficult if a Hoyer-type lift system is not available. Consequently, examining DMD patients out of their wheelchair may be impossible, as it is often very difficult to lift the heavier patients. It should also be kept in mind that these patients are non-ambulatory and may be or have been on steroids, both contributing to osteopenia and heightened risk of long-bone fracture. In fact, the complaint of hip pain in a patient with DMD would warrant radiographic evaluation for possible stress fracture.

Physical examination findings in DMD patients include a hip flexion contracture by Thomas test. Typically these patients will also have an abduction contracture that would limit adduction of the hip. The Ober test is used to document the hip's abduction contracture (see Chapter 2). In the rare patients with hip subluxation or instability, the typical findings of a Galeazzi sign, limited abduction or femoral head instability may be present.

Radiographic Evaluation

Standard anteroposterior and frog lateral radiographs of the hips and pelvis are usually sufficient to satisfactorily evaluate the hips in a DMD patient. Since the patients are non-ambulatory, the radiographs of the pelvis are always done supine. Because flexion contractures of the hips are often present, a 20–25° cephalad-angled view may be more advantageous for assessing the femoral head position in the acetabulum.

Management

Prevention of hip flexion contractures is the first step in maintaining functional and painless hips in this population. Oral steroids such as prednisone or Deflazacort have been shown to maintain muscle strength and preserve functional status including standing. Preservation of standing can delay or minimize the development of both hip subluxation/dislocation and scoliosis (Sussman 2002).

Once contractures become fixed, hip flexor tenotomy may be included as part of a package of lower-extremity soft tissue releases in DMD patients (Smith *et al.* 1993). Iliotibial band tenotomy or resection is done to minimize the development of hip abduction contractures, which can sometimes be severe enough to make positioning in the wheelchair difficult.

Although the hip abduction contracture may cause some seating issues, it has a beneficial side-effect in that the femoral head is well directed into the acetabulum. The long-term prognosis for hip stability in these patients is favorable based on the tendency for abduction contractures of the hip.

This generally good prognosis for hips in DMD was countered in a recent study from the UK that reviewed the incidence of hip dislocation or subluxation in patients with DMD (Chan *et al.* 2001). In this study, 15 out of 54 patients were found on serial radiographs to have hip subluxation or dislocation. The authors speculated that pelvic obliquity may be one possible cause of subluxation, and recommended early spinal fusion for scoliosis as a means to minimize pelvic tilt. The recommendation from this study was for the periodic radiologic evaluation of hips in DMD patients. Femoral head dislocation can occur in these patients, but it is very rare in the experience of this practitioner. Since scoliosis occurs in 90% of patients with DMD (Sussman 2002), spinal deformity and hip flexion contractures seem to be the driving forces that contribute to hip instability in these patients.

LIMB–GIRDLE AND OTHER MUSCULAR DYSTROPHIES
Limb–girdle muscular dystrophy is a term used to designate a group of progressive muscle weakness disorders (Sussman 2002). These disorders include facio-scapulo-humeral dystrophy and Emery–Dreifuss dystrophy. These are much less common types of muscular dystrophy, and seldom involve children since the age at presentation is often the second or third decade of life. They are distinguished from DMD by significantly lower CPK levels, and the lack of pseudohypertrophy of the calves (Sussman 2002). Hip involvement is rare in these disorders, since patients often remain ambulatory well into adult life.

MYOTONIC MUSCULAR DYSTROPHY
Myotonic disorders are characterized by difficulty relaxing a muscle after contraction. Since the condition is usually inherited via autosomal dominant transmission, the severity of the clinical findings may be quite variable. Likewise, the age at presentation may vary from shortly after birth until the second decade of life (Drennan 1990).

Myotonic patients may present with heelcord contractures, and other clinical findings include scoliosis or kyphosis, cataracts, muscle hypertrophy and weakness, and cardiac conduction abnormalities. An expressionless face is also characteristic, and mild mental retardation may be present (Drennan 1990). Hip dysplasia is rare in these patients, most of whom remain ambulatory well into adult life.

Charcot–Marie–Tooth disease
Charco–Marie–Tooth disease (CMT) or hereditary sensory motor neuropathy (HSMN) is a disorder of peripheral neuropathy causing primarily distal motor weakness. Previously known as peroneal muscular atrophy, CMT is a characterized by variable clinical manifestations, heterogeneity of inheritance patterns, and varied levels of disability. The lower extremities are more commonly affected than the upper extremities, involvement is usually symmetric, and the weakness is slowly progressive during the patient's lifetime. Often transmitted via autosomal dominant inheritance, CMT may affect generations of an

involved family. Distal muscle weakness and subsequent contractures are present based on the pattern and level of involvement and may be quite variable even within the same family.

ETIOLOGY

Demyelination of peripheral nerves is the primary defect in the CMT/HSMN disorders. Demyelination occurs because of abnormalities in the protein myelin or its adherence to peripheral nerves. Myelin is the primary protein comprising the peripheral nerve sheath. In CMT, the abnormal myelin disrupts the nerve sheath, causing decreased neuronal input to the peripheral skeletal muscles. This is manifested in electrophysiology testing as decreased nerve conduction velocity, resulting clinically in muscular atrophy and eventually fibrosis (Smith 2002).

PREVALENCE AND CLASSIFICATION OF CMT NEUROPATHIES

The incidence of CMT is about 1 per 2500 births, with an estimated 125,000 affected individuals in the USA (Ionasescu 1995).

Initial designation of CMT types was based on electrophysiology findings including nerve conduction velocity (NCV). Disorders with excessively slow NCV were identified as demyelinating, while those with minimally decreased NCV were termed axonal.

The most common type is the demyelinating neuropathy CMT or HSMN type 1, affecting approximately 60% of patients. The axonal or "neuronal" CMT or HSMN type 2 may have a similar clinical presentation to type 1.

Recent advances in molecular genetics have resulted in an enhanced understanding of the CMT disorders. Duplications of gene 17p11.2 have been identified in CMT 1A and the severity of the clinical manifestations can be correlated in the number of duplications at the genetic locus (Ionasescu 1995). This gene regulates production of the peripheral myelin protein (PMP) 22. Genetic research has identified abnormalities on chromosomes 1 (CMT 1B and 2) and X (CMT X) that account for different forms of the disease.

PRESENTATION AND DIAGNOSIS

Since over 75% of HSMN/CMT cases are autosomal dominant, evaluation of a patient for possible CMT starts with a good history, specifically seeking a family history of similar disorders. Presenting symptoms may include frequent falling or stumbling, difficulty with shoe wear or fitting, repeated ankle inversions and toe or foot deformities. Often new patients may not present until the second decade of life.

Physical examination findings often include lower-extremity weakness with foot deformities such as pes cavus and hindfoot varus and diminished or absent deep tendon and vibratory reflexes. Most CMT patients have difficulty standing on their heels.

Patients presenting with ankle instability or foot deformities usually require referral to an orthopedic surgeon for evaluation. The orthopedist in turn may seek neurologic consultation with the finding of cavus feet, diminished reflexes and weakness.

Genetic tests confirming CMT 1A or X are now available, but the characteristic findings of delay in NCV and reduced compound muscle action potentials on EMG studies confirm the diagnosis of CMT/HSMN.

CLINICAL ASPECTS
Patients with CMT/HSMN manifest the characteristics of lower-extremity weakness including muscle atrophy and imbalance. Impaired strength results in tendon contractures and gait disturbance. Characteristic foot deformities include the high-arched cavus foot, with hindfoot varus and claw toes. Upper-extremity involvement occurs sometimes decades later and is often milder than lower-extremity involvement, but manifests as intrinsic weakness causing difficulty with grip and fine motor control. The degree of involvement can be quite variable, but as many as 20% of patients are so severely affected as to be non-ambulatory (Smith 2002).

HIP INVOLVEMENT
Several recent studies have documented the presence and incidence of hip dysplasia in patients with CMT. The original report in 1985 described hip dysplasia in three families with CMT (Kumar *et al.* 1985). A subsequent review of 74 children with CMT found an incidence of hip dysplasia of nearly 10% and an average age at diagnosis of about 10.5 years (Walker *et al.* 1994). Screening radiographs of patients with CMT may permit earlier diagnosis of hip dysplasia, although they may not result in a change in the management.

The dysplasia of the hip in these patients seems to be acquired and not present at birth according to a recent study from the Netherlands (Van Erve and Driessen 1999). Two patients with normal X-rays in childhood who subsequently developed hip dysplasia of a secondary nature related to their neuromuscular disorder were documented in this study.

The etiology of the hip dysplasia is unclear, since CMT is a disorder causing distal but not proximal muscle weakness. Subtle proximal weakness around the hip girdle may contribute to the development of dysplasia.

HIP PHYSICAL AND RADIOGRAPHIC FINDINGS
Since hip dysplasia can be clinically silent and have no significant physical examination findings, radiographic assessment remains the sole means of diagnosis of hip disorders in these patients. Therefore, in patients with CMT, a screening radiograph of the hips is often appropriate around the age of 10, or the time of diagnosis if later. Since CMT often presents in the second decade of life, radiographs of the hips should accompany the diagnosis. The radiographic findings of hip dysplasia in CMT patients include subluxation of the femoral head and acetabular dysplasia (Fig. 14.2).

TREATMENT
Treatment for hip dysplasia is determined by the age of the patient at presentation, the severity of the dysplasia and the presence of additional symptoms. Bracing may be utilized for hip dysplasia in children under 5 years, but nonoperative management of hip dysplasia in older patients is not possible. Based on symptoms and radiographic findings, hip osteotomy may be necessary to optimize hip anatomy and minimize long-term disability from degenerative arthritis. Standard osteotomies of the proximal femur or pelvis are usually performed to normalize the hip, with outcome dependent on the degree of dysplasia at the time of diagnosis.

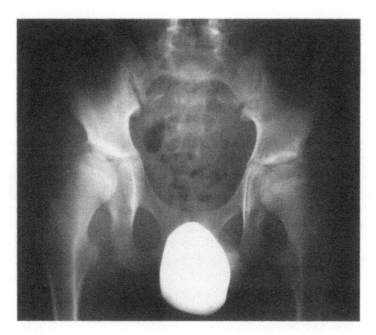

Fig. 14.2. Anteroposterior radiograph of the pelvis of a 12-year-old patient with CMT/HSMN and dysplasia of both hips.

Spinal muscular atrophy

Spinal muscular atrophy (SMA) is a progressive neuromuscular disorder caused by degeneration of the anterior column of the spinal cord and lower nuclei. Affected patients manifest variable symmetric weakness of the trunk and extremities, and fasciculations of the tongue are characteristic. Proximal muscles are the most severely affected (Shapiro and Specht 1993, Fisk and Hatfield 2002).

ETIOLOGY

SMA most commonly results from an autosomal recessive genetic defect on the fifth chromosome, typically a deletion in the 5q11.2–13.3 locus. This area is associated with production of the survival motor neuron and neuronal apoptosis inhibitor proteins. Persistence of programmed cell death of motor neurons is considered to be the reason for the progressive weakness of SMA (Shapiro and Specht 1993).

PREVALENCE

The incidence of SMA is approximately 1 in 20,000 births (Shapiro and Specht 1993). A functional classification system described by Evans *et al.* (1981) is appropriate as a predictor of hip subluxation. Type I, also known as Werding–Hoffman disease, is the most severe form of SMA and causes such profound weakness that children seldom survive beyond 1 year of age. Type II patients are able to sit but not stand, and type III patients stand but do no functional walking. Type IV patients ambulate for several decades but ultimately become wheelchair dependent. In the International SMA Consortium grading scheme (Munsat and Davies 1992). types III and IV are lumped together, leaving a total of three types. This scheme employs the onset of weakness as the defining characteristic of the three types: type I, onset before 6 months; type II, onset 6–18 months; type III, onset after 18 months.

HIP INVOLVEMENT

The incidence of lower extremity dysfunction, especially hip disorders, parallels the severity of the weakness in SMA patients.

Hip subluxation and dislocation are common in type II and III patients. One recent study found hip displacement in 20 of 24 type II patients and 7 of 17 type III patients (Sporer and Smith 2003). Dislocations/subluxations tended to occur around age 8 years in the type II patients and around age 11 in the type III group. The same study documented few if any symptoms of pain, impaired seating, difficulty with perineal care or skin ulceration in these patients who typically have normal cognitive and unimpaired sensation. Previous studies have documented a high incidence of resubluxation following surgery to stabilize the hips in these patients (Granata *et al.* 1989, Thompson and Larsen 1990).

PRESENTATION AND DIFFERENTIAL DIAGNOSIS

Patients with SMA may present in infancy with significant hypotonia and generalized muscle weakness. Proximal muscle weakness is more prominent than distal.

Less involved children will present with significant delay in acquistion of gross motor skills. Generally, SMA children have no impairment in sensation or cognition, and typically are bright and articulate. "Floppy" infants with low muscle tone, generalized weakness and significant gross motor delay should be referred to a pediatric neurologist for further work-up.

Differential diagnoses include muscular dystrophy and congenital myopathy syndromes.

The SMA child will often exhibit fine tremor of the fingers and tongue fasiculations, helping to distinguish SMA from these other conditions clinically (Fisk and Hatfield 2002).

HIP PHYSICAL EXAMINATION FINDINGS

Most SMA patients with hip involvement will demonstrate hip flexion contractures on physical examination, since they spend so much time sitting. The examination will reveal profound weakness about the hip, especially in the abductors. A positive Galeazzi sign will be noted in patients with unilateral dislocation.

RADIOGRAPHIC FINDINGS

Coxa valga is a common finding in SMA patients because of the significant abductor weakness typical of the disorder. Femoral head subluxation is also present, of variable severity depending on the extent of involvement of the patient (Fig. 14.3).

MANAGEMENT OF HIP DISORDERS

The consensus of a recent long-term follow-up study was that surgical intervention for hip

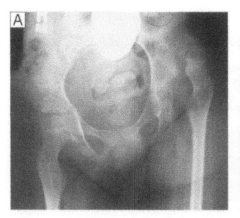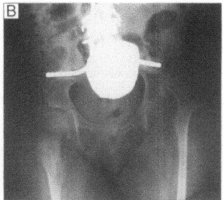

Fig. 14.3. Anteroposterior radiographs of the pelvis of a girl with SMA type II and chronic left hip dislocation for at least seven years: (A) aged 6 years; (B) following spinal fusion surgery at age 12 years. She remains asymptomatic.

subluxation or dislocation was unnecessary in the majority of these patients since they typically remain asymptomatic with no impairment in sitting (Sporer and Smith 2003). Other authors advocate restoration of the femoral head to the acetabulum with appropriate reconstructive operative techniques (Shapiro and Specht 1993).

The lack of symptoms related to hip instability is postulated to be secondary to the profound weakness of the hip musculature, such that there is little pressure on the femoral head to cause pain or discomfort. The diminished muscle strength available to stabilize a femoral head in the acetabulum often precludes a successful result from a reconstructive operative intervention. In non-ambulatory patients with dislocated hips, a stiff, located hip may be worse and more symptomatic than a flexible, dislocated one.

REFERENCES

Chan, K.G., Galasko, C.S., Delaney, C. (2001) 'Hip subluxation and dislocation in Duchenne muscular dystrophy.' *Journal of Pediatric Orthopaedics, Part B*, **10**, 219–225.
Drennan, J.C. (1990) 'Neuromuscular disorders.' *In:* Morrissy, R.T. (Ed.) *Lovell and Winter's Pediatric Orthopaedics.* Philadelphia: J.B. Lippincott, pp. 381–383.
Evans, G.A., Drennan, J.C., Russman, B.S. (1981) 'Functional classification and orthopaedic management of spinal musular atrophy.' *Journal of Bone and Joint Surgery, British Volume*, **63**, 516–522.
Fisk, J.R., Hatfield, M. (2002) 'Anterior horn cell diseases.' *In:* Fitzgerald, R.H., Kaufer, H., Malkani, A.L. (Eds) *Orthopaedics.* St. Louis, C.V. Mosby, pp. 1557–1558.
Granata, C., Merlini, L., Magni, E., Marini, M.L., Stagni, S.B. (1989) 'Spinal muscular atrophy: natural history and orthopaedic treatment of scoliosis.' *Spine*, **14**, 760–762.
Ionasescu, V. (1995) 'Charcot–Marie–Tooth neuropathies: from clinical description to molecular genetics.' *Muscle and Nerve*, **18**, 267–275.
Kumar, J., Marks, H., Bowen, J.R., MacEwen, G.D. (1985) 'Hip dysplasia associated with Charcot–Marie–Tooth disease in the older child and adolescent.' *Journal of Pediatric Orthopedics*, **5**, 511–514.
Munsat, T.L., Davies, K.E (1992) 'International SMA Consortium meeting (26–28 June 1992, Bonn, Germany).' *Neuromuscular Disorders*, **2**, 423–428.
Shapiro, F., Specht, L. (1993) 'The diagnosis and orthopaedic treatment of childhood spinal muscular atrophy,

peripheral neuropathy, Friedreich ataxia, and arthrogryposis.' *Journal of Bone and Joint Surgery, American Volume*, **75**, 1699–1714.

Smith, B.G. (2002) 'Heriditary sensory motor neuropathies.' *In:* Fitzgerald, R.H., Kaufer, H., Malkani, A.L. (Eds.) *Orthopaedics*. St. Louis: C.V. Mosby, pp. 1567–1573.

Smith, S.E., Green, N.E., Cole, R.J., Robison, J.D., Fenichel, G.M. (1993) 'Prolongation of ambulation in children with Duchenne muscular dystrophy by subcutaneous lower limb tenotomy,' *Journal of Pediatric Orthopedics*, **13**, 336–340.

Sporer, S.M., Smith, B.G. (2003) 'Hip dislocation in patients with spinal muscular atrophy.' *Journal of Pediatric Orthopedics*, **23**, 10–14.

Sussman, M. (2002) 'Duchenne muscular dystrophy,' *Journal of the American Academy of Orthopedic Surgery*, **10**, 138–151.

Thompson, C.E., Larsen, L.J. (1990) 'Recurrent hip dislocation in intermediate spinal muscular atrophy.' *Journal of Pediatric Orthopedics*, **10**, 638–641.

Thompson, G.H., Berenson, F.R. (2001) 'Other neuromuscular disorders.' *In:* Morrissy, R.T., Weinstein, S.L. (Eds.) *Pediatric Orthopaedics*. Philadelphia: Lippincott, pp. 637–639.

Van Erve, R.H., Driessen, A.P. (1999) 'Developmental hip dysplasia in heriditary sensory motor neuropathy type I.' *Journal of Pediatric Orthopedics*, **19**, 92–96.

Walker, J.L., Nelson, K.R., Heavilon, J.A., Stevens, D.B., Lubicky, J.P., Ogden, J.A., Vanden Brink, K.A. (1994) 'Hip abnormalities in children with Charcot–Marie–Tooth disease.' *Journal of Pediatric Orthopedics*, **14**, 54–59.

Younger, D.S. (Ed.) (1999) *Motor Disorders*. Philadelphia: Lippincott, Williams & Wilkins.

15
ORTHOTIC MANAGEMENT OF HIP PATHOLOGIES

Christopher Morris

Orthoses are externally applied devices used to modify the structural and functional characteristics of the neuromuscular and skeletal systems by applying forces to the body. Orthotists are health-care professionals trained in the clinical assessment, design and fitting of orthoses with an educational background in bioengineering and the medical sciences (International Organization for Standardization 1989a). The role of the orthotist is to translate the clinical prescription into a precise orthotic design, and then ensure that its construction and fit achieve these aims in practice.

This chapter will describe the contribution that orthoses can make to the management of the hip joint in childhood. We will consider first the fundamental principles of orthotic design, and then the role of orthoses in the management of hip disorders, using the WHO International Classification of Functioning (ICF) (World Health Organization 2001). Orthoses are designed with one of two primary aims: either to affect the body structure or to assist function, although as will be seen, an orthosis is frequently designed to achieve both of these aims.

Mechanical principles
FORCES AND VECTORS
Forces are *vector* quantities, that is they have both magnitude and direction. A single force acting on an object causes motion in the direction of the applied force. However, two forces acting on an object can cause compression, tension, shear or turning, and three forces can cause bending, depending on the direction in which the forces are acting (Fig. 15.1). When two forces are acting in different planes at right angles to each other then the magnitude and line of action of their combined effect can be calculated using geometry as the *resultant force*. Similarly, the magnitude of a single force acting in any direction can be resolved into its vertical and horizontal components (Fig. 15.2).

REACTION FORCES
All objects are affected by gravity. An object pushes down on the ground with a force (its weight) equal to its mass multiplied by gravity. As Newton stated, for every action there is an equal and opposite reaction. Therefore, the surface supporting an object, for example the ground supporting the body, pushes back with a reaction force equal to the weight of the object to prevent it from sinking (Fig. 15.3). Whilst this is perhaps a simple concept

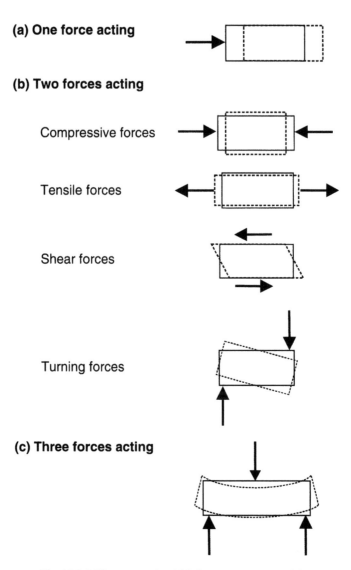

(a) One force acting

(b) Two forces acting

Compressive forces

Tensile forces

Shear forces

Turning forces

(c) Three forces acting

Fig. 15.1. Different ways in which forces can act on an object.

when static, during motion the reaction force on a body acts in all three planes. It can, however, still be calculated using geometry as the resultant *ground reaction force* if the vertical and horizontal components are known (Fig. 15.4). Nearly all forces applied by orthoses are *reaction forces*. Orthoses usually oppose forces applied to them by the body as a result of gravity, hypertonia or muscle imbalance, and in doing so oppose changes in body posture. Occasionally orthoses apply *active forces*. To create active forces, components such as springs, elastics or compressed gas pistons are used that release energy stored when the components are deformed.

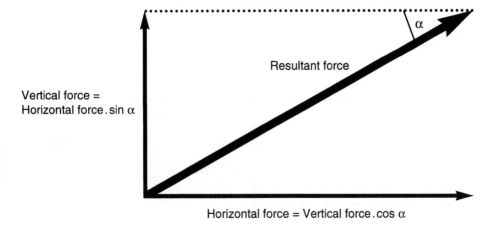

Vertical force =
Horizontal force . sin α

Resultant force

α

Horizontal force = Vertical force . cos α

Fig. 15.2. The magnitude and direction of the resultant force of two forces acting at a right angle to each other can be calculated using geometry. Similarly, the magnitude of a single force acting in any direction can be resolved into its vertical and horizontal components.

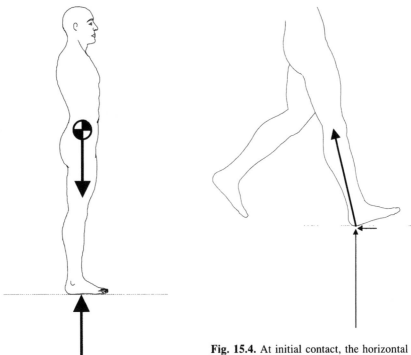

Fig. 15.3. The total body force acting downwards from its centre of mass is resisted by an equal and opposite reaction force from the support surface, following Newton's Third Law.

Fig. 15.4. At initial contact, the horizontal and vertical reaction forces create a resultant ground reaction force (GRF). The line of action of the GRF can effect moments around proximal joints, but usually remains close to the hip and knee joints during normal gait.

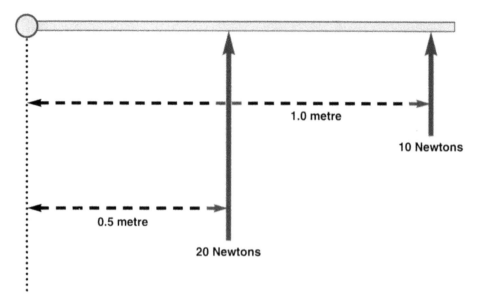

Fig. 15.5. A smaller force acting at a greater distance from the fulcrum, in this case a hinge on a door, will produce an equal moment to a greater force applied at a shorter distance (10 Newton metres in both cases). Therefore, with equal forces the longer the lever arm the greater the moment generated.

MOMENTS AND LEVERS

Forces acting around a fulcrum create a turning effect called the *moment*. Moments in any direction can be calculated from the magnitude of the force multiplied by the perpendicular distance at which the force is acting from the fulcrum point. This is why we are encouraged to push doors on the opposite side to the hinges reducing the force required to open them (Fig. 15.5). To prevent turning, the moments acting in one direction must be balanced by the moments acting in the other direction. This is the principle of the children's seesaw (or teeter-totter), where moments acting in one direction due to a force acting at a distance on one side of the fulcrum can be balanced by an equal moment acting in the opposite direction. The further a force acts from the fulcrum (measured at a right angle to the direction of the force), the less force is required to generate a moment; conversely, the shorter the distance the greater the force required to generate an equal moment (Fig. 15.6).

BENDING

When three forces act on an object as in Figure 15.6, the moments generated may cause bending. The resistance of the object to bending is dependent on its material and cross-sectional area, and on the distribution of the material about the bending axis. The bending resistance of an object such as a beam is known as the *second moment of area* (I) and increases in proportion to its thickness cubed (D^3), and directly with increases in its width (B) (Fig. 15.7). The importance of material distribution in resisting bending can be demonstrated by first flexing a plastic ruler across its flat plane, and then again after rotating it 90° along its axis.

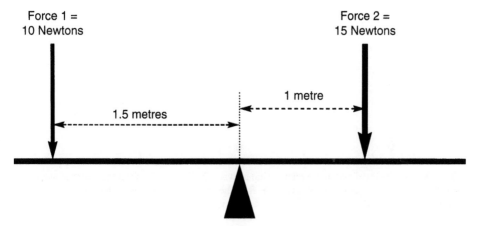

Reaction Force = Force 1 + Force 2 = 25 Newtons

Fig. 15.6. Moments acting in one direction on one side of the fulcrum are balanced by the moments acting in the other direction on the opposite side of the fulcrum (moment = 10 × 1.5 = 15 × 1 = 15 Newton metres). Note that the shorter the distance from the fulcrum at which the force acts (lever arm), the greater the magnitude of force required to generate the same moment.

Bending Resistance

$$I = \frac{BD^3}{12}$$

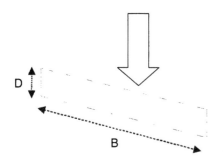

Fig. 15.7. The resistance of an object to bending is dependent on its cross-sectional area and the distribution of the material about the bending axis. The bending resistance of a beam is known as the second moment of area (I).

The ruler will allow large deflection about the flat plane, whereas it is not possible to notice any deflection having rotated it, even though the cross-sectional area is the same (Major and Stallard 1985). The length of an object such as a lever or beam will also influence its resistance to bending. As we have seen, the greater the distance a force is applied from the supporting points the greater the moments that will be generated, but there will also be greater bending with increasing length.

When designing structures to resist bending, the distance between the supporting points will influence the size and shape of the cross-sectional area and the choice of material. It

213

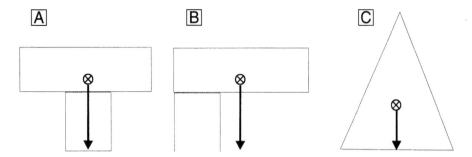

Fig. 15.8. Stability is defined by the relationship between the line of force from the centre of mass of an object and its base of support. (A) When the line from the centre of gravity falls within the base of support, stability is achieved. (B) When the line from the centre of gravity falls outside the base of support, the object is unstable. (C) Maximum stability is achieved with a wide base of support and a low centre of gravity.

is also more efficient to have the material distributed as far from the bending axis as possible, such as in the I-shaped metal girders used in buildings.

PRESSURE

Forces acting on an object must have an area over which they are applied. The pressure on the surface of the object is proportional to the size of the area over which the force acts. The larger the contact area, the lower the pressure created at the contact surface. Needles and nails have very small contact areas, which means that even with the application of low forces the pressure is sufficient to penetrate objects. Conversely, we can use a soft cushion on hard chairs to increase the contact surface area and hence appreciably decrease the pressure at the contact surface.

STABILITY

Stability describes the relationship between the position of the centre of mass (often called the centre of gravity) and its base of support. The distribution of material that constitutes an object influences the position of the centre of mass of that object. The weight of the object, that is its mass multiplied by gravity, acts vertically downward from the centre of mass. When the line from the centre of mass falls within the base of support then stability is achieved. However, when the line from the centre of mass falls outside the base of support, then the object is unstable (Fig. 15.8). Stability can be increased by having a wide base of support, as in the Eiffel Tower for example, and by keeping the centre of mass as low as possible.

Biomechanics of the hip joint

To understand the application of mechanics to the body and hence the principles of orthotic management, it is necessary to consider the body as a system of rigid segments hinged at joints and linked by muscles and ligaments. The angle between these segments is altered,

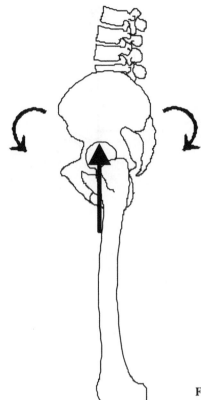

Fig. 15.9. In the sagittal plane the pelvis is balanced on the femurs with the hip joint acting like the fulcrum of a seesaw.

or controlled, through the action of external forces (gravitational or orthotic) or internal forces (muscular, ligamentous or inertial). From a mechanical standpoint, the hip joint is a difficult joint to control. In the introduction the levers described had adequate length and acted in a single plane, for instance similar to the femur and tibia either side of the knee joint. However, the pelvis is irregular in shape and the hip joint moves in all three planes, and frequently one hip joint cannot be considered separately from the spine and the opposite hip.

Looked at from the side (in the sagittal plane), the pelvis is balanced on the femur with the hip joint acting like the fulcrum of a seesaw (Fig. 15.9). The pelvis is naturally tilted slightly anteriorly as the foundation for the lumbar lordosis. It requires precise postural control to prevent it tilting excessively anteriorly which will cause lumbar hyperlordosis, or tilting excessively posteriorly causing lumbar kyphosis. Viewed from the front (in the coronal plane), it appears a more stable structure as long as both legs are supported. However, in single-limb stance the supporting hip joint again appears like a seesaw, and the moment caused by the weight of the body acting about the hip will cause the pelvis to drop on the unsupported side unless the hip abductor muscles can generate an equal moment. The muscle force

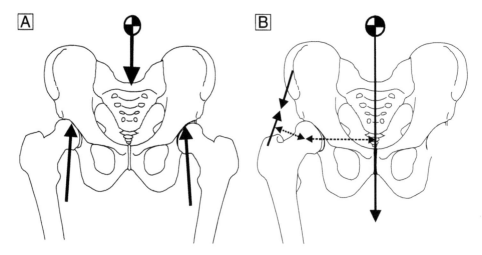

Fig. 15.10. In the coronal plane (A) the pelvis is stable when supported by both legs. However, during single limb support (B) the pelvis is unstable and the hip abductor muscles must generate sufficient force to produce a moment equal to the total body force acting about the fulcrum at the supporting hip joint.

required will be high because of the short and limited length of their lever arm (Fig. 15.10). In the presence of weak hip abductors, the lever arm of the body weight around the supporting hip can be reduced by laterally flexing the trunk towards the supporting side, thus reducing the moment and the demand on the hip abductor muscles.

In neither the sagittal nor the coronal planes is it easy to apply the forces necessary to control the pelvis with orthoses, simply because its shape does not allow it. The length of lever that can be achieved at the pelvis is always limited, so the forces needed are large and create high pressures at the orthosis–body interface. Consequently, in seeking acceptable interface pressures, the longer lever arm of the trunk can be utilized, providing the spine can be stabilized to act as a single segment. An example of this is seen in the sagittal plane when opposing forward trunk collapse for a standing child with paralysed hip extensors. In this instance forces can be applied posteriorly at the buttocks and anteriorly at the knees and chest to maintain erect posture, a force system often called three-point pressure (Figs. 15.1C, 15.6 and 15.11). If, however, there are hip flexion contractures, excessive extension of the trunk segment will merely result in hyperlordosis of the spine while the pelvis remains anteriorly tilted at the hips.

In the coronal plane, for an orthosis to maintain hip abduction and prevent adduction, forces applied on the distal thigh close to the femoral condyles will be lower than those applied at a point proximally (Fig. 15.12). Note that the length of the lever arm above the hip at the pelvis is again limited by the short structure of the pelvic segment. Applying forces to the trunk, without adequate stabilization of the pelvis and spine, will result in compensatory trunk side flexion (Fig. 15.13). Similarly, if there is hip adduction contracture, attempts to achieve greater abduction than is possible will result in pelvic obliquity and trunk side flexion.

216

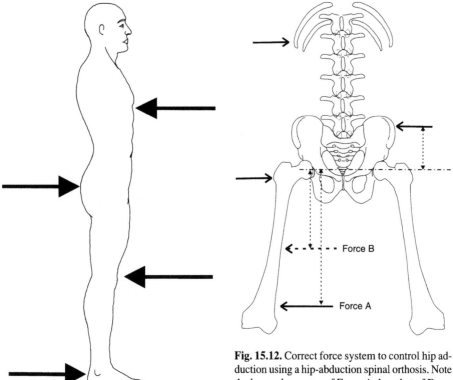

Fig. 15.11. A combination of three-point pressure force systems can be used to prevent hip and knee flexion and maintain an upright posture in hip–knee–ankle–foot orthoses.

Fig. 15.12. Correct force system to control hip adduction using a hip-abduction spinal orthosis. Note the longer lever arm of Force A than that of Force B; and note also the limited length of the lever arm above the hip at the pelvis. The spine has been stabilized as one segment to prevent lateral flexion. The displayed force system is mirrored for control of the opposite hip.

In the horizontal plane the problem of controlling rotation about the vertical axis is also difficult. The width of the pelvis now provides a reasonable length of lever; the difficulty is the absence of a lever to rotate the femur. To some degree, it may be possible to harness shear forces from the skin and the shape of the soft tissues to gain some control. In general, however, rotational control of the hip joint using orthoses requires extension to the foot, which unfortunately means transmitting the turning force, or *torque*, through the knee joint.

The hip joint's role in transmitting loads between the spine and lower limbs is crucial to achieve a mechanically efficient posture in sitting, standing or walking. In the presence of pathology, deforming internal forces can affect the angular relationships between the pelvis, thighs and spinal segments due to bony abnormality, muscle weakness or spasticity, or ligamentous insufficiency. If an orthosis aims to exert control of the angular motion of the hip joint, then the pelvis must be prevented from tilting in the sagittal plane, shifting obliquely in the coronal plane or rotating in the transverse plane, otherwise the corrective

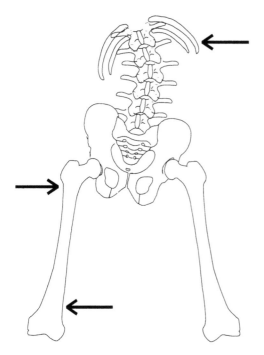

Fig. 15.13. If the position of the pelvis is not well controlled in a hip-abduction spinal orthosis and the spine is not adequately stabilized the resulting posture will be pelvic obliquity and trunk side flexion; note also that the right hip remains adducted even though the thigh segments appear symmetrically abducted. Hence it may be important to obtain an X-ray of the pelvis when delivering a hip abduction orthosis as containment of the femoral head in the acetabulum may be compromised.

moment will be lost. Careful assessment is necessary to ascertain the range of hip motion that can be achieved passively without changing the posture of the pelvis and spine.

Terminology

Acronyms proliferate in the description of orthoses; however, it can often be confusing to know what these abbreviations really mean. Three systems for naming and describing orthoses are commonly used:

(i) *Anatomical*. The correct terminology for describing an orthosis is generally accepted to be an indication of the joints that a device encompasses (International Organization for Standardization 1989b). Hence, for example, an ankle–foot orthosis (AFO) extends from below the knee to include the ankle and foot, and a knee–ankle–foot orthosis (KAFO) would further extend more proximally to the thigh and include the knee joint. Orthoses may be designed to affect the hip joint only (HO) or be part of more complex devices such as hip–knee–ankle–foot orthoses (HKAFO) or used in conjunction with thoracolumbar–sacral spinal orthoses (TLSO).

(ii) *Functional*. It is also useful to know what biomechanical effect the orthosis is designed to achieve. For this reason descriptive terms such as hip-abduction spinal orthoses (HASO) have also been adopted.

(iii) *Nominal*. There is often confusion when orthoses are named after people or places and this practice should in general be avoided. However, a few eponymous titles are included in this text where references to specific orthoses are made.

Materials

In the past most orthoses were constructed from materials such as metal and leather. Moulded leather spinal or thigh components required extensive metal reinforcement or subframes. These were often heavy and unsightly and took a long time for skilled technicians to fabricate. Although for some orthoses metal components are preferred because of their resistance to bending, modern fabrication methods often make much more use of plastic materials and modern production techniques. Thermoplastics are preferred to leather because of their reduced weight and fabrication time, and their improved appearance and hygiene, being easy to wipe clean.

The problems caused by the excessive heat that can be generated within plastic orthoses can be overcome by incorporating ventilation holes and using standard undergarments that can be changed as necessary. Contemporary orthoses are therefore usually made from thermoplastics such as polypropylene, polythene or heat-mouldable foams. These can be formed either at lower temperatures directly onto the body or at higher temperatures onto plaster models of the body which have been modified to avoid pressure on bony prominences and apply pressure to compliant soft tissues.

Different materials, different thickness of material, and the way in which orthoses are trimmed can alter the flexibility of the orthosis (Major and Stallard 1985). Plastics are available in a wide variety of colours and can also be patterned using special paper, making them more attractive to children and acceptable to families. Components such as steel, aluminium or synthetic hinges can be incorporated into the design of an orthosis to permit controlled ranges of movement between body segments.

Natural materials such as leather and sheepskin are often used for finishing orthoses with linings, covers and straps. Velcro has revolutionized the fastening of orthoses to the body and has largely replaced straps and buckles, although plastic or metal clips may be preferred for some applications.

Supply process

ASSESSMENT AND PRESCRIPTION

A prescription for orthoses will describe the overall treatment goals and orthotic objectives, but before designing an orthosis for a child a thorough assessment of the child's needs is essential. In the case of hip orthoses, this must include: range of hip joint motion, strength of hip muscles, and hip-joint congruency judged by radiological investigation. These factors must be evaluated together with sympathetic consideration of the concerns of the child and the parents or caregivers, as no orthosis can work if it is not worn. The choice of a specific orthotic design depends upon the physical characteristics of the child, other therapeutic or associated interventions such as the need for gastrostomy feeding tube access, and the goals and expectations of the clinicians and family. Whatever the treatment objectives, a family-centred approach will encourage appropriate use of an orthosis within the prescribed treatment regimen. The health-care team must therefore be well coordinated, work in partnership with the family, provide adequate general and specific information about the condition and the role of the prescribed orthosis, and support the family to ensure the orthosis is used correctly (King *et al.* 1996).

MEASUREMENT
Once the treatment goals have been defined these are interpreted by the orthotist into biomechanical objectives and the design of a specific orthosis. Accurate measurement of widths, lengths and circumferences, and the taking of plaster-cast models of the body if required, are vital to the quality of the finished orthosis. Following a comprehensive assessment of a child, this initial part of the process in supplying an orthosis must be afforded adequate time and the appropriate facilities. Together with orthotic technicians, the orthotist will fabricate the orthosis to the required specification. Occasionally, for more simple hip orthoses it may be more expedient to use a ready-made commercially available orthosis that can be modified in clinic.

FITTING AND EVALUATION
Orthoses often require fine tuning or small adjustments by the orthotist at the fitting stage, or at subsequent follow-up visits, and ready access to a suitably equipped workshop will reduce the time a child is without their orthosis and hence treatment. Evaluation of the effectiveness of the orthosis will often be conducted in collaboration with other members of the team. If an orthosis fails to achieve the treatment goals, it should be established whether this was caused by the orthotic design, incorrect manufacture or fitting, poor family compliance with the treatment regimen, or unrealistic expectations of orthotic intervention. A more detailed examination of the orthotic supply process is provided by Condie and Stewart (1997).

Indications for hip orthoses
The International Classification of Function (World Health Organization 2001) distinguishes between interventions that aim to affect impairments of body structure and those that aim to overcome activity limitations. Hip orthoses are prescribed either to affect the body structure by increasing containment of the femoral head in the acetabulum during growth or healing, or to facilitate activities that are limited by neuromuscular impairments. In some instances, such as for non-ambulant children with cerebral palsy, both objectives may be relevant.

Orthoses for impairments of hip joint structure
PROMOTING HIP-JOINT CONGRUENCY
Orthoses are used to encourage hip-joint congruency soon after birth for children with developmental dysplasia of the hip (DDH) and at any age following surgical intervention as an alternative to casting. In either case, the treatment goal of increasing containment of the femoral head in the acetabulum is achieved by holding the hip in a position of flexion and abduction.

Most designs rely on a shoulder harness to provide anchorage and counter-forces proximally at the trunk, and thigh cuffs to provide distal corrective hip abduction and flexion forces to maintain the desired position, for example the Von Rosen orthosis (Hadlow 1979) (Fig. 15.14). Variations on these principles include the commonly used Pavlik harness, which encloses the feet in soft bootees and by attaching these to the shoulder harness similarly achieves hip abduction and flexion (Ramsey et al. 1976) (Fig. 15.15). The advantage of

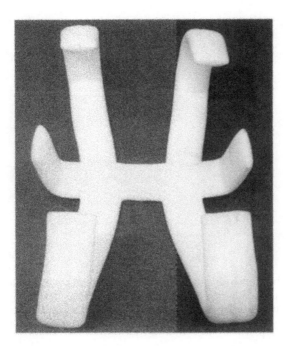

Fig. 15.14. The Von Rosen orthosis consists of a malleable aluminium frame coated in a vinyl covering, which can be shaped under the thighs and over the shoulder and around the waist of the child.

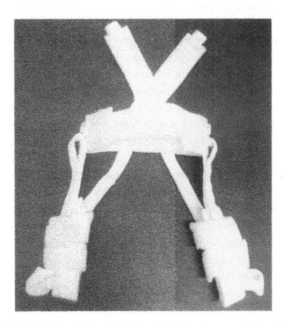

Fig. 15.15. The Pavlik harness is a fabric orthosis in which the straps connecting the soft bootees to the shoulder harness can be shortened, creating hip flexion and abduction.

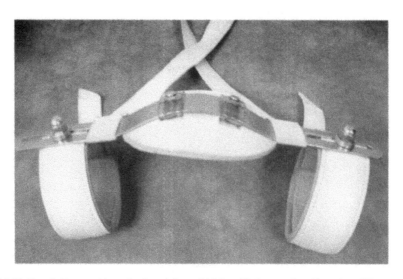

Fig. 15.16. Dennis Browne hip orthosis consists of thigh cuffs that can be adjusted to different widths within slots along a posteriorly placed aluminium bar. The reaction force of this three-point pressure orthosis is applied to the sacrum by the large central pad to maintain abduction. The shoulder straps fasten to the front of the thigh cuffs to maintain hip flexion and also prevent the bar rotating posteriorly.

this design is that it allows the child freedom to kick their legs within a controlled range of abducted and flexed hip motion and is therefore often preferred for children under 6 months whose hips are more easily reduced. Checking hip containment with ultrasound is recommended (Hangen *et al.* 1995, Taylor and Clarke 1997, Lerman *et al.* 2001). More rigid designs, such as the Dennis Browne abduction orthosis (Browne 1948), are indicated for stronger children over six months or perhaps following early surgical reduction. The Dennis Browne design better resists posterior subluxation of the hip and requires the shoulder harness component to prevent the pelvic section rotating in the sagittal plane (Fig. 15.16).

Traditionally, following hip reconstruction surgery 'broomstick' hip spica plaster casts have been set at 30° of unilateral hip abduction (combined 60° angle) and 30° of hip flexion, with the wooden broomstick bound into the cast across the thighs to provide extra rigidity. Hip spicas take considerable time to apply at the end of often already lengthy surgery, preclude visual inspection of the surgical wounds during the postoperative period, and can cause complications such as pressure sores. Another disadvantage of hip spicas is the need for intensive physiotherapy, and usually readmission to the ward, to mobilize the hip and knee joints to regain range of motion that will have stiffened from immobility in the cast. The use of an orthosis in these instances may overcome some of the complications associated with using hip spica casts. Orthoses used for children undergoing hip surgery can simply be thigh cuffs joined by a connecting bar sufficiently wide to create abduction. The problem with this design is that, without rigid attachment proximally to the trunk, the child can move one leg into adduction by allowing the other leg to abduct, tipping the pelvis obliquely with associated lateral trunk flexion; this is sometimes called the windsweeping effect. The

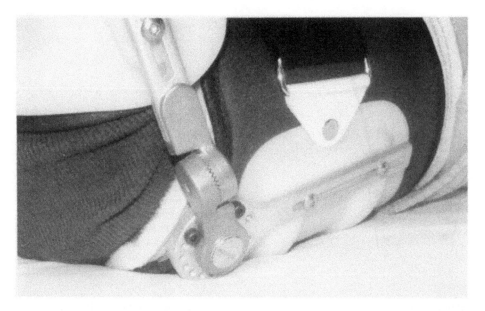

Fig. 15.17. The orthotic hip joint of the Maple Leaf orthosis allows incremental adjustment of hip flexion and abduction between modular pelvic and thigh components. It can be used as an alternative to the hip spica cast following hip reconstruction surgery.

design is therefore particularly inappropriate for children with asymmetrical muscle disorders, spasticity or behavioural problems.

An alternative to the hip spica is to use a custom moulded, one-piece plastic trough that with Velcro straps encases the posterior pelvis and thighs in the desired position. The disadvantage of this design is that the hip position is not adjustable once the orthosis is made. The most suitable design in these instances includes a pelvic section connected rigidly to the thigh cuffs. To provide adjustment an orthotic joint is fitted between the pelvic and thigh components. The ideal orthotic joint must allow incremental adjustment, and allow locking of the hip in the variable fixed positions in the sagittal and coronal planes. If the orthotic joint is sufficiently robust to resist the bending forces of adduction then the bar connecting the thighs will not be necessary. Such designs of hip orthosis have recently become available as modular systems such as the Maple Leaf™ (Fig. 15.17). Although initial experiences have promised faster postoperative mobilization, further clinical evaluation is necessary to test their efficacy in ensuring that surgically corrected hip containment is not compromised.

REDUCING FORCES ACTING THROUGH THE HIP JOINT
Theoretically, it is possible to unload the hip joint of the forces caused during weight bearing and walking. This may be indicated in destructive conditions where the upper femoral epiphysis is being impaired by inflammatory arthritis or ischaemic necrosis. Historically, various devices to unload the hip joint were developed for the treatment of Perthes' disease. These include the Snyder sling (Snyder 1947), which has an adjustable strap connecting a

223

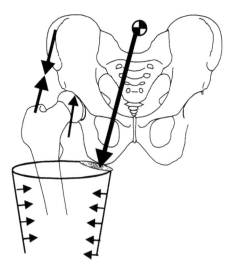

Fig. 15.18. An ischial weight-bearing knee–ankle–foot orthosis made longer than the leg can transfer some of the total body force from the pelvis to the ground through the orthosis and reduce forces acting on the hip joint. However, the effect of the hip abductor muscles and containment of the thigh segment still create a hip-joint reaction force.

shoulder and trunk harness to a metal loop on the back of the shoe heel which, when tensioned, prevents weight bearing and creates hip flexion, abduction and internal rotation. The Birmingham hip orthosis similarly holds the hip in flexion and abduction by containment in a plastic or leather orthosis from the nipple line to the knee, custom made to a cast of the child in the desired position (Harrison *et al.* 1982). The heel is suspended from the trunk section with a strap or chain, the line of action of which also creates internal rotation. A removable steel knee stirrup was added to prevent loading during kneeling. As children were forced to walk with crutches with both of these orthoses, the trend in managing Perthes' disease moved to weight-bearing abduction orthoses, maintaining a position of up to 45° abduction. These designs include the Scottish Rite (Meehan *et al.* 1992), Newington (Curtis *et al.* 1974) and Toronto orthoses (Bobechko *et al.* 1968), which allow hip flexion and extension in abduction and therefore reciprocal walking. This is achieved in the orthosis either by including multi-axial joints, such as in the Toronto orthosis, or a telescopic connecting bar between the thigh cuffs, as in the Scottish Rite orthosis. However, whilst these devices may indeed reduce the forces acting on the hip, the evidence for their effectiveness is equivocal and combined with the negative psychosocial effects (Price *et al.* 1988), their prescription has reduced considerably.

The weight of the body in standing and walking can be transmitted directly from the pelvis to the floor, bypassing the hip joint, using an ischial weight-relieving KAFO made several centimetres longer than the leg. The foot is therefore suspended off the floor and a raised shoe is required for the other limb to restore equilibrium at the pelvis. Although ground reaction forces are reduced, it must be remembered that some forces will still be applied to the hip by the surrounding muscles, especially hip abductors during the stance phase of gait, and because some load is transmitted to the orthosis by containment of the thigh segment (Fig. 15.18). Simply using a viscoelastic heel pad or insole can dissipate the ground reaction forces during gait and consequently reduce forces acting on the hip joint. Wedging a shoe or insole can change the line of action of the ground reaction force; this usually aims to align the force close to the hip joint thereby reducing the forces required of supporting muscles and ligaments.

Orthoses are not designed solely to treat impairments of body structure but also to overcome activity limitations. However, as a child's skeleton is being modified during growth partly by the forces that act upon it, the integrity of their body structure can be improved by enabling children to participate in activities with benefits that may last throughout their lives.

Orthoses to overcome activity limitations

Neuromuscular impairments such as cerebral palsy, spina bifida, the muscular dystrophies and atrophies, or arthrogryposis, affecting the bones, muscles and ligaments of the hip, can limit activities and restrict cognitive and social development. The Chailey Scales of 'levels of ability' in lying, sitting and standing (Pountney *et al.* 2000) and the principles of gait analysis (Gage 1991) are useful frameworks for identifying individual functional limitations and measuring change. Orthoses can provide stability and symmetry around the hips to enable children to have postural and movement opportunities otherwise denied them.

LYING

Being the position of maximum rest, lying needs to be either comfortable for several hours or a position that can be independently changed by the child. Lying is also the position in which we all first experience the environment. In terms of orthotic management, the biomechanical principles for prone and supine lying are very similar. However, the surface is important. High pressures at the body–orthosis interface can be avoided by maximizing the surface area of contact, avoiding forces on bony prominences and using compliant materials. The simplest orthoses for improving the symmetry and comfort in the lying posture are appropriately placed cushions or pillows on a regular firm bed. Some children with poor motor control, perhaps with cerebral palsy, may be able to alter their lying position using a custom modified lying orthosis such as the Chailey lying board (Pountney *et al.* 2000). Other children who are simply weak, such as those with muscular dystrophy or spinal muscular atrophy, may be able to alter their own lying posture only if provided with a bed with adjustable pneumatic remotely controlled sections under the mattress. The desired position of the hip joint will usually be slightly abducted and flexed, while the pelvis will be tilted anteriorly. Care should be taken to ensure the pelvis is not excessively tilted, which will happen if there is hip flexion contracture or spasticity, as this will cause a hyperlordotic posture of the lumbar spine and discomfort. Fixed deformities should therefore be accommodated in lying orthoses to ensure it is a restful position.

SITTING

Moving from lying to sitting changes the orientation of the body with respect to gravity, and the weight of the head, arms and trunk is now transmitted through the spine to the pelvis and thighs. Abducting the hips to increase the size of the base of support and anterior tilting of the pelvis, so that the centre of gravity of the upper body falls within the support area,

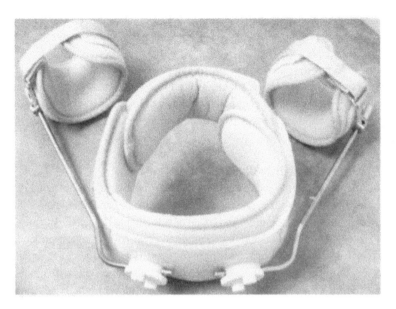

Fig. 15.19. The SWASH™ orthosis abducts the hips when flexed to provide a wider base of support for sitting enabling the child to focus on postural control of the trunk.

greatly improves sitting stability. Some children can sit independently and control their own trunk posture only if the hips and pelvis are positioned and supported to provide a stable base, for example using the Standing, Walking and Sitting Hip abduction orthosis (SWASH™) (Fig. 15.19). As the thigh cuffs are joined to the pelvic section by a posteriorly mounted curved connecting bar that facilitates polyplanar motion, the SWASH facilitates wider hip abduction when the hip is flexed, but when the hip is extended the joint is permitted to move in a slightly less abducted position. Although useful in helping children who are weak to gain sitting balance, the SWASH may not maintain hip abduction in children with spasticity because of its limited control of pelvic tilt, rotation and obliquity, or internal rotation of the hip. The SWASH orthosis was, however, reported useful in a single case study of a child with weak hip abductors rehabilitating following a septic hip (Torpey and Herle 2000).

Thoracolumbar–sacral orthoses (TLSOs) can improve sitting posture for children with scoliosis or kyphosis by maintaining the centre of gravity over the pelvis and hip base of support. Ideally, TLSOs are made from rigid thermoplastics such as polypropylene, closely moulded to maintain optimum posture of the pelvis and trunk as one segment. Soft designs, made from polythene foams rather than rigid thermoplastics, have been used for children with cerebral palsy without compromising respiratory function (Leopando *et al.* 1999). Rigid designs can incorporate cut out windows to facilitate breathing, but no orthosis is able to prevent progressive deformity (Miller *et al.* 1996, Terjesen *et al.* 2000).

For non-ambulant children, the benefits of the TLSO in controlling the position of the centre of gravity and stabilizing the trunk as a single segment can be combined with hip

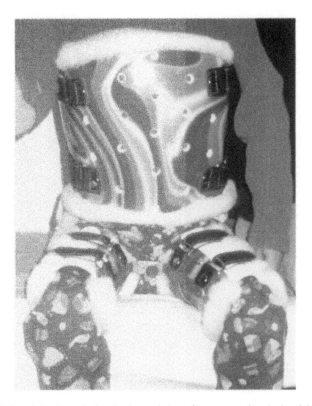

Fig. 15.20. Plastic hip abduction spinal orthosis consisting of custom-made spinal and thigh components connected with an orthotic hip joint that can be locked either at 90° of flexion for sitting or extended (zero flexion) for lying or standing.

abduction orthosis providing a stable base. Hip abduction spinal orthoses (HASOs) may be used in conjunction with a wheelchair seating system, or as an alternative to the wheelchair allowing the child to sit in regular furniture. The HASO (Fig. 15.20) consists of a bivalved custom-made plastic TLSO, closely moulded around the waist and pelvis, connected to thigh cuffs with an orthotic hip joint that can be locked at 90° of hip flexion (Drake and Boyd 1993). In this orthosis, maximum external control of sitting posture is provided. As the same hip joint can also be locked with the hip extended straight, the HASO can be useful for all the activities of lying, sitting and standing (Bower 1990, Boyd and Drake 1993). A similar conventional metal and leather design can be fabricated using the same orthotic hip joint (Hopkins 1992) (Fig. 15.21). However, the efficacy of the conventional non-moulded design is undermined by its limited control of the multisegmental pelvis and spine. It is also worth noting that although these HASOs will preferably hold the child in a symmetrical posture, fixed deformities must be accommodated. Therefore it may be necessary to provide an asymmetrical hip position to maintain neutral pelvic posture. Sitting posture may also be complicated by tightness of the hip extensors, as significant tightness in these muscles

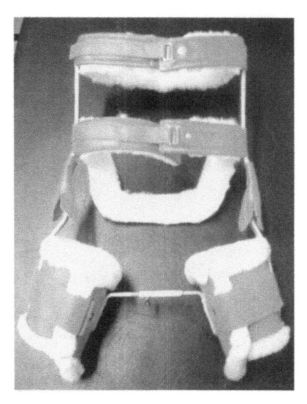

Fig. 15.21. This metal and leather hip abduction spinal orthosis does not adequately control pelvis and spine but can be used in conjunction with separate spinal orthosis or for children who have independent control of their trunk.

will tilt the pelvis posteriorly causing lumbar kyphosis (sometimes called sacral sitting). In some seating systems, knee blocks are additionally used to apply an axial force along the femur to the hip in a further effort to prevent pelvic rotation (Scrutton 1978). HASOs were initially designed for children with cerebral palsy but the design has also been used for other impairments where hip and spinal postural management is required, such as children with intermediate spinal muscular atrophy. Despite the efficacy of the HASO as a sitting orthosis, there is not yet evidence that it can alter the natural history of progressive hip migration and subluxation.

STANDING

Standing, even for the non-ambulant child, may be beneficial for the body structure by stretching muscles and other periarticular tissues and increasing bone density (Chad *et al.* 1999). The activity of standing is also important to allow children to experience the world from the same eye-level as their peers (Stuberg 1992, Chad *et al.* 1999).

Intrinsic stability in standing can be achieved using three-point pressure, the hip being

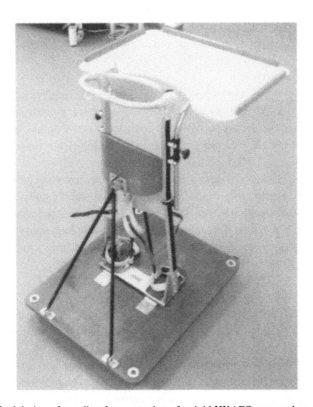

Fig. 15.22. Salford design of standing frame consists of a rigid HKAFO mounted on a broad wooden base. The HKAFO is hinged on the base allowing the child to be carefully positioned while lying supine, then brought to an upright position and secured to the posterior supports using a split pin. A table can be added to make standing more interesting. The base rests on castors, which means the frame can be moved without lifting.

extended by force applied to the buttocks that is simultaneously resisted by other forces applied anteriorly at the knees and chest (see Fig. 15.11). External stability in standing frames is usually provided by a heavy and broad support base to which the hip–knee–ankle–foot orthosis (HKAFO) is securely fixed. An early version of these HKAFOs was the parapodium (Motloch 1971), and there are now a variety of modular and custom-made standing frame designs available. Ideally the hips will be slightly abducted to widen the standing base and enhance hip-joint containment as in the Salford design (Fig. 15.22). It is possible to accommodate fixed hip and knee contractures of up to 30° but in these situations heel raises should be included so that the feet are supported on a flat surface. Also, as the reaction forces required to support the body in standing increase dramatically with increasing hip and knee flexion, the orthosis–body interfaces must be closely moulded to the anatomy to reduce interface pressures, and padding such as sheepskin may be necessary to make them tolerable to the child. Leg-length discrepancy must be accommodated to prevent pelvic obliquity. The forces acting on the body during standing may help a more located hip joint to be modelled and form appropriately. Provision of a table at the correct height can also make standing an enjoyable and stimulating activity as well as providing physiological benefits.

UPRIGHT LOCOMOTION

Upright locomotion is a worthwhile goal for children who achieve standing as it is an activity that offers a different perception of the environment, greater independence and a useful form of exercise. Weakness of the hip abductor or extensor muscles, for example in children with paraplegia, or fixed contractures of the hip flexor muscles, may limit or prevent a functional gait. The most important determinants of efficient walking for children with lower-level spina bifida lesions, in terms of energy expenditure and gaining independence on level surfaces, appear to be control of pelvic rotation and obliquity and hip abduction by functioning hip abductor muscles (Duffy *et al.* 1996). Once stabilization of the hip joint has been accomplished, with similar force systems as in standing, then upright locomotion is possible providing the child has some control of their head, arms and trunk. This will be a swing-through gait, swivel walking, or reciprocal ambulation.

Swivel walkers

Swivel walkers comprise a standing frame fixed to a broad, heavy baseplate (Fig. 15.23). The weight of the baseplate lowers the centre of gravity and the frame supporting the body maintains the position of the centre of gravity over the base of support. Underneath the base are two footplates mounted on bearings and offset so that either one can be flat on the floor at any time while being large enough to still provide extrinsic stability in this position. Providing the centre of gravity is forward of the bearing centre, when the child leans or rotates their head, arms and trunk so that only one footplate is on the supporting surface, the baseplate will rotate forward on the unsupported side (Stallard *et al.* 1978). Using this method only minimal coordination is required to facilitate locomotion and no walking aid is required. Swivel walking is therefore appropriate for very young children and those with weak upper-limb strength or poor hand function, such as in arthrogryposis.

Reciprocal walking orthoses

Swing-through and reciprocal gaits require adequate upper-limb and trunk strength, especially the latissimus dorsi muscles, and coordination to use crutches or other walking aids. Swing-through gait can be facilitated by orthoses that prevent hip flexion and maintain knee extension so that the whole lower body can transmit loads in weight bearing and be lifted off the floor as one segment. The considerable energy expenditure involved in swing-through gait renders it impossible for many children, especially when encumbered with even lightweight orthoses. The most energy-efficient and appropriate orthosis for children with inadequate hip control will usually be one of the designs of reciprocating gait orthoses.

In essence, reciprocal gait requires the hip of the stance limb to be extending while the hip of the swing limb is flexing. Pelvic rotation is also an important prerequisite of normal gait to increase step length (Gage 1991). In an early attempt to overcome the limitations of orthotic joints which prevent pelvic rotation a polyplanar hip joint was developed (Scrutton *et al.* 1967). Following this, the first attempts were made to experiment with connecting

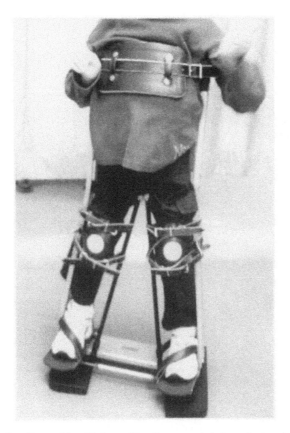

Fig. 15.23. A swivel walker enables this boy with arthrogryposis independent upright locomotion. He had tried a Parawalker™ but struggled to use a walking aid because of poor upper-limb and hand function.

the left and right hinges using single and twin cables (Scrutton 1969). At the same time, working independently in North America, Wally Motloch was also developing reciprocal walking orthoses using nylon cord pulley systems and gearbox mechanisms. The twin-cable system eventually became known as the Reciprocating Gait Orthosis (RGO™) (Douglas *et al.* 1983). The moulded plastic leg sections provide close anatomical control, fit inside ordinary footwear and can be concealed under loose clothing. More advanced versions of the RGO achieve adequate propulsion using a stiffer single cable (Advanced RGO™) or rigid bars (Isocentric RGO™), and, for children without fixed contractures or deformities, the medial sidebars can be discarded without compromising intrinsic stability (Fig. 15.24). In all the interconnected RGOs, the power to flex the swinging leg comes from the ground reaction of the walking aid causing extension of the standing hip and hence flexion of the opposite hip to advance the body.

In the UK, at the Orthotic Research and Locomotion Assessment Unit (ORLAU) of the Robert Jones and Agnes Hunt Hospital, Oswestry, the Hip Guidance Orthosis (HGO),

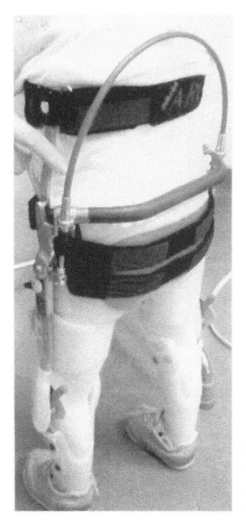

Fig. 15.24. Junior Advanced Reciprocating Gait Orthosis (ARGO™) interconnects left and right hip joints with a single cable to facilitate reciprocal hip flexion and extension. The Junior ARGO is an ideal first walking orthosis for infants under 25 kg, but larger hip joints are required for heavier children.

later commercially renamed the Parawalker™, was developed to overcome the same activity limitation using a different orthotic solution (Rose 1979) (Fig. 15.25). The HGO does not use cables and does not directly interconnect the motions of the orthotic hip joints. Instead, the unloaded limb of the HGO swings forward due to the extra weight afforded by heavy footplates together with hip extension of the stance limb powered by the reaction of the ground through the walking aid and upper limbs (Butler *et al.* 1984). The hip joints themselves are rigidly connected, and adduction of the stance and swinging limb due to bending is resisted by the rigidity of the sidebars. As the HGO is worn over clothes it is relatively easy for children to move into position and fasten it themselves.

The biomechanical requirements of the orthotic joints used in the RGO and HGO are the same, notably, resistance of adduction and limited range of low-friction hip flexion–ex-

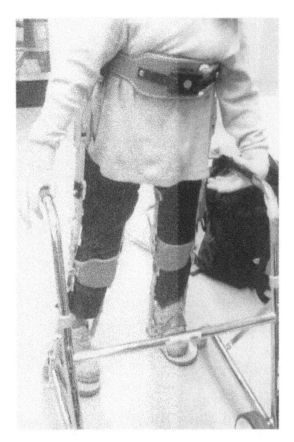

Fig. 15.25. The extra rigidity afforded by the large hip joints of the Parawalker™ or Hip Guidance Orthosis (HGO) better resist hip adduction, enabling greater clearance of the swinging limb.

tension that can be unlocked to permit sitting (Stallard 1993). Intrinsic stability is afforded by the HKAFO design, and using crutches or other walking aids provides extrinsic stability. A recent prospective comparison of the systems did not discern any advantage of one design over the other; the study did highlight that although initial motivation was high, only a quarter of children chose this form of mobility in the longer term (Robb *et al.* 1999). The advantages of cosmesis and close control provided by moulded plastic leg sections were combined with the low-friction hip joints and more rigid sidebars of the HGO for a girl with osteogenesis imperfecta who had become very weak following internal fixation for repeated fractures of the femoral neck (Fig. 15.26). Fuller descriptions of the biomechanics of walking orthoses can be found in Rowley and Rose (1991) and Stallard (1993).

Internal hip rotation in standing and walking
Internal rotation of the hips in the transverse plane is usually seen as an internal foot-progression angle, or in-toeing, during gait. The causes of in-toeing are many, and to some

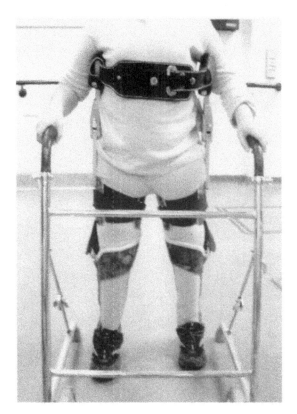

Fig. 15.26. Hybrid hip–knee–ankle–foot orthosis for a girl with osteogenesis imperfecta with lower limb weakness and skeletal malalignment following fractures and a long period of immobility. The lightweight moulded plastic leg sections provide correction of knee and ankle valgus and maintain knee extension. The hip joints from the Parawalker compensate for her weak hip abductor muscles and allow low-friction flexion and extension using a mixture of her own muscle power and the ground reaction force through the walking aid.

degree they may occur as part of normal development in children. In-toeing can also result from excessive pelvic rotation, a strategy to increase step length, or foot, ankle or tibial deformity during gait rather than internal hip rotation (Gage 1991). Conversely, real internal rotation of the semi-flexed hip causing the knees to come together, or 'scissor' gait, can be confused for hip adduction when viewed in the coronal plane. This is frequently seen in children with cerebral palsy because of persistent skeletal anteversion of the femur (Gage 1991), and for ambulant children is more common than true hip adduction or internal rotation at the hip joint.

    Although it may be possible to harness shear forces from the skin and the shape of the soft tissues to gain some control using a moulded thigh cuff, in general rotational control of the hip joint using orthoses requires extension to the foot. This is an intrinsic component of the designs of HKAFOs, where the foot progression angle is fixed by the torsional setting

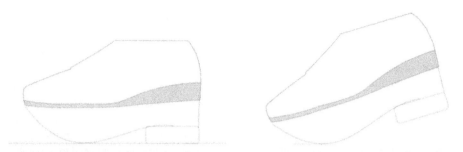

Fig. 15.27. The external raise is tapered off towards the toe-end of the shoe to facilitate heel-rise and tibial advancement during gait. Up to 15 mm of heel raise can be accommodated inside the shoe, shown as the shaded area in the drawings.

of the orthosis. A design of 'twister' orthosis incorporating either a flexible torque cable within the thigh segment of a HKAFO or elastic bands wound around the limb can create active rotational forces. However, when the cause of internal hip rotation is persistent femoral anteversion or spasticity, such as in cerebral palsy, twister orthoses are not advised because the applied torque can lead to excessive strain on the soft tissues of the knee joint.

ACCOMMODATING LEG-LENGTH DISCREPANCY
The most common lifelong sequela of hip-joint pathology is that of leg-length discrepancy (LLD). One leg can be shorter because of migration of the femoral head away from containment in the acetabulum or secondary to impaired growth of the femur following destructive disease or surgery. In order to maintain symmetrical posture it is necessary to accommodate the LLD using some form of levelling raise or foot orthosis. A difference of up to 15mm can be hidden inside the shoe using an internal heel elevator or insole. When the LLD exceeds this height or if the shoe is too low cut to accommodate an internal shoe raise then the additional material can be fixed to the underside of the shoe. Modern orthotic materials and techniques facilitate modification of most types of ordinary shoes in an aesthetically pleasing and lightweight fashion, often inserting the raise within the original sole of the shoe. The height of the heel of the shoe, or pitch, will also influence the exact dimensions of the shoe raise. In order to avoid excessive pressure under the forefoot, material is added to both the sole and heel. However, because the added material will stiffen the shoe and restrict the heel from rising during gait, the raise is tapered off towards the toe end of the shoe to facilitate heel rise and tibial advancement (Fig. 15.27).

Summary and conclusions
There are a wide variety of orthotic interventions that can help children to overcome activity limitations imposed by pathologies affecting the hip, and perhaps improve the structure of the hip joint. As we have seen in this chapter, orthoses can enable children to walk, stand and sit, who would otherwise be unable to accomplish these tasks. By enabling children to adopt upright postures, bone density may be increased. Orthoses can be used to limit the progression of hip deformity by stretching periarticular tissues, or by holding the growing

skeleton in positions that increase containment of the femoral head in the acetabulum. Orthoses may also improve postoperative care by replacing conventional plaster casts.

Successful use of hip orthoses requires thorough assessment of the child's needs and an understanding of the basic principles of biomechanics and postural management presented in this chapter. Orthotic prescription should be part of a comprehensive physical management programme designed to meet the needs of the child and family. For many of the orthoses described, even when the biomechanical objectives are met, successfully achieving the treatment goals depends on adequate medical supervision and support from therapists, helpers and caregivers. The hip is not an easy joint to control, and the team need to remember that the theoretical advantages of orthoses, particularly to enable function, may be outweighed by the difficulties of incorporating the orthosis into family life. It may therefore not be worth persevering with something that was initially well worth attempting.

REFERENCES

Bobechko, W.P., McLaurin, C.A., Motloch, W.M. (1968) 'Toronto orthosis for Legg–Perthes disease.' *Artificial Limbs*, **12** (2), 36–41.

Bower, E. (1990) 'Hip abduction and spinal orthosis in cerebral palsy (an alternative to the use of special seating, lying boards and standing frames).' *Physiotherapy*, **76**, 658–659.

Bowker, P., Condie, D.N., Bader, D.L., Pratt, D.J. (1993) *Biomechanical Basis of Orthotic Management.* Oxford: Butterworth-Heinemann.

Boyd, R., Drake, C. (1993) 'Effectiveness of the hip abduction and spinal orthosis for postural management in a group of non ambulant bilateral cerebral palsy children.' *ISPO UK Newsletter*, Summer, 26–27.

Browne, D. (1948) 'The treatment of congenital dislocation of the hip.' *Proceedings of the Royal Society of Medicine*, **41**, 388–390.

Butler, P.B., Major, R.E., Patrick, J.H. (1984) 'The technique of reciprocal walking using the hip guidance orthosis (HGO) with crutches.' *Prosthetics and Orthotics International*, **8**, 33–38.

Chad, K.E., Bailey, D.A., McKay, H.A., Zello, G.A., Snyder, R.E. (1999) 'The effect of a weight-bearing physical activity program on bone mineral content and estimated volumetric density in children with spastic cerebral palsy.' *Journal of Pediatrics*, **135**, 115–117.

Condie, D.N., Stewart, C.P.U. (1997) *The Supply Process.* Dundee: Distance Learning Section, Department of Orthopaedic & Trauma Surgery, University of Dundee.

Curtis, B.H., Gunther, S.F., Gossling, H.R., Paul, S.W. (1974) 'Treatment for Legg–Perthes disease with the Newington ambulation– abduction brace.' *Journal of Bone and Joint Surgery, American Volume*, **56**, 1135–1146.

Douglas, R., Larson, P.F., D'ambrosia, R., McCall, R.E. (1983) 'The LSU reciprocating-gait orthosis.' *Orthopedics*, **6**, 834–839.

Drake, C., Boyd, R. (1993) 'The design and manufacture of a thermoplastic hip abduction/spinal orthosis for bilateral non ambulant cerebral palsy children.' *ISPO UK Newsletter*, Summer, 25–26.

Duffy, C.M., Hill, A.E., Cosgrove, A.P., Corry, I.S., Graham, H.K. (1996) 'The influence of abductor weakness on gait in spina bifida.' *Gait and Posture*, **4**, 34–38.

Gage, J.R. (1991) *Gait Analysis in Cerebral Palsy. Clinics in Developmental Medicine No. 121.* London: Mac Keith Press.

Hadlow, V.D. (1979) 'Congenital dislocation of the hip over a ten-year period.' *New Zealand Medical Journal*, **89**, 126–128.

Hangen, D.H., Kasser, J.R., Emans, J.B., Millis, M.B. (1995) 'The Pavlik harness and developmental dysplasia of the hip: Has ultrasound changed treatment patterns?' *Journal of Pediatric Orthopedics*, **15**, 729–735.

Harrison, M.H., Turner, M.H., Smith, D.N. (1982) 'Perthes' disease. Treatment with the Birmingham splint.' *Journal of Bone and Joint Surgery, British Volume*, **64**, 3–11.

Hopkins, B.P. (1992) 'The development of a symmetrical hip orthosis.' *Physiotherapy*, **78**, 428–432.

International Organization for Standardization (1989a) *ISO 8549–1: Prosthetics and Orthotics—Vocabulary, Part 1: General Terms for External Limb Prostheses and External Orthoses.* Geneva: IOS.

International Organization for Standardization (1989b) *ISO 8549–3: Prosthetics and Orthotics—Vocabulary, Part 3: Terms Relating to External Orthoses.* Geneva: IOS.

King, G., King, S., Rosenbaum, P. (1996) 'Interpersonal aspects of care-giving and client outcomes: a review of the literature.' *Ambulatory Child Health*, **2**, 151–160.

Leopando, M.T., Moussavi, Z., Holbrow, J., Chernick, V., Pasterkamp, H., Rempel, G. (1999) 'Effect of a soft Boston orthosis on pulmonary mechanics in severe cerebral palsy.' *Pediatric Pulmonology*, **28**, 53–58.

Lerman, J.A., Emans, J.B., Millis, M.B., Share, J., Zurakowski, D., Kasser, J.R. (2001) 'Early failure of Pavlik harness treatment for developmental hip dysplasia: Clinical and ultrasound predictors.' *Journal of Pediatric Orthopedics*, **21**, 348–353.

Major, J., Stallard, J. (1993) 'Hip–knee–ankle–foot orthoses.' *In:* Bowker, P., Condie, D.N., Bader, D.L., Pratt, D.J. (Eds.) *Biomechanical Basis of Orthotic Management.* Oxford: Butterworth-Heinemann, pp. 168–190.

Meehan, P.L., Angel, D., Nelson, J.M. (1992) 'The Scottish Rite abduction orthosis for the treatment of Legg–Perthes disease. A radiographic analysis.' *Journal of Bone and Joint Surgery, American Volume*, **74**, 2–12.

Miller, A., Temple, T., Miller, F. (1996) 'Impact of orthoses on the rate of scoliosis progression in children with cerebral palsy.' *Journal of Pediatric Orthopedics*, **16**, 332–335.

Motloch, W. (1971) 'The parapodium: an orthotic device for neuromuscular disorders.' *Artificial Limbs*, **15**, 36–47.

Pountney, T.E., Mulcahy, C.M., Clarke, S.M., Green, E.M. (2000) *The Chailey Approach to Postural Management.* Birmingham, England: Active Design.

Price, C.T., Day, D.D., Flynn, J.C. (1988) 'Behavioral sequelae of bracing versus surgery for Legg–Calve–Perthes disease.' *Journal of Pediatric Orthopedics*, **8**, 285–287.

Ramsey, P.L., Lasser, S., MacEwen, G.D. (1976) 'Congenital dislocation of the hip. Use of the Pavlik harness in the child during the first six months of life.' *Journal of Bone and Joint Surgery, American Volume*, **58**, 1000–1004.

Robb, J.E., Gordon, L., Ferguson, D., Dunhill, Z., Elton, R.A., Minns, R.A. (1999) 'A comparison of hip guidance with reciprocating gait orthoses in children with spinal paraplegia: results of a ten-year prospective study.' *European Journal of Pediatric Surgery*, **9**, Suppl. 1, 15–18.

Rowley, D.I., Rose, G.K. (1991) 'Walking aids.' In: Bannister, C.M., Tew, B. (Eds.) *Current Concepts in Spina Bifida and Hydrocephalus. Clinics in Developmental Medicine No. 122.* London: Mac Keith Press, pp. 104–118.

Rose, G.K. (1979) 'The principles and practice of hip guidance articulations.' *Prosthetics and Orthotics International*, **3**, 37–43.

Scrutton, D. (1969) 'Interconnected hip hinge in lower limb bracing.' MSc thesis, University of Surrey.

Scrutton, D. (1978) 'Developmental deformity and the profoundly retarded child.' *In:* Apley, J. (Ed.) *Care of the Handicapped Child. Clinics in Developmental Medicine No. 67.* London: Mac Keith Press, pp. 83–91.

Scrutton, D.R., Robson, P., Davies, R.M. (1967) 'Polyplanar hip joint for use in lower limb bracing.' *Nature*, **213**, 950–952.

Snyder, C.H. (1947) 'A sling for use in Legg–Perthes' disease.' *Journal of Bone and Joint Surgery*, **29**, 524–526.

Stallard, J., Rose, G.K., Farmer, I.R. (1978) 'The ORLAU swivel walker.' *Prosthetics and Orthotics International*, **2**, 35–42.

Stallard, J. (1985) *Structures and Materials: An Introduction Based on Orthotics.* Oswestry: Orthotic Research and Locomotion Assessment Unit, Robert Jones & Agnes Hunt Hospital.

Stuberg, W.A. (1992) 'Considerations related to weight-bearing programs in children with developmental disabilities.' *Physical Therapy*, **72**, 35–40.

Taylor, G.R., Clarke, N.M. (1997) 'Monitoring the treatment of developmental dysplasia of the hip with the Pavlik harness. The role of ultrasound.' *Journal of Bone and Joint Surgery, British Volume*, **79**, 719–723.

Terjesen, T., Lange, J.E., Steen, H. (2000) 'Treatment of scoliosis with spinal bracing in quadriplegic cerebral palsy.' *Developmental Medicine and Child Neurology*, **42**, 448–454.

Torpey, P.C., Herle, S.E. (2000) 'Use of the SWASH orthosis for sitting and gait function in a child with sequelae of septic hip.' *Physiotherapy Case Reports*, **3**, 45–56.

World Health Organization (2001) *International Classification of Functioning, Disability and Health (ICF).* Geneva, WHO.

16
UNUSUAL DISORDERS

Durgesh Nagarkatti

In this chapter I will discuss some unusual disorders of the hip, including their etiology and pathogenesis, presentation, management and treatment. Unusual disorders in this context encompass several conditions of different etiology including disorders of hematology and disorders associated with various syndromes.

Arthrogryposis
Arthrogryposis comprises a large spectrum of heterogeneous disorders characterized by joint contractures at birth. Alman and Goldberg (2001) have grouped these contracture disorders into the following categories based on their clinical manifestation:
1. Syndromes involving all four extremities, including amyoplasia (arthrogryposis multiplex congenita) and Larsen syndrome.
2. Distal arthrogryposis involving mainly the hands and feet, with facial involvement in some of these syndromes.
3. Pterygia syndromes, including multiple pterygias and popliteal pterygia, which have extensive skin webbing crossing flexion creases of multiple joints.
    Several studies have looked at the inheritance of arthrogryposis. Hall (1985) concluded that arthrogryposis was the result of a birth defect occurring in 1 in 3000 births, with a hetero-geneous genetic basis. Wynne-Davis and coworkers in two separate studies, one an inter-national collaboration, concluded that arthrogryposis multiplex congenita is a non-genetic disease of early pregnancy, associated with a variety of unfavorable intrauterine factors including the possibility of an unknown viral agent (Wynne-Davies and Lloyd-Roberts 1976, Wynne-Davies *et al.* 1981). Shohat *et al.* (1997), in a genetic study of one large Arab-Israeli family, placed the gene causing amyoplasia between D5S1456 and D5S498. Davidson and Beighton (1976) in their study in South Africa also postulated an unknown environmental agent for a spurt in the incidence of arthrogryposis. Decreased fetal move-ments in the third trimester with oligohydramnios due to possibly diminished fetal mobility have been reported (Sarwark *et al.* 1990). Histology of muscle in arthrogryposis shows a small muscle mass with fibrosis and often with neuropathic and myopathic features (Alman and Goldberg 2001).

PRESENTATION
Amyoplasia, first described as a separate disorder by Hall (1997), is characterized by multiple contractures, decreased limb girth and typical positioning of extremities. Hall reported that amyoplasia comprised 38% of all cases of arthrogryposis in his study. The

features include adduction and internally rotated shoulders, extended elbows with severe wrist flexion and ulnar deviation. The lower extremities demonstrate hips typically flexed, abducted and externally rotated, the knees in extension, and usually club feet.

The incidence of hip involvement ranges from 51% to 85%, with hip dislocation occurring in 15–31% (Sarwark et al. 1990, Hall 1997, Alman and Goldberg 2001). Hip contractures have been reported in most patients with amyoplasia, with approximately one-third of the patients having unilateral or bilateral dislocation (Shapiro and Bresnan 1982). Hoffer et al. (1983) described the common hip contracture resulting in flexion, abduction and external rotation deformity (Buddha-like position). The extreme flexed position of the extremity leads to uncovering of the femoral head posteriorly and thus dislocation (Huurman and Jacobsen 1985).

TREATMENT

The initial approach to managing a child with arthrogryposis should be multidisciplinary, involving the orthopedic surgeon, neurologist, geneticist, therapists and counselors. With regard to the musculoskeletal problems, an emphasis should be made to start early passive range of motion exercises to correct the joint contractures and maintain position with splinting (Carlson et al. 1985).

The primary goal for the hip joint is also the same, namely a pain-free and stable joint in a functional position. However, with regard to the lower extremity attention must first be given to correction of the feet and knees before tackling the hips, and all corrections should be completed preferably before the child starts to walk (Huurman and Jacobsen 1985). In the presence of a hip contracture without dislocation, which is a more frequent finding, gentle manipulations are advocated, followed by splinting in the corrected position. With a mobile lumbar spine, up to 35° of flexion deformity is acceptable (Hoffer et al. 1983). In the absence of any improvement, soft-tissue releases by age 2 years may be necessary. Care must be taken at the time of capsulotomy to preserve the blood supply to the femoral head by releasing the capsule anteriorly, superiorly and close to the acetabulum with or without a subtrochanteric extension osteotomy (Huurman and Jacobsen 1985).

Management of a dislocated hip by closed reduction is rarely successful. Studies of untreated bilateral dislocations have shown most patients to be pain-free with a satisfactory range of motion (Williams 1978, Huurman and Jacobsen 1985, Staheli et al. 1987). Children with untreated unilateral dislocations did fare worse, with limited mobility and a higher incidence of scoliosis compared to bilateral dislocations, attributed to the fixed pelvic obliquity in the unilateral dislocations (Sarwark et al. 1990). Therefore, all authors advocate aggressive management of unilateral dislocation to reduce the problems associated with unreduced dislocations. Some studies showed high rates of complication and worse function with open reduction of bilateral hip dislocations and thus recommended leaving bilateral dislocations alone (Williams 1978, Hoffer et al. 1983, Sarwark et al. 1990). Other studies involving early hip reduction and decreased duration of immobilization have shown better results with low complications (Staheli et al. 1987, Szoke et al. 1996, Akasawa et al. 1998). The better results by these authors may be attributed to the earlier age of surgery and reduced periods of immobilization. Most authors have advocated using an anterior approach to reduction of the hip dislocation. However, recent studies have shown equally good results with the medial approach for reduction (Carlson *et al*. 1985, St Clair and Zimbler 1985).

The complications of surgery include joint stiffness, failure to achieve reduction, and redislocation. Redislocation, however, is uncommon after a stable concentric reduction (Huurman and Jacobsen 1985). Early case reports of total joint replacement in adult patients with arthrogryposis have shown a good range of motion in the early postoperative period. However, this range of motion returned to the preoperative status within two years of surgery (Cameron 1998).

Hemophilia

Hemophilia comprises a group of disorders of hemostasis characterized by a deficiency in coagulation factors. The only disorders associated with sufficient bleeding to cause hemophilic arthropathy include the classic hemophilia (hemophilia A) in which a deficiency of factor VIII is present, and Christmas disease (hemophilia B) in which there is a deficiency of factor IX (Arnold and Hilgartner 1977, Greene 2001). Both these disorders are sex-linked recessive and thus are largely restricted to the male population with the female being the carrier. A study by Soucie *et al*. (1988) on the occurrence of hemophilia in the USA found that 79% of patients had a factor VIII deficiency. The age-adjusted prevalence of hemophilia A and B was 13.4 cases per 100,000 males, and the incidence was 1 in 5032 live male births.

Diagnosis of hemophilia at an early age is suspected when infants have abnormally increased bruising from immunization sites and bleeding from circumcisions, and in the older child with unusual bruising when learning to walk (Greene 2001). A history of affected males on the maternal side is often seen. Laboratory diagnosis demonstrates an elevated partial thromboplastin time, and specific factor assays establish the diagnosis and severity (Greene 2001). Coagulation factor deficiencies are graded as severe (<1% activity), moderate (1–5% activity), or mild (>5% activity) (Greene and McMillan1989). Soucie and coworkers in their study showed a severe involvement in 43%, moderate in 26% and mild in 31% of the population. Prior to 1965, nonsurgical management of hemophiliacs involved large volumes of transfusions to compensate for the factor deficiencies. With the discovery of cryoprecipitate and concentrates, factor replacement with transfusion therapy at home became much easier (Greene 2001). Initial preparations of the factor concentrate involved pooling of the plasma from several donors and this was associated with transmission of hepatitis and HIV. With increasing surveillance, this has not been seen in hemophiliacs receiving transfusion since 1984 (Greene and McMillan 1989). Currently, using recombinant technology both factors VIII and IX are being produced and used, negating the risk of transmission of hepatitis and HIV viruses.

Antibodies to the transfused factors develop in 15% of patients with severe factor VIII hemophilia, with the incidence being lower in factor IX deficiency (Shapiro 1979). Development of these antibodies or inhibitors severely restricts the options in these patients. The level of antibody titers in patients makes them either high or low responders. Low responders can undergo elective surgery with high doses of factor VIII, while the high responders require sequential transfusions to induce immune tolerance. Newer modalities including

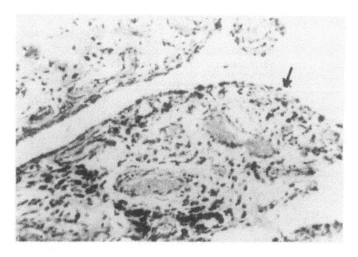

Fig. 16.1. Knee synovium demonstrating inflammatory changes. (Reproduced by permission from Rodriguez-Merchan 1996.)

activated factor VIIa are being tried in these patients as they bypass the factor VIII step in the coagulation cascade (Greene 2001).

The pathogenesis of hemophilic arthropathy starts with bleeding episodes in the joint over a short period. The hemarthrosis in the joint causes synovial tissue inflammation as a result of the breakdown products of the blood that exceed the capacity of the synovial cells. Arnold *et al.* (1977) found an increase in hydrolytic enzymes in the joint fluid and synovium. Stein and Duthie (1981) demonstrated well-defined cytoplasmic deposits of iron, termed siderosomes, in synovial cells, synovial tissue and chondrocytes. These cells then disintegrate, releasing lysosomes that exacerbate the inflammation and joint destruction. Thus a vicious cycle is set up with the synovium being hypervascular, hypertrophic, friable and with a tendency to bleed easily, causing further episodes of hemarthrosis to occur (Fig. 16.1). With progression of hemophilia, the synovium loses its villous formation and is replaced with fibrous tissue that manifests as early disabling arthritis when combined with the joint destruction.

JOINT INVOLVEMENT
Jordan (1958) clearly described the typical radiographic abnormalities associated with hemophilic arthropathy. Radiographic features of early-stage hemophilia include soft-tissue swelling, osteopenia, and in the immature skeleton an overgrowth of the epiphysis. The excessive growth may lead to limb-length discrepancy, angular deviations and alteration in the skeletal structure (Rodriguez-Merchan 1996). With disease progression, subchondral cysts, subchondral irregularity, patellar squaring, marginal erosions, radial head and trochlear notch widening are characteristic (Greene 2001). End-stage arthritis is characterized by joint-space narrowing and sclerotic subchondral bone. Based on the typical changes seen on knee radiographs initially Arnold and Hilgartner (1977) and then Petterson *et al.* (1990)

241

TABLE 16.1
Radiographic grading of hemophilic arthropathy*

Classification	Score
Subchondral irregularity	
Absent	0
Mild (< 50% of joint surface)	1
Pronounced	2
Joint space narrowing	
Absent	
<50%	1
>50%	2
Joint margin erosion	
Absent	0
Present	1
Joint surface incongruity	
Absent	0
Mild	1
Pronounced	2

*Reproduced by permission from Greene (1989).

classified the stages of hemophilic arthropathy. Greene *et al.* (1989) in a study involving 105 knees compared a new classification developed by them to the two earlier systems. They found their new four-sign, seven-point classification to be better and simpler than the earlier classifications (Table 16.1).

The most common joints involved with hemophilic arthropathy include the knee, elbow and ankle, accounting for almost 80% of the cases The hip, shoulder and wrist are rarely involved and thus rarely progress to significant arthropathy. One of the reasons postulated for the infrequent involvement of the hip is the distribution of the synovium in the joint (Rodriguez-Mercahn 1996). In the immature skeleton, hemarthrosis in the hip may result in changes similar to Perthe's disease as was seen in studies by Pettersson *et al.* (1990) and Rodriguez-Merchan (1996). Unlike Perthe's disease these changes always involve the entire epiphysis with relative sparing of the metaphysis. Kilcoyne and Nuss (1999) described a femoral head osteonecrosis developing in a child with hemophilia. In a rare case, repeated hemarthrosis in a child leading to hip dislocation has been reported. The reduced hip then went on to bony ankylosis (Floman and Niska 1983).

Studies by Winston (1952), Teitelbaum (1977) and Post (1980) had shown recurrent intra-articular bleeding producing chronic synovitis and early degenerative arthritis. Goodman *et al.* (1987) in a large study involving 102 mature hemophilic hips with a mean follow-up of seven years showed that 59% of the patients had at least one bleeding episode during the study period. Forty-nine patients (64 hips) showed at least a 15° change in range of motion at some time. In their final review, 34 of the 64 hips suffered loss of motion. Their data also suggested that early loss of hip motion after an acute bleed is usually regained within a year except for a minimal reduction in hip rotation. In a case report, Ishiguru *et al.* (2001)

242

described a 48-year-old male hemophiliac who exhibited hip arthropathy that was similar to rapidly destructive arthropathy. His hip joint was destroyed six months after the onset of symptoms. All studies failed to reveal any neuropathic, inflammatory or septic arthropathy, except for coagulopathy. MRI revealed an expansive joint capsule with synovial proliferation in the affected hip joint, and a histological examination after surgery revealed bone necrosis, nonspecific inflammation, hemosiderosis and synovial hypertrophy.

Patients with severe factor deficiency develop muscle hemorrhages after minor trauma. Sites in the lower extremity include the iliopsoas, iliacus, quadriceps and posterior calf muscles. Hemarthrosis into the hip joint can be differentiated from bleed in the iliopsoas by flexing the hip. Rotation of the hip in this position in the case of an iliopsoas bleed will be relatively normal whereas with joint hemarthrosis it would be restricted. Bleeding into the iliacus can also cause a femoral nerve paralysis because of the tight compartment.

It is known that repeated bleeding into joints or muscles in patients with moderate or severe hemophilia leads to hemophilic arthropathy. Greene and McMillan (1989) recommend regular prophylactic infusions of the factor to prevent spontaneous bleeding by maintaining a plasma factor level above 1%. This plasma factor level should prevent bleeds that occur with trivial injuries.

Management of minor and major hemarthrosis differs significantly. Minor hemarthrosis can be successfully managed at home with transfusions, ice packs, splints and crutches with analgesics. A major hemarthrosis requires aspiration, splinting, a rehabilitation program and repeated transfusions to minimize the risk of hypertrophic synovitis. Greene and McMillan (1989) have shown that aspiration, by removing blood, reduces the amount of iron exposed to the synovial cells and therefore decreases the synovial hypertrophy and reduces the severe pain.

In the presence of synovitis, joint motion is not particularly restricted. The principle of treating the synovitis is to decrease the chances of further joint bleeds. Storti *et al.* (1969) were the first to report the use of synovectomy in hemophiliacs. It has been seen in further studies that synovectomy consistently reduces the rate of hemarthrosis. Greene (2001) believes that the procedure delays but does not eliminate the progression of arthritis. Recent advances include arthroscopic synovectomy followed by a brief period of functional splinting and continuous passive motion to maintain or regain the range of motion. Nonsurgical synovectomy using radioactive isotopes may be a useful alternative in patients with antibodies. The radioactive isotopes cause fibrosis of the synovial tissue, while maintaining the integrity of the articular cartilage and bone.

Pseudotumors or hemophiliac cysts are the result of bleeding that may be intramuscular, subperiosteal or intraosseous. These grow large in size with repeated bleeding and can be frequently mistaken for aneurysmal bone cyst, osteomyelitis or sarcomas. Greene (2001) has observed most pseudotumors involving the pelvic girdle and recommends early excision if possible (Fig. 16.2). Fractures of the lower extremity are common due to the osteopenia and contractures especially involving the femoral neck and supracondylar regions of the femur. These should be treated expeditiously to restore function and decrease morbidity.

Joint deformities in hemophiliacs should be detected early and treated aggressively to maintain function. Use of ultrasonography and CT can help differentiate from hemarthrosis

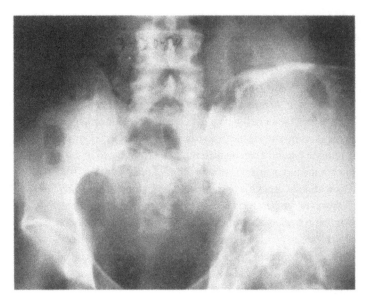

Fig. 16.2. Anteroposterior X-ray of the pelvis of an adult male hemophiliac with a massive pseudotumor involving the entire left ilium. In addition there is osteonecrosis of the left femoral head and severe degenerative changes involving the articular cartilage. (Reproduced by permission from Greene 2001.)

from a muscular bleed. Heim *et al.* (1998) used these techniques to treat hip hemarthrosis by aspiration of the hematoma after confirming diagnosis with sonography.

Several studies have looked at the efficacy of total hip replacement in hemophiliacs. Nelson *et al.* (1992), Kelley *et al.* (1995), Lofqvist *et al.* (1996) and Takedani *et al.* (2000), evaluating the effectiveness and suitability of joint replacement in this population, found that the patients experienced relief from pain and intra-articular bleeding in affected joints but only marginal improvement in the range of motion. There was a significant improvement in quality of life for these patients. However, Kelley *et al.* and Lofqvist *et al.* found a higher revision rate in these patients when compared to patients with primary osteoarthritis. It must also be noted that a high number of hemophiliacs undergoing total joint replacement have hepatitis and/or HIV that places them at a greater risk for infection and failure.

Down syndrome

Down syndrome is the most common chromosomal abnormality in humans. Besides the characteristic facies, children with Down syndrome have short stature and delayed milestones, with most not walking until the age of 2–3 years with a classic wide-based, waddling gait (Cronk *et al.* 1988).

The inheritance pattern demonstrated by cytogenetic testing shows that complete trisomy 21 accounts for 95% of the cases, followed by 2% mosaics and 3% translocations (Brock 1993). The overall incidence is 1 per 660 births, this figure rising with increasing maternal age to 1 in 250 for mothers aged over 35 years.

The non-orthopedic involvement of children with Down syndrome typically includes mental retardation, congenital heart disease in one-half of patients, duodenal atresia, leukemia in 1%, endocrinopathies with hypothyroidism in particular, and infection (Alman and Golberg 2001). Twenty per cent of the children develop orthopedic abnormalities including cervical spine instabilities in 10–30%, scoliosis in one-half especially in the institutionalized with severe mental retardation, and lower lumbar spine spondylolisthesis. There is also a high incidence of patellar instability, pes planus, metatarsus primus varus and hip dysplasia (Diamond *et al.* 1981).

The etiology for these orthopedic findings has been postulated as joint laxity and muscle hypotonia. Based on criteria laid out by Carter and Wilkinson (1964), Semine *et al.* (1978) demonstrated generalized joint laxity in 65 of 85 Down syndrome children and correlated it with cervical spine instability (Brock, 1993, Diamond, 1981). However, Livingstone and Hirst (1986) using the same criteria did not find any joint laxity and instead proposed muscle hypotonia as the underlying etiology for the skeletal manifestations.

HIP DISORDERS
There is an increased incidence of hip disorders with Down syndrome in published data, including slipped capital femoral epiphysis of 1.3%, Perthes' disease in 2%, acetabular dysplasia or dislocation in 2.9%, and an overall incidence of childhood hip disease of 6.2–7.9% (Semine *et al.* 1978, Cronk *et al.* 1988). However, Bennet *et al.* (1982) in a study of 220 institutionalized patients found that 5% developed a dislocated or dislocatable hip.

HIP DISLOCATION
Dislocation is the most common hip disorder in Down syndrome. It is rarely present at birth and usually occurs between the ages of 2 and 13 years as either an acute or an habitual event (Livingstone and Hirst 1986, Shaw and Beals 1992). Untreated dislocations go on to develop into a fixed subluxation, progressive dysplasia, antalgic gait and finally a painful arthritis (Semine *et al.* 1978, Bennet *et al.* 1982, Livingstone and Hirst 1986, Cronk *et al.* 1988). Hybpermobility, ligamentous laxity, and pelvic and acetabular abnormalities are some of the factors responsible for recurrent hip dislocation. Gore (1981) demonstrated a thin, attenuated and poorly developed fibrous posterior capsule without any tear or detachment in a child with Down syndrome with recurrent hip dislocation. There are distinct features to the pelvis in infancy, including broad iliac wings, reduced iliac angles and reduced acetabular angles, which are diagnostic and may contribute to the hip instability (Gore 1981, Hresko *et al.* 1993). Greene (1998) postulated that hip dislocation can cause a redundant, patulous posterior hip capsule, which coupled with ligamentous laxity and muscle hypotonia results in recurrent dislocation. Shaw and Beals (1992) in their study of older children and adults (228 hips) found a deepened acetabulum with decreased anteversion and a horizontal roof, a normal neck–shaft angle, and a moderately increased femoral anteversion that would be expected to create an intrinsically stable joint. There was also an increase in external rotation at the hip on examination of these patients, contributing to the characteristic gait.

Management of the unstable hip in these children is difficult and fraught with a high rate of treatment failures. Both nonoperative and operative methods have been reported.

An initial prolonged trial of immobilization followed by bracing has shown success in children less than 6 years of age. Greene (1998) in a study of three hips successfully treated his patients with closed reduction followed by a prolonged course of immobilization or bracing initially full-time for a period of four to six months, and then ambulatory abduction orthoses for four to eight months. He believed immobilization to be critical towards reversing the pathologic patulous posterior capsule.

Operative treatment is recommended for the hips that fail a prolonged trial of immo-bilization and in older patients. The surgical procedure includes femoral or pelvic osteotomies with imbrication of the redundant capsule. The hip is usually dislocated posteriorly and may be approached through the anterior or posterior approach. Bennet *et al.* (1982) and Aprin *et al.* (1985) preferred an anterior capsular imbrication, while Gore (1981) in contrast ap-proached the hip posteriorly and reported successful treatment of a recurrent hip dislocation with posterior capsular imbrication and reinforcement of the deficient posterior capsule with the short external rotators. Aprin *et al.* classified their hips in two groups based on the morphology of the acetabulum: group I with a normal acetabulum, and group II with an insufficient and abnormal acetabulum. The authors recommended a femoral osteotomy with anterior capsular imbrication in cases with normal acetabulum and including a pelvic osteotomy for the dysplastic acetabula.

However, surgery is technically demanding and is associated with a high rate of com-plications and recurrence. Bennet *et al.* in their study of 22 hips managed operatively had eight redislocations, two subluxations and five infections, while in Aprin *et al.*'s study the complications included osteomyelitis of the ilium in one, fracture of the proximal femur in one, three recurrent subluxations and three patients with a limp.

ADULT HIP PROBLEMS

The life expectancy of children with Down syndrome has increased with improvements in the medical and surgical care of congenital heart disease, leukemia and infections. This has led to survival of less involved patients well into their sixties, experiencing debilitating hip problems. Hresko *et al.* (1993), in their study of 130 hips in patients with a mean age of 40 years, found radiographic abnormalities in 22%; Cristofaro *et al.* (1986) reported an incidence of osteoarthritis of 10%; and Shaw and Beals (1992) found radiographic abnormalities in 8%. Hresko *et al.*, in a subgroup of 18 patients followed by serial examination, showed that hip instability occurred in adulthood and became worse with time and in some patients, hip instability started after skeletal maturity. A study by Kioschos *et al.* (1999) showed a high incidence of avascular necrosis leading to osteoarthritis with the possible etiology being an increased number of acute slips and late diagnosis.

A few studies have shown total hip arthroplasty to be a satisfactory treatment for severe hip disease in these patients. Kioschos *et al.* carried out total hip replacement in six adult patients (nine hips) with severe arthritis of the hip; after a mean follow-up of 7.75 years all had relief of pain and full hip function. Skoff and Keggi (1987) in their eight total hip replacements had excellent results with no infection, loosening or dislocation at a mean follow-up of 4.3 years. Most of the reported cases have been treated with an ingrowth femoral stem.

The high incidence of complications and the systemic involvement of patients with Down syndrome at all ages require a complete preoperative preparation followed by careful post-operative monitoring.

Sickle cell disease

Sickle cell disease is a disorder of erythrocytes and includes SS disease, which is homozygous for hemoglobin S; SC disease, which is heterozygous for hemoglobin S and hemoglobin C; and Sb, which is heterozygous for hemoglobin S and hemoglobin b-thalassemia. In a study by Schneider *et al.* (1976) of almost a quarter million African-Americans, the frequency of sickle cell disease was 1.4 per thousand and the gene for hemoglobin S occurred in 8%. Hemoglobin S results from an abnormality of b-globulin on chromosome 11, causing sub-stitution of valine for glutamic acid at the sixth codon from the amino-terminus (Greene 2001). Hemoglobin C is the result of lysine substituting the same glutamic acid in hemoglobin S. After SS disease, SC disease is the second most common type of sickle cell disease in the USA (Schneider *et al.* 1976).

The pathogenesis of sickle cell disease involves vasooclusion and hemolysis. Conditions of low oxygen tension and decreased blood flow cause hemoglobin S polymerization and conversion into a gel of intertwined fibers (Bunn 1997). Thus, erythrocytes become fragile and are destroyed. However, the erythrocytes are also rigid, clogging smaller blood vessels causing tissue infarction (Greene 2001). Several other factors also contribute, including erythrocyte adhesion to endothelium and cell dehydration.

PRESENTATION

There is great clinical variability in the manifestation of sickle cell disease, the reasons for which are not well understood. About 50% of people with sickle cell disease survive beyond the fifth decade in the USA compared to less than 2% surviving to age 5 in some areas of Africa (Schneider *et al.* 1976, Skoff and Keggi 1987). Advances in pediatric preventive care including vaccination against pneumococcus, hepatitis B and hemophilus influenza, and prophylactic penicillin use have reduced the complications in children with sickle cell disease (McKie 1998). A common non-orthopedic problem is a cerebrovascular accident in children, with the risk of recurrence being 50–70% if the disease is untreated (Platt *et al.* 1994, Pegelow *et al.* 1995, Steinberg 1999).

Musculoskeletal issues include dactylitis, sickle cell crises, osteomyelitis, osteonecrosis and septic arthritis. The hemolytic anemia in children with sickle cell disease leads to an increase in the size of the medullary spaces and osteopenia with classical changes in the spine of biconcave "fish" vertebrae (Fig. 16.3). The most common cause of extremity and back pain is sickle cell crises, which result from localized infarction in the bone marrow associated with elevated levels of substance P (Earley *et al.* 1998, McKie 1998). Keeley and Buchanan (1982) have shown the humerus, tibia and femur to be the most common sites of infarction. Infections are also more common in these patients and can be attributed to hypersplenism, defective opsonization and secondary bacteremia from bowel infarction (Greene 2001). In a study by Dalton *et al.* (1996) the incidence of osteomyelitis was 1.6% per admission for orthopedic complaints in children with sickle cell disease. It is extremely

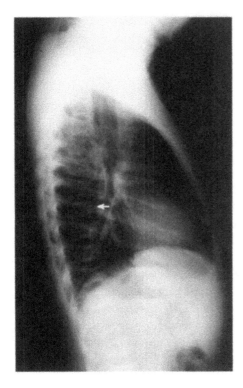

Fig. 16.3. Lateral X-ray of the thoracic spine in a child with sickle cell disease: early infarcts with vertebral collapse.

important to differentiate osteomyelitis from sickle crises to reduce the complications of osteomyelitis and multifocal infections. Clinical features and studies including a temperature greater than 39°C, more pain than usual, a left shift in the peripheral count, positive blood culture and biopsy are helpful in differentiating the two conditions. Sadat-Ali *et al.* (1998) have shown ultrasonography to be of use in detecting subperiosteal collections in osteomyelitis. Salmonella and gram-negative osteomyelitis are more common in children with sickle cell disease because of infarction of bowel mucosa leading to bacteremia (Burnett *et al.* 1998). Osteomyelitis when diagnosed should be treated with agent-specific and sensitive antibiotics.

HIP MANIFESTATIONS
Avascular necrosis of the femoral head is a common problem in sickle cell disease. Milner *et al.* (1991) in a large radiographic study involving 2890 patients over 5 years of age found an overall prevalence of 9.7% of osteonecrosis that was dependent on patient age and type of sickle cell disease, and bilateral disease was seen in 54% of the patients (Milner *et al.* 1991) (Table 16.2). Patients homozygous in the SS group for the a-thalassemia gene were 2.4 times more likely to have osteonecrosis compared to other groups. The patients with osteonecrosis may be asymptomatic for a long time. Hernigou *et al.* (1991) in a study of sickle cell children with avascular necrosis of the hip (95 hips) at a mean follow-up of 19 years demonstrated a better result in patients who developed the osteonecrosis before the

TABLE 16.2
Prevalence of osteonecrosis of the hip in sickle cell disease*

| Age group | Hemoglobin genotype | | | | Total |
	SS N (%)	SβO N (%)	SC N (%)	Sβ+ N (%)	N (%)
5–9	6 (1.7)	0	1 (0.9)	0	7 (1.3)
10–14	20 (5.8)	1 (3.2)	3 (2.6)	0	24 (4.6)
15–24	50 (8.5)	6 (13.0)	10 (8.1)	0	66 (8.2)
25–34	65 (18.5)	6 (24.0)	17 (18.5)	7 (20.0)	95 (18.8)
35–44	23 (23.0)	3 (50.0)	7 (17.5)	1 (11.1)	34 (21.9)
≥45	15 (34.9)	1 (25.0)	9 (29.0)	2 (40.0)	27 (32.5)
Total	179 (10.0)	17 (11.9)	47 (9.1)	10 (6.9)	253 (9.7)
Age-adjusted rate	10.2	13.1	8.8	5.8	—
95% CI	8.8–11.6	7.7–18.5	6.4–11.2	2.6–9.0	8.5–10.9

*Adapted by permission from Milner *et al.* (1991)—see source reference for denominators used for calculation of percentages.

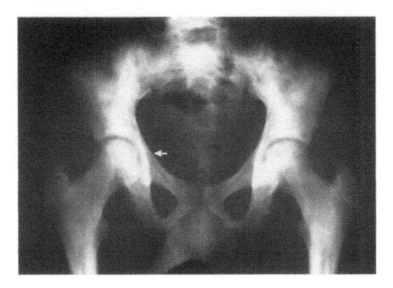

Fig. 16.4. Anteroposterior X-ray of the pelvis of a child with sickle cell disease: bone infarcts in the femoral head (arrow) leading to avascular necrosis.

age of 10 years than in those who developed it between 10 and 14 years of age. MRI is helpful in demonstrating the extent of involvement of osteonecrosis of the femoral head. Rao *et al.* (1988) have shown segments of the femoral head to be involved in varying degrees, implying that in the pathophysiology of osteonecrosis the segments are infarcted at different times (Fig. 16.4). Malizos *et al.* (2001) have shown the usefulness of MRI-based, semi-automated volumetric quantification in accurately defining the extent and site of

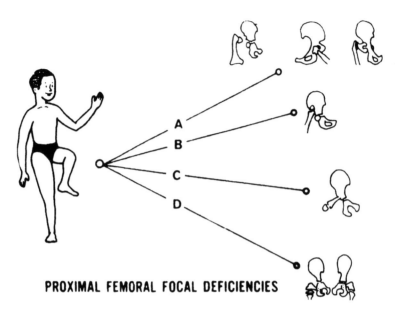

PROXIMAL FEMORAL FOCAL DEFICIENCIES

Fig. 16.5. Aitken classification of proximal femoral focal deficiencies. (Reproduced by permission f rom Morrissy and Weinstein 1996.)

necrosis in order to perform drilling and grafting. Washington *et al.* (1985) have shown the efficacy of conservative treatment in the presence of an intact lateral pillar. In the presence of extensive head involvement, femoral and acetabular osteotomies may be required.

Total hip arthroplasty is the final recourse for patients with extensive disease and severe restriction of activities of daily living. However, studies by Rand *et al.* (1987), Bishop *et al.* (1988), Hanker and Amstutz (1988) and Clark *et al.* (1989) have shown poor results. The incidence of postoperative infection was high, and in all series the revision rate was greater than 50% by four years postoperatively. In contrast to these disappointing results, most patients in the study by Chung and Ralston (1971) gained relief from their disabling symptoms and were functionally better after total joint arthroplasty. Thus before being offered this procedure, the children and their parents should be educated about the high risks involved.

Proximal focal femoral deficiency (PFFD)
PFFD is a term used to describe a condition with a short femur and an apparent absence of continuity between the neck and the shaft (Herring and Cummings 1996). The inheritance of femoral deficiency in most cases is unknown. However, a few cases have been associated in the past with the use of thalidomide, and with some autosomal dominant disorders with variable penetrance and expressivity (Kelly 1974, Herring and Cummings 1996, Kalaycioglu and Aynaci 2001).

Aitken (1969) proposed a classification into four categories based on radiographic findings, and this is still the most widely used system in practice today (Fig. 16.5). Class

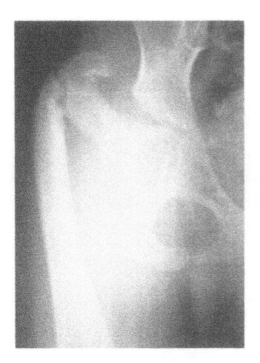

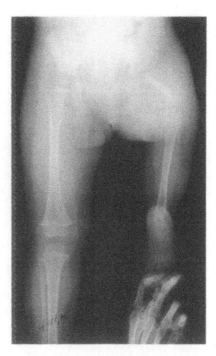

Fig. 16.6. Class A PFFD with short femur with femoral head present and within a well-formed acetabulum. Note the intertrochanteric pseudoarthrosis.

Fig. 16.7. Class B PFFD. The femur is shorter and the unossified femoral head is directed toward a well-formed acetabulum.

A presents as a short femur with a defect in the subtrochanteric region. The femoral head is present in a well-formed acetabulum, with the pseudarthrosis in the subtrochanteric region healing in a varus deformity by maturity. The femoral shaft may lie proximal to the acetabulum (Fig. 16.6). In class B, the femoral shaft is shorter than in class A, with the femoral head being absent at birth in the presence of a normal acetabulum. The femoral head appears as the child matures. The proximal end of the femur has a bony tuft and lies above the level of the acetabulum. At maturity, however, there is no contact between the shaft and the head segment (Fig. 16.7). Class C presents with a much shorter femoral segment than class B with an absent femoral head and a severely dysplastic acetabulum. Class D has an extremely short or even absent femoral segment with a flat lateral pelvic wall in place of the acetabulum (Fig. 16.8).

Hamanishi (1980) in another classification graded the femoral abnormalities along a spectrum with 10 gradations from a shortened femur to complete absence of the femur. He also observed congenital coxa vara to be a distinct entity unrelated to PFFD.

Gillespie (1998) classified these abnormalities into three groups based on the treatment options. Group A consisted of patients with a short femur and a stable hip that could be treated with limb lengthening; group B included Aitken A, B and C; and Group C was equivalent to Aitken D. Gillespie recommended prosthetic treatment for groups B and C.

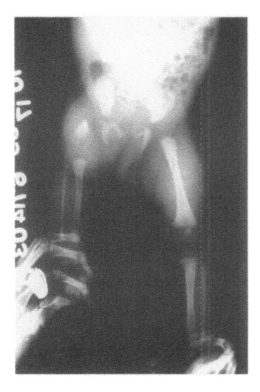

Fig. 16.8. Class D PFFD. The entire proximal two-thirds of the femur is absent and the acetabulum is effaced with no socket.

PRESENTATION

The PFFDs have characteristic features with bilateral involvement in 15% of cases (Morrissy *et al.* 2001). The femur is short and bulbous, with the hip being flexed, abducted and externally rotated. There is frequently a flexion deformity present at the hip and knee that adds to the already shortened extremity. Fibular deficiencies are present in almost 70–80% of PFFD patients, and they clinically have tibial shortening and equinovalgus at the foot (Bevan-Thomas and Millar 1967). Examination of these children is difficult because of the short, bulbous thigh and the knee being at the level of the groin. There is usually knee instability in the anteroposterior plane associated with cruciate deficiencies (Johansson and Aparisi 1983). Johansson and Aparisi describe a related disorder with congenital shortening of femur that presents with an anterolateral bow of the femur, valgus deformity of the knee and anteroposterior instability due to absent cruciate ligaments. The children often have an ipsilateral fibular hemimelia and limited straight leg raise due to shortened hamstrings.

TREATMENT

Several options exist for the treatment of PFFD and these can be postponed until age 2–3 years, as this is the best age for surgical options. Having determined the extent of leg-length discrepancy at maturity, one of the first decisions to be made is whether the child is a candidate for limb lengthening. The selection criteria for limb lengthening are that the length discrepancy is no greater than 20 cm, the hip joint is stable, and the knee, ankle and foot are good (Morrissy *et al.* 2001). In cases where the estimated discrepancy is greater than 20 cm, a decision for prosthetic fitting is made along with a choice of surgical options.

PROSTHETIC MANAGEMENT
When the child with PFFD is ready to stand, the initial prosthetic management would begin with an extension or nonstandard prosthesis. The sole purpose of this prosthesis is to prepare the child for early ambulation by equalizing the limb lengths. McCollough (1963) has identified four indications for using nonstandard prostheses: (1) awaiting the proper age for surgery; (2) patient refuses surgery and a prosthesis is necessary for ambulation; (3) in bilateral cases, to achieve extra height or better balance; (4) in the event of absence of bilateral upper extremity, thus requiring the feet for daily living activities.

The definitive prostheses required after various surgical procedures like Syme amputation or a Van Nes rotationplasty are very specific and tailored to provide the best function for the child (Friscia *et al.* 1989). Several studies have shown better functional results and gait with a rotationplasty and prosthesis in comparison to an amputation (Bevan-Thomas and Millar 1967, Morrissy *et al.* 2001).

SURGICAL MANAGEMENT
There are several choices for surgery in a child with PFFD including knee arthrodesis, foot amputation, Van Nes rotationplasty, hip stabilization and iliofemoral arthrodesis. These procedures are dependent on the clinical and radiographic findings.

Knee arthrodesis is a standard procedure usually performed in conjunction with amputation of the foot. It creates a long and efficient lever arm that is easier to control in prosthesis. Fusion is usually performed between 2 and 3 years of age and may include removal of one or both growth plates (Epps 1983). A foot amputation is best performed at the time of knee fusion, since the foot adds unnecessary length and is difficult to accommodate in a socket.

Van Nes rotationplasty rotates the limb 180° through the knee arthrodesis and/or the tibia (Van Nes 1950). The goal of rotationplasty is to have the now rotated ankle joint at the level of the opposite knee joint and function as a below-knee amputee. Several authors have shown significant advantages of performing a rotationplasty in children with limb-sparing surgery for tumors and congenital deficiencies (Bevan-Thomas and Millar 1967, Torode and Gillespie 1983, Morrissy *et al.* 2001). The selection criterion for this surgery is a normal functioning ankle joint and it is contraindicated in cases with extensive ankle abnormalities. The one drawback to this procedure is the cosmetic aspect of a backward foot, and all concerned should meet other families with similar problems to get a better understanding.

There has been controversy regarding the need to stabilize the involved hip or not, with studies showing equally good results with both treatments (Aitken 1969, Eps 1983, Johansson and Aparisi 1983, Murray *et al.* 1985, Goddard *et al.* 1995). Morrissy *et al.* (2001) are of the opinion that surgery benefits patients with Aitken class A or B with correction of the pseudarthrosis and varus deformity. Pirani *et al.* (1991) in a study of the soft tissues around

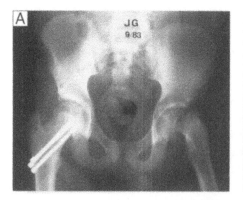

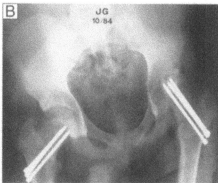

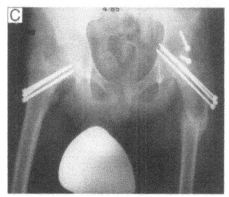

Fig. 16.9. X-rays of a young male with bilateral slipped capital femoral epiphysis.

(A) The right femur has been prophylactically pinned; however, there is an acute slip of the left femur.

(B) The left femoral epiphysis has been reduced and pinned, but there is early aseptic necrosis with collapse of the left femoral head. The cartilage space of the right hip is beginning to narrow.

(C) The right hip demonstrates further chondrolysis with further decreased articular cartilage space. The left hip joint required arthrodesis due to progressive femoral head necrosis.

the hip have shown that all the muscles are present but much smaller, with the exception of the obturator externus and sartorius, which are hypertrophied and muscular. The lack of soft tissue also compromises all hip stabilization procedures. Iliofemoral arthrodesis has been used to address the problem of hip instability. Steel *et al.* (1987) have described a technique of fusing the distal femoral segment to the pelvis at the level of the acetabulum with the femur flexed 90°, so that the knee joint functions as the hip joint. Brown In a recent study, Brown (2001) combined the iliofemoral arthrodesis with rotationplasty, such that the knee functions as the hip joint and the ankle functions as the knee.

PFFD fortunately is not very common and there exist several choices both surgical and nonsurgical to improve the functioning of the involved child. Excellent nursing is central in the care of these children and their families both for psychosocial support and teaching during the decision-making process and to help meet the rehabilitation goals (Stormer 1997).

Chondrolysis of the hip

Chondrolysis or progressive loss of the articular cartilage is most frequently reported as a complication occasionally encountered during treatment for slipped capital femoral epiphysis (SCFE) (Fig. 16.9). This complication is reported to occur in approximately 8% of treated cases of SCFE. Much less common is the condition of idiopathic chondrolysis of the hip, the incidence of which is not known. The patient presents with a painful hip with limp and reduced range of motion. The synovium becomes edematous, and there is loss of articular synovial fluid, and progressive fibrillation of the cartilage leading to erosion and loss of joint space (Cruess 1983). A thorough evaluation is necessary to differentiate this condition from juvenile rheumatoid arthritis, tuberculosis, pyogenic arthritis and pigmented villinodular synovitis. Early reports suggested that the changes were irreversible, leading to progressive stiffness and fibrous or bony ankylosis. More recently, more favorable outcomes have been reported with aggressive treatment with nonsteroidal anti-inflammatory medicines, vigorous physical therapy to maintain range of motion, and restriction from weight bearing (Daluga and Millar 1989). In selected cases a more vigorous approach consisting of subtotal capsulotomy of the hip joint in combination with vigorous physical therapy, traction and non-weight-bearing have shown full recovery of joint articular cartilage and range of motion (Roy and Crawford 1988).

Conclusion
The clinician must become familiar with the basic concepts of acquiring a thorough history and performing a complete physical examination before proceeding with appropriate laboratory evaluations and routine X-ray examinations. It is evident from this overview of unusual conditions that many different childhood afflictions may first present as a painful hip or an abnormal gait pattern.

REFERENCES

Aitken, G.T. (1969) 'Proximal femoral deficiency.' *In: A Symposium on Proximal Femoral Focal Deficiency – A Congenital Anomaly.* Washington, DC: National Academy of Sciences, p. 1.

Akazawa, H., Oda, K., Mitani, S., Yoshitaka, T., Asaumi, K., Inoue, H. (1998) 'Surgical management of hip dislocation in children with arthrogryposis multiplex congenita.' *Journal of Bone and Joint Surgery, British Volume,* **80**, 636–640.

Alman, B.A., Goldberg, M.J. (2001) 'Syndromes of orthopaedic importance.' *In:* Morrissy, R.T., Weinstein, S.L. (Eds.) *Lovell and Winter's Pediatric Orthopaedics. 5th Edn.* Philadelphia: Lippincott-Raven, pp. 305–310.

Aprin, H., Zink, W.P., Hall, J.E. (1985) 'Management of dislocation of the hip in Down syndrome.' *Journal of Pediatric Orthopedics,* **5**, 428–431.

Arnold, W.D., Hilgartner, M.W. (1977) 'Hemophilic arthropathy. Current concepts of pathogenesis and management.' *Journal of Bone and Joint Surgery, American Volume,* **59**, 287–305.

Bennet, G.C., Rang, M., Roye, D.P., Aprin, H. (1982) 'Dislocation of the hip in trisomy 21.' *Journal of Bone and Joint Surgery, British Volume,* **64**, 289–294.

Bevan-Thomas, W.H., Millar, E.A. (1967) 'A review of proximal focal femoral deficiencies.' *Journal of Bone and Joint Surgery, American Volume,* **49**, 1376–1388.

Bishop, A.R., Roberson, J.R., Eckman, J.R., Fleming, L.L. (1988) 'Total hip arthroplasty in patients who have sickle-cell hemoglobinopathy.' *Journal of Bone and Joint Surgery, American Volume,* 70, 853–855.

Brock, D. (1993) *Molecular Genetics for the Clinician.* Cambridge: Cambridge University Press.

Brown, K.L. (2001) 'Resection, rotationplasty, and femoropelvic arthrodesis in severe congenital femoral deficiency. A report of the surgical technique and three cases.' *Journal of Bone and Joint Surgery, American Volume,* **83**, 78–85.

Bunn, H.F. (1997) 'Pathogenesis and treatment of sickle cell disease.' *New England Journal of Medicine,* **337**, 762–769.

Burnett, M.W., Bass, J.W., Cook, B.A. (1998) 'Etiology of osteomyelitis complicating sickle cell disease.' *Pediatrics,* **101**, 296–297.

Cameron, H.U. (1998) 'Total joint replacement in multiplex congenita contractures: a case report.' *Canadian Journal of Surgery*, **41**, 245–247.

Carlson, W.O., Speck, G.J., Vicari, V., Wenger, D.R. (1985) 'Arthrogryposis multiplex congenita. A long-term follow-up study.' *Clinical Orthopaedics and Related Research*, **194**, 115–123.

Carter, C.O., Wilkinson, J.A. (1964) 'Genetic and environmental factors in the etiology of congenital dislocation of the hip.' *Clinical Orthopaedics and Related Research*, **33**, 119–128.

Chung, S.M., Ralston, E.L. (1971) 'Necrosis of the humeral head associated with sickle cell anemia and its genetic variants.' *Clinical Orthopaedics and Related Research*, **80**, 105–117.

Clarke, H.J., Jinnah, R.H., Brooker, A.F., Michaelson, J.D. (1989) 'Total replacement of the hip for avascular necrosis in sickle cell disease.' *Journal of Bone and Joint Surgery, British Volume*, **71**, 465–470.

Cristofaro, R.L., Donovan, R., Cristofaro, J. (1986) 'Orthopedic abnormalities in an adult population with Down's syndrome.' *Orthopaedic Transactions*, **10**, 150.

Cronk, C., Crocker, A.C., Pueschel, S.M., Shea, A.M., Zackai, E., Pickens, G., Reed, R.B. (1988) 'Growth charts for children with Down syndrome: 1 month to 18 years of age.' *Pediatrics*, **81**, 102–110.

Cruess, R.L. (1983) 'The pathology of acute chondrolysis of the hip.' *Journal of Bone and Joint Surgery, American Volume*, **65**, 1266–1275.

Dalton, G.P., Drummond, D.S., Davidson, R.S., Robertson, W.W. (1996) 'Bone infarction versus infection in sickle cell disease in children.' *Journal of Pediatric Orthopedics*, **16**, 540–544.

Daluga, D.T., Millar, E.A. (1989) 'Idiopathic chondrolysis of the hip.' *Journal of Pediatric Orthopedics*, **9**, 405–411.

Davidson, J., Beighton, P. (1976) 'Whence the arthrogrypotics?' *Journal of Bone and Joint Surgery, British Volume*, **58**, 492–495.

Diamond, L.S., Lynne, D., Sigman, B. (1981) 'Orthopedic disorders in patients with Down's syndrome.' *Orthopaedic Clinics of North America*, **12**, 57–71.

Earley, C.J., Kittner, S.J., Feeser, B.R., Gardner, J., Epstein, A., Wozniak, M.A., Wityk, R., Stern, B.J., Price, T.R., Macko, R.F., Johnson, C., Sloan, M.A., Buchholz, D. (1998) 'Stroke in children and sickle-cell disease: Baltimore–Washington Cooperative Young Stroke Study.' *Neurology*, **51**, 169–176.

Epps, C.H. (1983) 'Proximal femoral focal deficiency.' *Journal of Bone and Joint Surgery, American Volume*, **65**, 867–870.

Floman, Y., Niska, M. (1983) 'Dislocation of the hip joint complicating repeated hemarthrosis in hemophilia.' *Journal of Pediatric Orthopedics*, **3**, 99–100.

Friscia, D.A., Moseley, C.F., Oppenheim, W.L. (1989) 'Rotational osteotomy for proximal femoral focal deficiency.' *Journal of Bone and Joint Surgery, American Volume*, **71**, 1386–1392.

Gillespie, R. (1998) 'Classification of congenital abnormalities of the femur.' *In:* Hering, J.A., Birch, J.G. (Eds.) *The Child with a Limb Deficiency.* Rosemont, IL: American Academy of Orthopedic Surgeons. p. 63.

Goddard, N.J., Hashemi-Nejad, A., Fixsen, J.A. (1995) 'Natural history and treatment of instability of the hip in proximal femoral focal deficiency.' *Journal of Pediatric Orthopaedics, Part B*, **4**, 145–149.

Goodman, S., Gamble, J.G., Dilley, M. (1987) 'Hip motion changes in hemophilia.' *Journal of Pediatric Orthopedics*, **7**, 664–666.

Gore, D.R. (1981) 'Recurrent dislocation of the hip in a child with Down's syndrome. A case report.' *Journal of Bone and Joint Surgery, American Volume*, **63**, 823–825.

Greene, W.B. (1998) 'Closed treatment of hip dislocation in Down syndrome.' *Journal of Pediatric Orthopedics*, **18**, 643–647.

Greene, W.B. (2001) 'Diseases related to the hematopoietic system.' *In:* Morrissy, R.T., Weinstein, S.L. (Eds.) *Lovell and Winter's Pediatric Orthopaedics. 5th Edn.* Philadelphia: Lippincott-Raven, pp. 379–389.

Greene, W.B., McMillan, C.W. (1989) 'Nonsurgical management of hemophilic arthropathy.' *Instructional Course Lectures*, **38**, 367–381.

Greene, W.B., Yankaskas, B.C., Guilford, W.B. (1989) 'Roentgenographic classifications of hemophilic arthropathy. Comparison of three systems and correlation with clinical parameters.' *Journal of Bone and Joint Surgery, American Volume*, **71**, 237–244.

Hall, J.G. (1985) 'Genetic aspects of arthrogryposis.' Clinical Orthopaedics and Related Research, 194, 44–53.

Hall, J.G. (1997) 'Arthrogryposis multiplex congenita: etiology, genetics, classification, diagnostic approach, and general aspects.' *Journal of Pediatric Orthopaedics, Part B*, **6**, 159–166.

Hamanishi, C. (1980) 'Congenital short femur. Clinical, genetic and epidemiological comparison of the naturally occurring condition with that caused by thalidomide.' *Journal of Bone and Joint Surgery, British Volume*, **62**, 307–320.

Hanker, G.J., Amstutz, H.C. (1988) 'Osteonecrosis of the hip in the sickle-cell diseases. Treatment and complications.' *Journal of Bone and Joint Surgery, American Volume*, **70**, 499–506.

Heim, M., Varon, D., Strauss, S., Martinowitz, U. (1998) 'The management of a person with haemophilia who has a fixed flexed hip and intractable pain.' *Haemophilia*, **4**, 842–844.

Hernigou, P., Galacteros, F., Bachir, D., Goutallier, D. (1991) Deformities of the hip in adults who have sickle-cell disease and had avascular necrosis in childhood. A natural history of fifty-two patients.' *Journal of Bone and Joint Surgery, American Volume*, **73**, 81–92.

Herring, J.A., Cummings, D.R. (1996) 'The limb deficient child.' *In:* Morrissy, R.T., Weinstein, S.L. (Eds.) *Pediatric Orthopaedics. 4th Edn.* Philadelphia: Lippincott-Raven, pp. 1137–1180.

Hoffer, M.M., Swank, S., Eastman, F., Clark, D., Teitge, R. (1983) 'Ambulation in severe arthrogryposis.' *Journal of Pediatric Orthopedics*, **3**, 293–296.

Hresko, M.T., McCarthy, J.C., Goldberg, M.J. (1993) 'Hip disease in adults with Down syndrome.' *Journal of Bone and Joint Surgery, British Volume*, **75**, 604–607.

Huurman, W.W., Jacobsen, S.T. (1985) 'The hip in arthrogryposis multiplex congenita.' *Clinical Orthopaedics and Related Research*, **194**, 81–86.

Ishiguro, N., Takagi, H., Ito, T., Oguchi, T., Takamatsu, J., Iwata, H. (2001) 'Rapidly destructive arthropathy of the hip in haemophilia.' *Haemophilia*, **7**, 127–130.

Johansson, E., Aparisi, T. (1983) 'Missing cruciate ligament in congenital short femur.' *Journal of Bone and Joint Surgery, American Volume*, **65**, 1109–1115.

Jordan, H.H. (1958) *Hemophilic Arthropathies*. Springfield, IL: Charles C. Thomas.

Kalaycioglu, A., Aynaci, O. (2001) 'Proximal focal femoral deficiency, contralateral hip dysplasia in association with contralateral ulnar hypoplasia and clefthand: a case report and review of literatures of PFFD and/or FFU.' *Okajimas Folia Anatomica Japonica*, **78**, 83–89.

Keeley, K., Buchanan, G.R. (1982) 'Acute infarction of long bones in children with sickle cell anemia.' *Journal of Pediatrics*, **101**, 170–175.

Kelley, S.S., Lachiewicz, P.F., Gilbert, M.S., Bolander, M.E., Jankiewicz, J.J. (1995) 'Total hip and knee arthroplasty for arthropathy in a hemophiliac.' *Journal of Bone and Joint Surgery, American Volume*, **77**, 828–834.

Kelly, T.E. (1974) 'A—familial proximal focal femoral deficiency (PFFD).' *Birth Defects Original Article Series*, **10** (5), 195.

Kilcoyne, R.F., Nuss, R. (1999) 'Femoral head osteonecrosis in a child with hemophilia.' *Arthritis and Rheumatism*, **42**, 1550–1551.

Kioschos, M., Shaw, E.D., Beals, R.K. (1999) 'Total hip arthroplasty in patients with Down's syndrome.' *Journal of Bone and Joint Surgery, British Volume*, **81**, 436–439.

Livingstone, B., Hirst, P. (1986) 'Orthopedic disorders in school children with Down's syndrome with special reference to the incidence of joint laxity.' *Clinical Orthopaedics and Related Research*, **207**, 74–76.

Lofqvist, T., Sanzen, L., Petersson, C., Nilsson, I.M. (1996) 'Total hip replacement in patients with hemophilia. 13 hips in 11 patients followed for 1–16 years.' *Acta Orthopaedica Scandinavica*, **67**, 321–324.

Malizos, K.N., Siafakas, M.S., Fotiadis, D.I., Karachalios, T.S., Soucacos, P.N. (2001) 'An MRI-based semi-automated volumetric quantification of hip osteonecrosis.' *Skeletal Radiology*, **30**, 686–693.

McCollough, N.C. (1963) 'Non-standard prosthetic applications for juvenile amputees.' *Inter-Clinic Information Bulletin*, **2**, 7.

McKie, V.C. (1998) 'Sickle cell anemia in children: practical issues for the pediatrician.' *Pediatric Annals*, **27**, 521–524.

Milner, P.F., Kraus, A.P., Sebes, J.I., Sleeper, L.A., Dukes, K.A., Embury, S.H., Bellevue, R., Kosy, M., Moohr, J.W., Smith J. (1991) 'Sickle cell disease as a cause of osteonecrosis of the femoral head.' *New England Journal of Medicine*, **325**, 1476–1481.

Morrissy, R.T., Weinstein, S.L. (Eds.) (1996) *Lovell and Winter's Pediatric Orthopaedics. 4th Edn.* Philadelphia: Lippincott-Raven

Morrissy, R.T., Giavedoni, B.J., Coulter-O'Berry, C. (2001) 'The limb deficient child.' *In:* Morrissy, R.T., Weinstein, S.L. (Eds.) *Lovell and Winter's Pediatric Orthopaedics. 5th Edn.* Philadelphia: Lippincott-Raven, pp. 1237–1246.

Murray, M.P., Jacobs, P.A., Gore, D.R., Gardner, G.M., Mollinger, L.A. (1985) 'Functional performance after tibial rotationplasty.' *Journal of Bone and Joint Surgery, American Volume*, **67**, 392–399.

Nelson, I.W., Sivamurugan, S., Latham, P.D., Matthews, J., Bulstrode, C.J. (1992) 'Total hip arthroplasty for hemophilic arthropathy.' *Clinical Orthopaedics and Related Research*, **276**, 210–213.

Pegelow, C.H., Adams, R.J., McKie, V., Abboud, M., Berman, B., Miller, S.T., Olivieri, N., Vichinsky, E.,

Wang W., Brambilla D. (1995) 'Risk of recurrent stroke in patients with sickle cell disease treated with erythrocyte transfusions.' *Journal of Pediatrics*, **126**, 896–899.

Pettersson, H., Wingstrand, H., Thambert, C., Nilsson, I.M., Jonsson, K. (1990) 'Legg–Calvé–Perthes disease in hemophilia: incidence and etiologic considerations.' *Journal of Pediatric Orthopedics*, **10**, 28–32.

Pirani, S., Beauchamp, R.D., Li, D., Sawatzky, B. (1991) 'Soft tissue anatomy of proximal femoral focal deficiency.' *Journal of Pediatric Orthopedics*, **11**, 563–570.

Platt, O.S., Brambilla, D.J., Rosse, W.F., Milner, P.F., Castro, O., Steinberg, M.H., Klug, P.P. (1994) 'Mortality in sickle cell disease. Life expectancy and risk factors for early death.' *New England Journal of Medicine*, **330**, 1639–1644.

Post, M. (1980) 'Hemophilic arthropathy of the hip.' *Orthopedic Clinics of North America*, **1**, 65–67.

Rand, C., Pearson, T.C., Heatley, F.W. (1987) 'Avascular necrosis of the femoral head in sickle cell syndrome: a report of 5 cases.' *Acta Haematologica*, **78**, 186–192.

Rao, V.M., Mitchell, D.G., Steiner, R.M., Rifkin, M.D., Burk, D.L., Levy, D., Ballas, S.K. (1988) 'Femoral head avascular necrosis in sickle cell anemia: MR characteristics.' *Magnetic Resonance Imaging*, **6**, 661–667.

Rodriguez-Merchan, E.C. (1996) 'Effects of hemophilia on articulations of children and adults.' *Clinical Orthopaedics and Related Research*, **328**, 7–13.

Roy, D.R., Crawford, A. (1988) 'Idopathic chondrolysis of the hip. Management by subtotal capsulectomy and aggressive rehabilitation.' *Journal of Pediatric Orthopedics*, **8**, 203–207.

Sadat-Ali, M., al-Umran, K., al-Habdan, I., al-Mulhim, F. (1998) 'Ultrasonography: can it differentiate between vasoocclusive crisis and acute osteomyelitis in sickle cell disease?' *Journal of Pediatric Orthopedics*, **18**, 552–554.

Sarwark, J.F., MacEwen, G.D., Scott, C.I. (1990) 'Amyoplasia (a common form of arthrogryposis).' *Journal of Bone and Joint Surgery, American Volume*, **72**, 465–469.

Schneider, R.G., Hightower, B., Hosty, T.S., Ryder, H., Tomlin, G., Atkins, R., Brimhall, B., Jones, R.T. (1976) 'Abnormal hemoglobins in a quarter million people.' *Blood*, **48**, 629–637.

Semine, A.A., Ertel, A.N., Goldberg, M.J., Bull, M.J. (1978) 'Cervical-spine instability in children with Down syndrome (trisomy 21).' *Journal of Bone and Joint Surgery, American Volume*, **60**, 649–652.

Shapiro, F., Bresnan, M.J. (1982) 'Orthopaedic management of childhood neuromuscular disease. Part II: Peripheral neuropathies, Friedreich's ataxia, and arthrogryposis multiplex congenita.' *Journal of Bone and Joint Surgery, American Volume*, **64**, 949–953.

Shapiro, S.S. (1979) 'Antibodies to blood coagulation factors.' *Clinical Haematology*, **8**, 207–214.

Shaw, E.D., Beals, R.K. (1992) 'The hip joint in Down's syndrome. A study of its structure and associated disease.' *Clinical Orthopaedics and Related Research*, **278**, 101–107.

Shohat, M., Lotan, R., Magal, N., Shohat, T., Fischel-Ghodsian, N., Rotter, J.I., Jaber, L. (1997) 'A gene for arthrogryposis multiplex congenita neuropathic type is linked to D5S394 on chromosome 5qter.' *American Journal of Human Genetics*, **61**, 1139–1143.

Skoff, H.D., Keggi, K. (1987) 'Total hip replacement in Down's syndrome.' *Orthopedics*, **10**, 485–489.

Soucie, J.M., Evatt, B., Jackson, D. (1998) 'Occurrence of hemophilia in the United States. The Hemophilia Surveillance System Project Investigators.' *American Journal of Hematology*, **59**, 288–294.

St Clair, H.S., Zimbler, S. (1985) 'A plan of management and treatment results in the arthrogrypotic hip.' *Clinical Orthopaedics and Related Research*, **194**, 74–80.

Staheli, L.T., Chew, D.E., Elliott, J.S., Mosca, V.S. (1987) 'Management of hip dislocations in children with arthrogryposis.' *Journal of Pediatric Orthopedics*, **7**, 681–685.

Steel, H.H., Lin, P.S., Betz, R.R., Kalamchi, A., Clancy, M. (1987) 'Iliofemoral fusion for proximal femoral focal deficiency.' *Journal of Bone and Joint Surgery, American Volume*, **69**, 837–843.

Stein, H., Duthie, R.B. (1981) 'The pathogenesis of chronic haemophilic arthropathy.' *Journal of Bone and Joint Surgery, British Volume*, **4**, 601–609.

Steinberg, M.H. (1999) 'Management of sickle cell disease.' *New England Journal of Medicine*, **340**, 1021–1030.

Stormer, S.V. (1997) 'Proximal femoral focal deficiency.' *Orthopaedic Nursing*, **16** (5), 25–31.

Storti, E., Traldi, A., Tosatti, E., Davoli, P.G. (1969) 'Synovectomy, a new approach to haemophilic arthropathy.' *Acta Haematologica*, **41**, 193–205.

Szoke, G., Staheli, L.T., Jaffe, K., Hall, J.G. (1996) 'Medial-approach open reduction of hip dislocation in amyoplasia-type arthrogryposis.' *Journal of Pediatric Orthopedics*, **16**, 127–130.

Takedani, H., Mikami, S., Abe, Y., Kin, H., Kawasaki, N. (2000) [Total hip and knee arthroplasty for arthropathy in a hemophiliac.] *Rinsho Ketsueki*, **41**, 97–102.

258

Teitelbaum, S. (1977) 'Radiologic evaluation of the hemophilic hip.' *Mount Sinai Journal of Medicine*, **44**, 400–401.

Torode, I.P., Gillespie, R. (1983) 'Rotationplasty of the lower limb for congenital defects of the femur.' *Journal of Bone and Joint Surgery, British Volume*, **65**, 569–573.

Van Nes, C.P. (1950) 'Rotation-plasty for congenital defects of the femur: making use of the ankle of the shortened limb to control the knee joint of the prosthesis.' *Journal of Bone and Joint Surgery, British Volume*, **32**, 12–15.

Washington, E.R., Root, L. (1985) 'Conservative treatment of sickle cell avascular necrosis of the femoral head.' *Journal of Pediatric Orthopedics*, **5**, 192–194.

Williams, P. (1978) 'The management of arthrogryposis.' *Orthopedic Clinics of North America*, **9**, 67–88.

Winston, M.E. (1952) 'Haemophiliac arthropathy of the hip.' *Journal of Bone and Joint Surgery, British Volume*, **34**, 412–420.

Wynne-Davies, R., Lloyd-Roberts, G.C. (1976) 'Arthrogryposis multiplex congenita. Search for prenatal factors in 66 sporadic cases.' *Archives of Disease in Childhood*, **51**, 618–623.

Wynne-Davies, R., Williams, P.F., O'Connor, J.C. (1981) 'The 1960s epidemic of arthrogryposis multiplex congenita: a survey from the United Kingdom, Australia and the United States of America.' *Journal of Bone and Joint Surgery, British Volume*, **63**, 76–82.

INDEX

(Page numbers in *italics* refer to figures/tables.)

262

trauma, 125, 126, 127
Nuclear scintigraphy, *see* Scintigraphy

O

Ober test, 33–34, *34*, 201
Obesity, slipped capital femoral epiphysis and, 64–65, 74
Odontoid hypoplasia, 116
Oestrogen, physeal strength, 75
Open bone graft epiphysiodesis, 82
Orthopaedic specialist referral
  achondroplasia, 109
  developmental dysplasia, 53
  pseudoachondroplasia, 112–113
  slipped capital femoral epiphysis, 79–80, 85
  spondyloepiphyseal dysplasia tarda, 116
Orthoses, 209–237
  applications/indications, 220
    cerebral palsy, 169, *170*
    Charcot–Marie–Tooth disease, 204
    Down syndrome, 246
    impairments of hip structure, 220–225
    leg-length discrepancy, 235, *235*
    myelomeningocele, 184, *184*, 188, *189*
    Perthes' disease, 98
    proximal focal femoral deficiency, 253
    spina bifida, 225
  hip joint biomechanics, 214–218
  lying, 225
  materials, 219
  mechanical principles, 209–214
    active forces, 210
    bending, 212–214, *213*
    forces and vectors, 209, *211*
    ground reaction force, 210, *211*
    moments and levers, 212, *212*, *213*
    pressure, 214
    reaction forces, 209–210, *211*
    stability, 214, *214*
  overcoming activity limitations, 225–235
  promoting hip-joint congruency, 220–223, *221*, *222*, *223*
  reciprocal walking, 230–233, *232*
  reducing forces acting through hip joint, 223–225, *224*
  sitting, 225–226, *226*
  standing, 228–230, *229*
  supply process, 219–220
    assessment and prescription, 219
    fitting and evaluation, 220
    measurement, 220
  swivel walkers, 230, *231*
  terminology, 218
  upright locomotion, 230–235, *231*, *232*
Orthotic Research and Locomotion Assessment Unit (ORLAU), 231–232

Orthotists, role, 209
Ortolani manoeuvre, 36–37, *38*, *52*
  positive result, 52, 55
  risk factors, *49*, 53
Ortolani negative dislocation, 56
Ortolani positive hip, 52, 55
Ossification, 10
  coalescence, 90
  delayed, 112, *112*, 113, 116
  pelvis, 119, 125
  primary centers, 119
Ossific nucleus, embryological development, *4*, 6, 9
Osteoarthritis, 104
  achondroplasia, 110
  Down syndrome adult, 246
  multiple epiphyseal dysplasia, 113
  pseudoachondroplasia, 112
Osteochondrodysplasias, *see* Skeletal dysplasias
Osteochondromas, 66–67, *67*
Osteoid osteoma, 20
  diagnosis, 43–44, *66*
  treatment, 66
Osteomyelitis, diagnosis, 42, 63
Osteonecrosis, 81
  screw fixation, 84–85
  sickle cell disease, prevalence, 248–249, *249*
  see also Avascular necrosis
Osteopaenia
  Duchenne's muscular dystrophy, 201
  juvenile idiopathic arthritis, *133*, 141–142
Osteoporosis, periarticular, 133
Osteosarcoma, 44, 71, *71*
Osteotomies
  cerebral palsy, 174–176, *175*, *176*
  Charcot–Marie–Tooth disease, 204
  Down syndrome, 246
  myelomeningocele, 188, *189*, 190
  Perthes' disease, 99, *100*, 100–102
  slipped capital femoral epiphysis, 82–83

P

Pain, 19
  back, 24, 35, 110
  bone, 20
  buttock, 125
  groin, 77, 91
  "growing", 59
  hip, 43, 59–73
    decision matrix, 62, *63*
    diagnosis, 59, 77
    differential diagnosis, 62–72, *72*, 124
    Duchenne's muscular dystrophy, 201
    imaging, 61, *62*, 67
    laboratory studies, 61–62
    physical examination, 59–61, 124
    slipped capital femoral epiphysis, 77

271